# Receptors and Ion Channels

# Receptors and Ion Channels

Proceedings of the Symposium on
Receptors and Ion Channels
Tashkent, USSR, October 2–5, 1986

Editors
Y. A. Ovchinnikov · F. Hucho

W DE G

Walter de Gruyter · Berlin · New York 1987

*Editors*

Yuri A. Ovchinnikov, D. Sc.
Professor
Shemyakin Institute of Bioorganic Chemistry
USSR Academy of Sciences
Moscow
USSR

Ferdinand Hucho, Dr. rer. nat.
Professor of Biochemistry
Free University Berlin
Department of Chemistry
Institute of Biochemistry
Thielallee 63
D-1000 Berlin 33
Germany

*Library of Congress Cataloging in Publication Data*

Symposium on Receptors and Ion Channels (1986 : Tashkent, Uzbek U.S.S.R.)
Receptors and ion channels.
Bibliography: p.
Includes indexes.
1. Cell receptors--Congresses. 2. Ion channels--Congresses.
I. Ovchinnikov, Jurij A. (Jurij Anatol'evich), 1934– .
II. Hucho, Ferdinand, 1939– . III. Title.
QH603.C43S95 1986 574.87'5 87-9003
ISBN 0-89925-375-X (U.S.)

*CIP-Kurztitelaufnahme der Deutschen Bibliothek*

**Receptors and ion channels** : proceedings of the Symposium on Receptors and Ion Channels, Tashkent, USSR, October 2–5, 1986 / ed. Y. A. Ovchinnikov ; F. Hucho. – Berlin ; New York : de Gruyter, 1987.
ISBN 3-11-010346-X
NE: Ovčinnikov, Jurij A. [Hrsg.]; Symposium on Receptors and Ion Channels <1986, Taškent>

 Printing: Gerike GmbH, Berlin. Binding: Dieter Mikolai, Berlin. – Printed in Germany.

# PREFACE

Few areas of modern biology are advancing as rapidly as the wide-ranging field of receptors and ion channels. Several model systems have been investigated in unprecedented detail. New techniques are available for investigating the molecular structures and mechanism of these membrane molecules which serve key functions in the nerve cell: recombinant DNA techniques, computer-aided high resolution electron microscopy, monoclonal antibodies, and patch clamp techniques, to name a few.

This volume presents recent results obtained by German and Soviet scientists. It contains the proceedings of a symposium held last fall in Tashkent/Usbekistan. The organizers felt it would be important to review the progress in this field and to discuss contributions made by scientists in East and West. Western neurobiologists may be surprised by the similarity of approaches and standards in such different systems.

The subdivision of this volume is somewhat arbitrary. There are receptors containing ion channels and second messenger systems interacting with both receptors and ion channels. Of necessity, there is also some overlap between chapters. Furthermore, the organizers considered it important to include active ion transport systems, and they also added a section on neurotoxins, the valuable tools of the neurobiologists.

The success of a symposium depends largely on its atmosphere and an organization favoring intellectual exchange. We would like to extend special thanks to the local organizers, especially to Professor Tashmukhamedov and his colleagues, who laid the groundwork for an exciting meeting with many new results and insights.

Berlin, January 1987

Y.A. Ovchinnikov
Ferdinand Hucho

CONTENTS

# I RECEPTORS

## A) NICOTINIC ACETYLCHOLINE RECEPTOR

# I Receptors

## a) Nicotinic Acetylcholine Receptor

# THE ION CHANNEL OF THE NICOTINIC ACETYLCHOLINE RECEPTOR

W. Oberthür, F. Lottspeich §, F. Hucho
Institut für Biochemie, Freie Universität Berlin, Thielallee 63, 1000 Berlin (West).
§ Max-Planck-Institut für Biochemie, Martinsried.

## Introduction

Ion channels consist of two functional moieties, a gating device and a selectivity filter (1). The former can react either to changes in the membrane potential or to chemical signals, e.g., changes in neurotransmitter concentration. The latter determines which type of ion may permeate through the gated channel. Well-characterized examples of voltage-dependent ion channels are the axonal $Na^+$- and $K^+$-channels (2). The best known chemically gated ion channel is the nicotinic acetylcholine receptor (AChR) (3).
The nicotinic acetylcholine receptor (fig. 1) is a heteropentamer with the quaternary structure $\alpha_2\beta\gamma\delta$ (4).

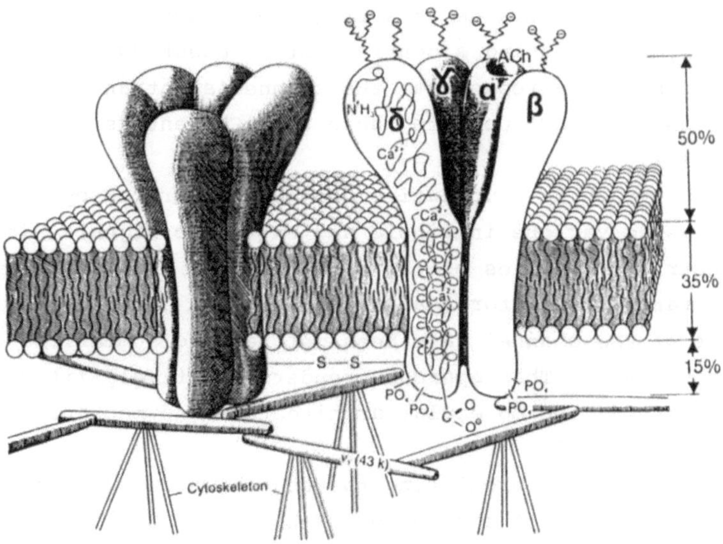


*Fig. 1: Biochemical model of the nicotinic acetylcholine receptor (nAChR) from Torpedo marmorata electric tissue*

Receptors and Ion Channels

It is a glycoprotein of $M_r$ 290,000 D. Its signal recognition-(acetylcholine-) binding sites and its ion channel are integral parts of the pentameric protein complex interacting in a way similar to allosteric enzymes where active sites and regulatory sites communicate via conformational changes within the tertiary structure (5). While the agonist binding sites are relatively well-characterized -- being located on the α-polypeptide chains -- relatively little is known about the location of the ion channel within the AChR. Here we describe several approaches for elucidating the channel structure and its mechansim of functioning.

Results

The first and most direct approach to obtaining information about the AChR ion channel is to 'look' at it. Electron microscopy, especially in connection with computer-aided image processing, is a powerful tool for getting insights into the ultrastructure of a molecule. This approach is the subject of another chapter in this volume. Electron microscopy identifies the receptor from *Torpedo marmorata* electric tissue as a ringlike structure with a fivefold axis of symmetry having a central pit of about 30 Å diameter. This most probably represents the channel's entrance. Its diameter is constant at least down to where the AChR enters the lipid bilayer (6).

Another approach is elucidating channel properties by kinetic methods using various intrinsic and extrinsic signals, including the electric properties of the receptor-rich membrane. By these methods various receptor states representing distinct ion conductivities of the channel have been defined and summarized in various kinetic schemes. This approach renders relatively little information concerning the molecular architecture and mechanism of action of the ion channel.

A third approach is predicting the channel structure from the known primary structures of the receptor subunits. One such prediction has been especially fruitful in stimulating experiments with the aim of proving or disproving a given model: Finer-Moore and Stroud (7) predicted that each of the five polypeptide chains spans the postsynaptic membrane with five helical hydrophobic sequences, one of which is amphipathic. The amphipathic helix, called helix A, comprises amino acids 425 - 458 (aligned sequences), which can be modeled into a helix with hydrophobic amino acid side chains on one side and charged residues on the other. According to this model, the charged side of helix A from each of the five subunits forms the ion channel. The obvious advantage of this model is that it gives a plausible explanation of how a charged particle may permeate through the lipid bilayer of the plasma membrane. The 'amphipathic-helix-model' has provoked scores of ingenious experiments with monoclonal antibodies (8 - 10), site-directed mutagenesis (11), and other methods of verifying its predicted consequences concerning the distribution of sequence-domains over the membrane and the amino acid residues involved in the channel structure. So far the results of all these experiments have been ambiguous. The location of the AChR-ion channel remained obscure.

The most promising approach is derived from the pharmacology of the AChR. There are three classes of cholinergic effectors affecting the AChR and its channel: agonists, competitive antagonists, and noncompetitive antagonists (12). The latter class, which is chemically very heterogeneous, contains compounds thought to block cholinergic transmission by sterically or allosterically blocking the AChR-ion channel (4,5). The binding site for these compounds should therefore be located either within the ion channel or at a domain of the receptor protein closely related to it.

One such noncompetitive antagonist is the lipophilic cation triphenylmethylphosphonium ($TPMP^+$). We have previously shown (13) that $TPMP^+$ blocks the ion flux through the AChR channel at concentrations at which no inhibition of agonist binding occurs. There is one $TPMP^+$-binding site/AChR, as compared to two acetylcholine binding sites. $TPMP^+$ competes for this site with the well-proven channel blockers phencyclidine (PCP) and histrionicotoxin (HTX). Like these, it blocks the ion channel at the endplate in a voltage-dependent manner (14).

Moreover, $TPMP^+$ can be used as a photoaffinity label: irradiation of an AChR/$^3H$-$TPMP^+$—complex with UV light causes irreversible incorporation of radioactivity into the receptor protein (15). The receptor subunits are photolabeled differently depending on the receptor state: in the resting state most of the radioactivity incorporated is found in the α-polypeptide chains, in the presence

of the agonist carbamoylcholine, i.e. in the desensitized state a significant shift occurs: now most of the label is found in the β- and δ-chains. Interestingly, a similar shift is observed when photolabeling is performed in presence of antagonists, including flaxedil. This indicates that the change in the labeling pattern is not simply correlated with desensitization of the receptor, since flaxedil as a pure competitive antagonist has no desensitizing activity. We have used these findings for monitoring structural changes in the receptor protein triggered by cholinergic effectors and for defining receptor functional states including an hitherto overlooked antagonist state (16).
By all criteria $TPMP^+$ is a highly specific inhibitor of the AChR-ion channel. We therefore used it as a probe for detecting sites in the protein contributing to the structure and activity of the receptor's ion channel.

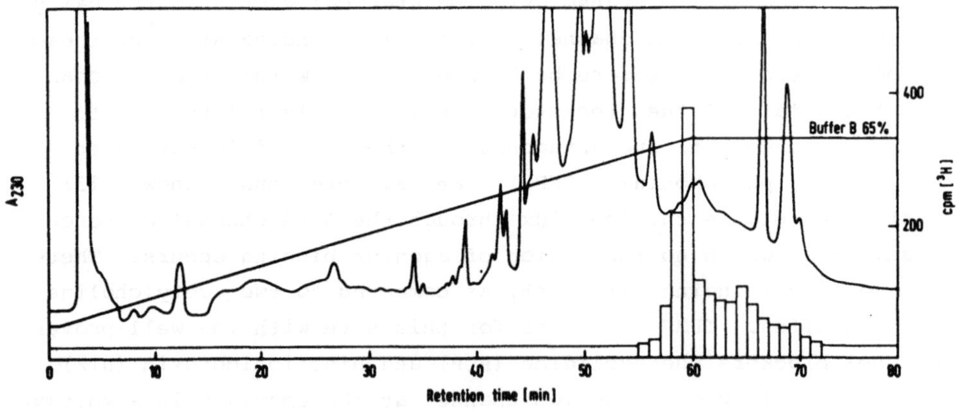


*Fig. 2: Purification of a $^3H$-$TPMP^+$-labeled CNBr-peptide. HPLC-chromatogram (Organogen-HP-Gel-RP7) of labeled δ-subunit*

After photolabeling of AChR from *Torpedo marmorata* with $^3$H-TPMP$^+$ we separated the receptor subunits by preparative SDS-polyacrylamide gel electrophoresis and cleaved them with CNBr or with trypsin. The cleavage products were separated on a reversed-phase HPLC column. Analysis of the HPLC fractions showed that even within the subunits labeling was highly specific: one major radioactivity peak occured (fig. 2), indicating that predominantly one site in the primary structure of the subunit was labeled (17).
Two main results should be mentioned: the distribution of label in the HPLC peptides obtained by tryptic cleavage of different receptor subunits shows a striking similarity. We have shown by microsequencing techniques that $^3$H-TPMP$^+$-labeled homologous positions in the α-, β-, and δ-polypeptide chains (α 248, β 254, δ 262).
The other important result is the following: position ser 262 in the δ-subunit was labeled irrespective of whether photolabeling was performed with AChR in the resting state (in absence of any other cholinergic effector besides TPMP$^+$), in the desensitized state (AChR equilibrated with 0.1 mM agonist), or in the presence of the competitive antagonist flaxedil which, as mentioned above, also stimulates photolabeling of the δ-subunit (fig. 3).
This indicates that it is probably not the open channel which reacts with TPMP$^+$. More likely an amino acid residue, located close to the entrance of the channel, is the target of the photoreaction.

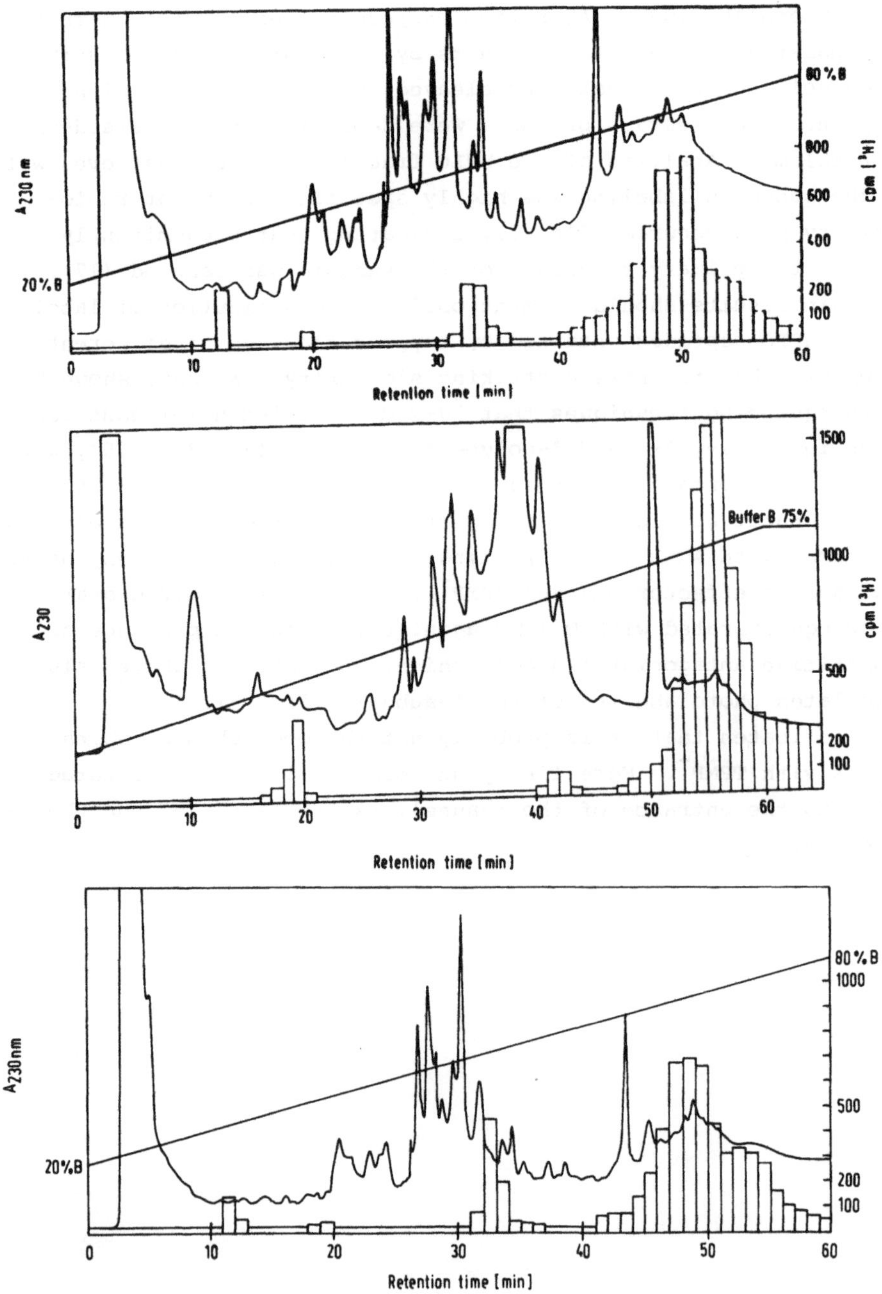


*Fig. 3:* *HPLC-chromatograms of $^{3}H$-$TPMP^{+}$-labeled δ-subunits. Labeling an absence of cholinergic effectors (top), in presence of 0.1 mM carbamoylcholine (middle), in presence of 0.1 mM flaxedil (bottom). Tryptic cleavage.*

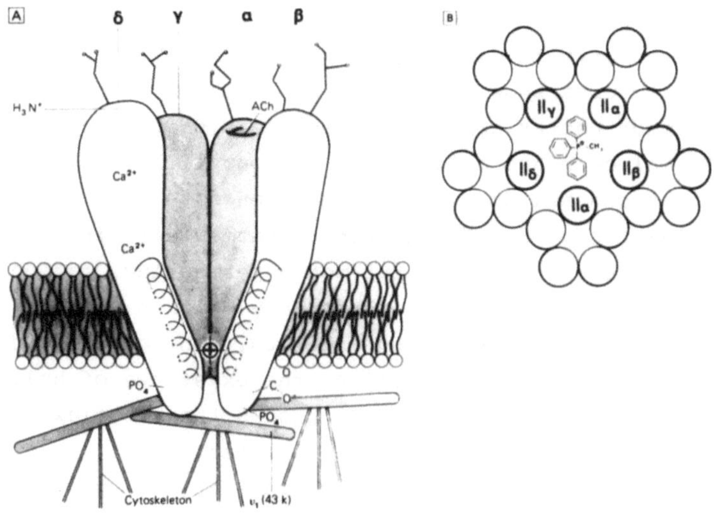


*Fig. 4: Helix II model of AChR-ion channel. Longitudinal section (left), cross section in the labeling plane.*

Discussion

The results of the photolabeling and microsequencing experiments are summarized in a model of the AChR-ion channel (fig. 4) which has the following features:

i) The ion channel is formed by the five homologous helices II, each one of which is contributed by the five receptor subunits.

ii) At the entrance (extracellular side) it is wide enough (30 Å) to be filled with water and to let the charged cation enter. It becomes narrow somewhere near to the membrane bilayer.

iii) The narrow part of the channel contains enough polar groups to make it permeable for cations.

The model is consistent with many experimental data from various laboratories: electron microscopy (ref. 18 and accompanying paper) showed the fivefold axis of symmetry and the dimensions of the channel entrance. Electrophysiological experiments have shown that the permeating cation is not in contact with charged amino acid side chains, but with dipoles, mainly water (19). Comparison of primary structures show that helix II is the best conserved sequence, much better conserved than the amphipathic helix A. The $TPMP^+$ molecule has a diameter of about 11 Å (20), allowing it to enter the channel down to its reaction site (ser 262). Cations up to a diameter of 6.4 Å are able to permeate (21); therefore $TPMP^+$ is a channel-blocking, but not a permeating, cation. While several of the other helices, especially helix A and helix V, are in dispute as membrane-spanning entities, none of the prediction models of subunit folding question the existence of helix II. The question remains whether $TPMP^+$ blocks the ion flux through the AChR-ion channel sterically or allosterically. In other words: is the site of the photoreaction (ser 262) part of the channel itself or is it a regulatory site? Since conformational changes related to receptor desensitization enhance the affinity for $TPMP^+$ and increase photolabeling of the δ-subunit, the binding site is probably a regulatory site; simultaneously, this site may well be within the channel, in a part of its funnel-shaped structure which is wide enough to let $TPMP^+$ enter. A noncompetitive inhibitor located here should inhibit ion flux through the channel effectively. Obviously this site is accessible in the closed-channel resting, desensitized, and antagonist states.

## Acknowledgements

This work would have been impossible without the help and hospitality of the Max-Planck-Institut für Biochemie, Martinsried. Financial support by the Deutsche Forschungsgemeinschaft (SFB 312), and the Fonds der Chemischen Industrie is gratefully acknowledged.

## References

1. Hille, B., 1984. Ionic Channels of Excitable Membranes. Sinauer Associates Inc., Sunderland.

2. Noda, M., et al. 1984. Nature 312, 121-127.

3. Changeux, J.-P., Devillers-Thiery, A., and Chemouille, P. 1984. Science 225, 1335-1345.

4. Hucho, F. 1986. Eur.J. Biochem. 158, 211-226.

5. Changeux, J.-P.. 1981. Harvey Lect. 75, 85-254.

6. Brisson, A., and Unwin, P.N.T.. 1985. Nature 315, 474-477.

7. Finer-Moore, J., and Stroud, R.M.. 1984. Proc. Natl. Acad. Sci. USA 81, 155-159.

8. Lindstrom, J., Criado, M., Hoch-Schwender, S., Fox, J.L., and Sarin, V.. 1984. Nature 311, 573-575.

9. Watters, D., and Maelicke, A.. 1983. Biochemistry 22, 1811.

10. Neumann, D., Gershoni, J.M., Fridkin, M. and Fuchs, S.. 1985. Proc. Natl. Acad. Sci. USA 82, 3490-3493.

11. Mishina, M., et al.. 1985. Nature 313, 364-369.

12. Heidmann, T., Oswald, R.E., and Changeux, J.-P.. 1983. Biochemistry 22, 3112-3127.

13. Lauffer, L., and Hucho, F.. 1982. Proc. Natl. Acad. Sci. USA 79, 2406-2409.

14. Fahr, A., Hellmann, S., Lauffer, L., Muhn, P., and Hucho, F.. 1985. 36. Mosbach-Colloquium, 103-112.

15. Muhn, P., and Hucho, F.. 1983. Biochemistry 22, 421-425.

16. Fahr, A., Lauffer, L., Schmidt, D., Heyn, M.P., and Hucho, F.. 1985. Eur. J. Biochem. 147, 483-487.

17. Oberthür, W., Muhn, P., Baumann, H., Lottspeich, F., Wittmann-Liebold, B., and Hucho, F.. 1986. EMBO J. 5. 1815-1819.

18. Brisson, A., and Unwin, P.N.T.. 1984. J.Cell. Biol. 99, 1202-1211.

19. Lewis, C.A., and Stevens, C.F. 1983. Proc. Natl. Acad. Sci. USA 80, 6110-6113.

20. McPhail, A.T., Semeniuk, G.M., and Chesnut, D.B.. 1971. J. Chem. Soc. (A), 2174-2180.

21. Huang, L.-Y., Catterall, W.A., and Ehrenstein, G.. 1978. J. Gen. Physiol. 71, 394-410.

# PATTERN RECOGNITION IN STRUCTURAL ANALYSIS OF THE ACETYLCHOLINE RECEPTOR

W. Kunath, H. Sack-Kongehl

Fritz-Haber-Institut der Max-Planck-Gesellschaft,
Faradayweg 4-6, D-1000 Berlin 33

M. Giersig, F. Hucho

Institut für Biochemie, Fachbereich Chemie, Freie Universität
Berlin, Thielallee 63, D-1000 Berlin 33.

## Introduction

In this paper we present a new method of pattern recognition applied to very noisy electron micrographs of acetylcholine receptor molecules (AChR). The micrographs are taken of AChR-rich membranes negatively stained with phosphotungstate. From biochemistry it is known that the AChR consists of five subunits from four different proteins (1). From electron microscopical investigations different structures have been obtained. Brisson and Unwin (2) detected a pentameric structure by a three-dimensional analysis of a tubular crystal. The analysis of two-dimensional crystals (3) or of single molecules (4) has so far not resulted in a pentameric, but in less symmetrical structures. In the meantime progress in image processing of single molecules has been achieved using multivariate analysis methods (5). This paper concerns rotationally invariant multivariate analysis of single AChR images.

## Image processing

Difficulties in pattern recognition of AChR images arise because of the variability of the surrounding stain distribution. The stain material has a granularity of about the same size as the structural details of interest. In fig. 1 an electron micrograph is shown exhibiting noisy ringlike structures of the AChR sticking

Receptors and Ion Channels

out of a membrane. After digitization of the micrograph, the individual AChR were extracted into small image fields of 32 by 32 pixels, corresponding to 90 Å by 90 Å. Multivariate analysis of a set of such images starts with an alignment to bring them into identical positions, translationally as well as rotationally. The translational alignment of the AChR can easily be done, because there is a central stain deposit. In the arrangement in fig. 2 the AChR are already centered by crosscorrelating them relative to a reference which was simply a gaussian shaped ring. The next computational step should be a rotational alignment, but as can be seen, the images are so noisy that it is not reasonable to choose one of them as a reference. To take an artificial structure as reference, on the other hand, means to put a priori information into the alignment. Thus we developed a multivariate analysis procedure which is independent of the rotational orientation of the molecules, making a rotational alignment unnecessary.

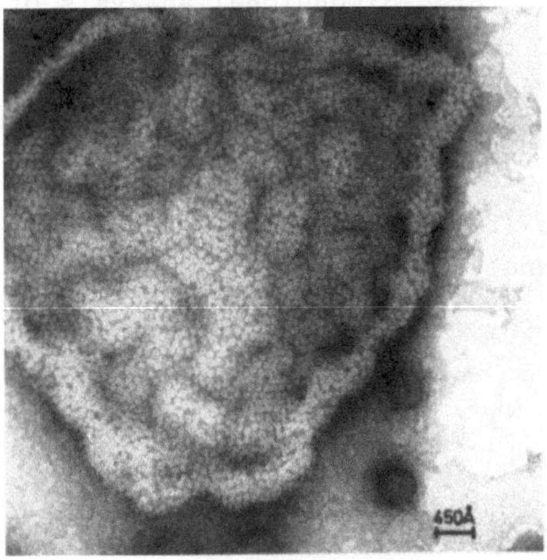


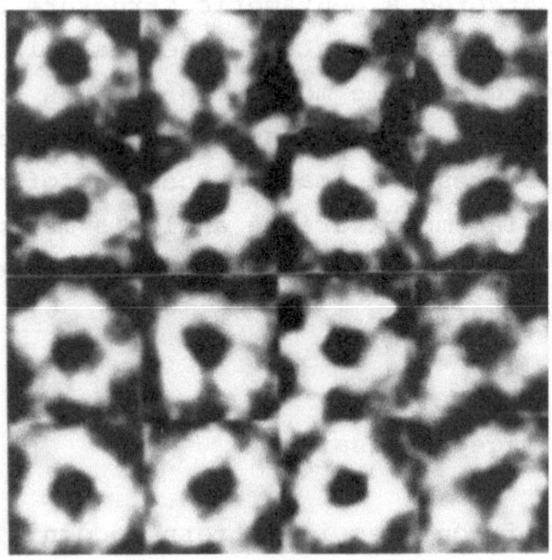

*Fig. 1:* *Electron micrograph of an AChR-rich membrane from Torpedo californica, negatively stained with phosphotungstate (pH = 7.4).*

*Fig. 2:* *Translationally aligned AChR images extracted from the micrographs shown in fig. 1.*

The basic idea is to encode the information about the molecular structure in a form which contains the orientation as a common phase factor, say exp(-iα) if α is the angle of orientation. At first we calculate a Fourier-ring function, which contains the most important information about the molecule, and then we look at its harmonics. This is illustrated in figs. 3 and 4.

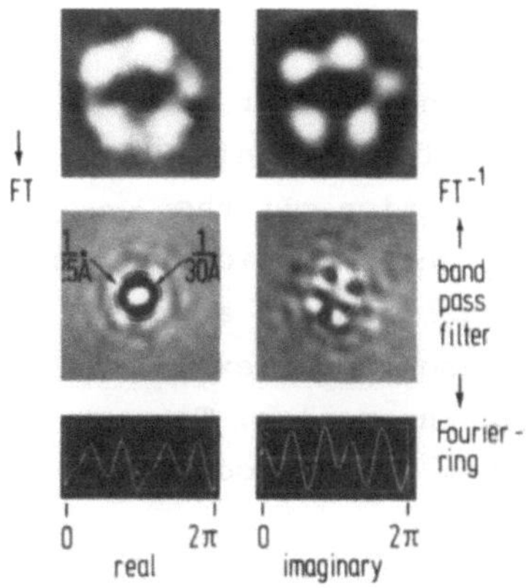


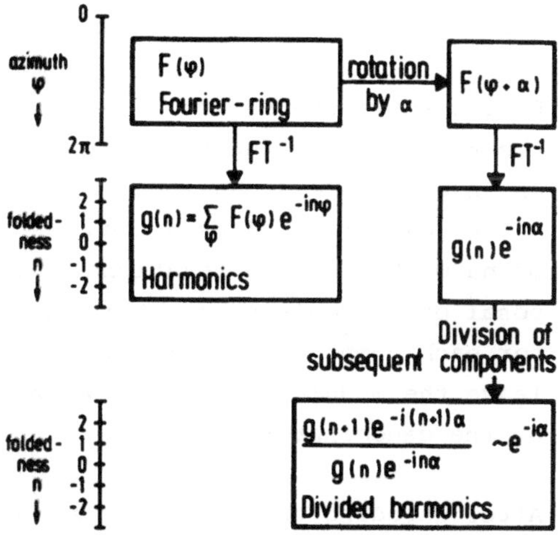


*Fig. 3: Upper row: AChR image before (left) and after (right) band pass filtering.*

*Middle row: Real and imaginary part of the Fourier-transform of the AChR image. The band pass according to the spatial frequency interval between 1/25 $Å^{-1}$ and 1/30 $Å^{-1}$ is indicated by white rings.*

*Lower row: One-dimensional real and imaginary part of the Fourier-ring function obtained by interpolating the Fourier coefficients within the selected frequency interval. The imaginary part indicates a five-fold rotational symmetry which is clearly resolved in the filtered image, too.*

*Fig. 4: Principle of encoding a rotation by the angle α as common phase factor exp(-iα) of the data set describing the molecular structure. The Fourier-ring function F(ϕ) as dependent of the azimuth ϕ in the Fourier-domain changes to F(ϕ+α). The decomposition of the rotated Fourier-ring function into its harmonics as dependent of the foldedness n results in a phase factor exp(-inα) for the n-th harmonic. The set of the quotients of subsequent harmonics has the common factor exp(-iα).*

Fig. 3 shows which structural details within the molecule are most important. After calculating the Fourier-transform of an image, all Fourier-coefficients which are outside a small spatial frequency band are set to zero. An inverse Fourier-transformation results in the band-pass filtered image, which obviously contains the most important structural details. The distances in this image lie between 25 and 30 Å. The Fourier-coefficients in the spatial-frequency band are interpolated to a one-dimensional Fourier-ring function.

Fig. 4 shows the effect of a rotation by an angle $\alpha$. At first the Fourier-ring function is decomposed into its harmonics by an inverse, one-dimensional Fourier-transformation. If the molecule is rotated by $\alpha$ then the phases of the harmonics change by $n\alpha$ with n as the rotational symmetry. According to a proposal of P. Schiske we obtain the common phase factor $\exp(-i\alpha)$ for each component by division of subsequent harmonics. To leave the modulus unchanged we still multiply by the modulus of the denominator.

After encoding the molecular structure into a vector of such modified harmonics we perform the multivariate analysis. For this the vectors of all molecules are arranged as columns of a rectangular matrix. Then the matrix is factorized by singular value decomposition. This is used to calculate the two sets of eigenvectors and the singular values (which are the roots of the corresponding eigenvalues) of the rectangular matrix. The idea of this decomposition is illustrated in fig. 5 for a simple example. We start with a set of images with identical structure but different orientations $\alpha_j$. The corresponding modified harmics are arranged in a rectangular matrix. $h_n$ indicates the n-th modified harmonic and $\exp(i\alpha_j)$ the phase factor due to the different orientations. By singular value decomposition we obtain a product of three matrices. The first one contains the vector of modified harmonics independent of the orientations.

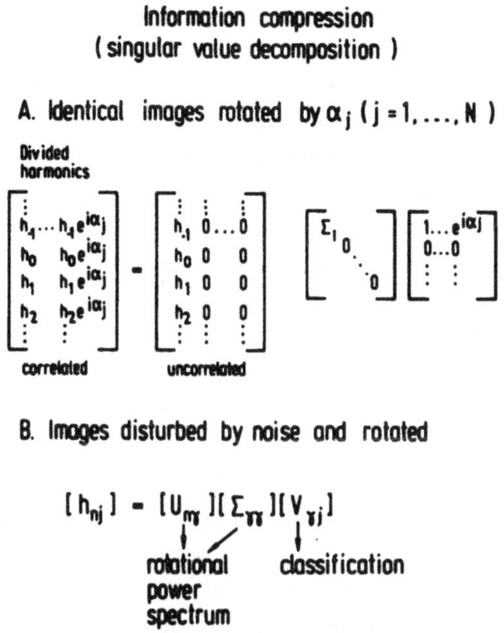


*Fig. 5: Principle of information compression by transformation of a set of correlated vectors (columns in the original matrix) into another set of uncorrelated vectors by singular value decomposition. It results in the product of two sets of eigenvectors (first and third, unitary matrix) and the singular values (the second, real, diagonal matrix).*

*A: In this example the correlated vectors differ by the phase factors* $\exp(i\alpha_j)$, $j = 1,2 \ldots, N-1$ *with N as the number of vectors (images). The common information is the modulus of the vectors which appears as the first uncorrelated eigenvector in the first matrix. The phase factors are the components of the first eigenvector in the third matrix.*

*B: The general form of singular value decomposition with h as the original matrix of modified harmonics. The matrix U is used to calculate the rotational power spectrum (squared modulus of the product* $U\Sigma$*). The matrix V is used to find similarities between the correlated vectors and to put them into different classes.*

This is the most common information inherent in the original matrix. The phase factors, i.e. the information about the orientations, are contained in the row vector in the third matrix. Thus the pattern which originally is distributed in different orientations is recognized uniquely in the first matrix of this decomposition. The general case of noisy patterns differing in rotational orientation is more complicated. But the essential feature of the decomposition is that starting from a set of correlated patterns, the result is a set of uncorrelated patterns. Thus if we start with a large set of AChR images and calculate the matrix of the modified harmonics, then after decomposition we obtain a set of modified harmonics which are uncorrelated. Because there is no redundancy in the uncorrelated set, the information about the molecular structure is contained in the first few uncorrelated harmonics only. The rest is noise. Because we are mainly interested in the question about the rotational symmetry of the AChR, we only need the squared modulus of the modified harmonics. This immediately gives the rotational power spectrum.

## Results

The result of the analysis of three idependent sets of 100 AChR images is shown in fig. 6. For each set the rotational power spectrum is shown for the symmetry components 1 to 7. The power spectra indicate a maximum for one-fold symmetry in the first eigenvector and maxima for two- and five-fold symmetry in the second as well as in the third eigenvectors. Other symmetry components, which we do not show here, are found with less importance in the next (4th, 5th, and so on) eigenvectors. The total power spectrum as the sum of spectra belonging to all eigenvectors is shown in the last row. Here again we observe maxima for two- and five-fold symmetry.
If we compare the results of the three independent sets of molecules, we find a very good agreement for the power spectra.

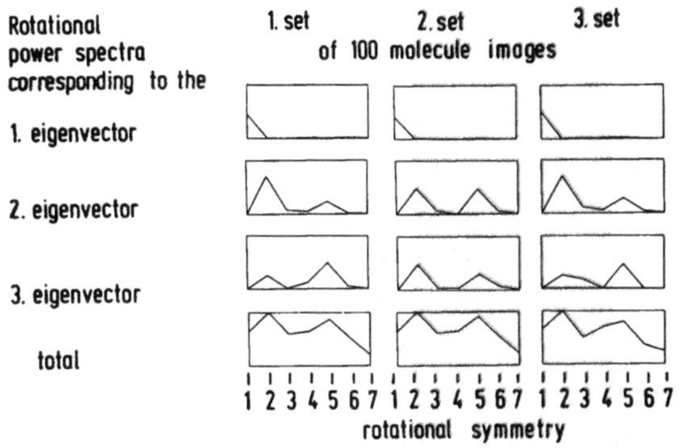


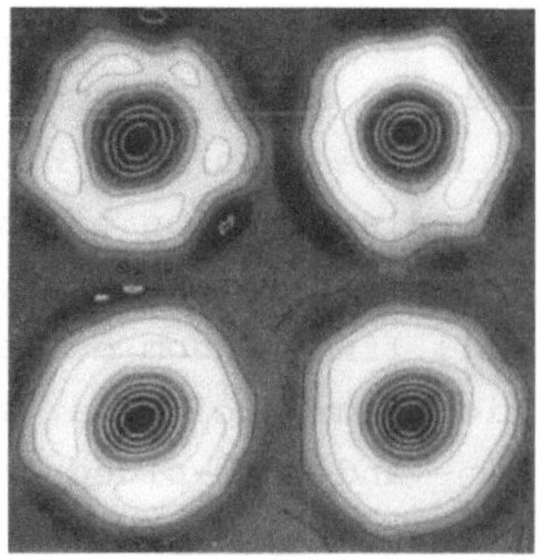

Fig. 6

Fig. 7

*Fig. 6:* *Rotational power spectra corresponding to the 1st, 2nd and 3rd uncorrelated modified harmonics (eigenvectors) and to their sum. The three columns of the curves are results obtained from independent sets of 100 molecules each.*

*Fig. 7:* *Averaged structures within a set of 100 AChR images separated into four classes according to their mutual similarity.*

Thus we can trust these results. What we have to dicuss is the meaning of the occurrence of one-, two- and five-fold symmetry elements. There is no doubt about the correlation of the five-fold symmetry with the pentameric structure of the molecule which is suggested for instance by Hucho in a biochemical model derived from biochemical considerations (1).

The interesting point about the power spectra is that the two- and five-fold symmetry appears in two eigenvectors. Because eigenvectors are uncorrelated, there must be a difference which we cannot detect in the power spectra and that is the phase. What we find is that in one eigenvector the orientation of the

two-fold symmetry lies just between two mirror planes. We do not believe that the AChR exists in two different structures according to these results. We interpret this difference as caused by random distribution of the stain material. If one assumes a ring-like structure which is surrounded statistically by stain material, one will find random deviations from a circular shape. But a deviation from a circular shape will have a strong one-sided and other two- and more-sided components with decreasing importance. We interpret the distinct maximum of the five-fold symmetric component as clear evidence for a pentameric structure.
In fig. 7 class averages are shown which have been found by comparison of 100 AChR images and summing them up into four different classes according to their similarity. The class average exhibiting the clearly resolved five-fold symmetry is the sum of only 15 of the 100 images, which is a small portion. On the other hand, in a separate analysis (6,7), we also found only 20% of the images with a predominant five-fold symmetry. This is the same portion which we obtain by comparing the rotational power of the five-fold symmetrical component with the power of all components. Thus the signal-to-noise ratio in the micrograph of the AChR is only about 1/5. The other three of the class averages in fig. 7 represent the noise part of the molecule images, one of them with a distinct two-fold symmetry.

## Acknowledgement

The authors thank Prof. E. Zeitler, Dr. P. Schiske, and M. van Heel for discussions and helpful suggestions.

## References

1. Hucho, F. 1986. Eur. J. Biochem. 158, 211-226.
2. Brisson, A., and Unwin, P.N.T. 1985. Nature 315, 474-477.
3. Kistler, J. and Stroud, R.M. 1981. Proc. Natl. Acad. Sci. USA 78, 3678-3682.
4. Zingsheim, H.P., Neugebauer, D.-Ch., Barrantes, F.J., and Frank, J. 1980. Proc. Natl. Acad. Sci. USA 77, 952-956.

5. van Heel, M., and Frank, J. 1981. Ultramicroscopy 6, 187-194.

6. Kunath, W., Giersig, M., Sack-Kongehl, H., and van Heel, M., 1986. In: XIth International Congress on Electron Microscopy, Kyoto, Japan. Vol 1.

7. Giersig, M., Kunath, W., Sack-Kongehl, H., and Hucho, F., 1986. In: "Nicotinic Acetylcholine Receptor", ed. A. Maelicke, pp. 7-17, Springer-Verlag, Berlin/Heidelberg.

# SELECTIVE LABELING STUDY ON TOPOGRAPHY OF ACETYLCHOLINE RECEPTOR AND BACTERIORHODOPSIN

V.I.Tsetlin, T.N.Alyonycheva, A.B.Kuryatov, K.A.Pluzhnikov
Shemyakin Institute of Bioorganic Chemistry, USSR Academy of Sciences, Moscow, USSR

## Introduction

Chemical modification of proteins is a recognized method for studying the relationships between their structure and biological activity. Nowadays genetic engineering and site directed mutagenesis appear to be the most direct way to understanding the functional role of specified amino acid residues. However, studies on the spatial structure of proteins and their binding to respective receptors require the incorporation of reporter groupings, isotopically labeled or unusual amino acids. These goals can be achieved by traditional chemical modification which, due to HPLC, has recently gained much in its potency and accuracy.

A series of chemically modified cobra neurotoxin derivatives containing spin, flourescence or photoactivable labels have been earlier prepared at our Institute (see reviews (1,2)). It is the maltitude of derivatives that allowed characterization of the binding surfaces of the neurotoxins and nicotinic acetylcholine receptor (AchR). The present report deals with some peculiarities of the neurotoxin binding to the membrane and solubilized AchR, as well as with modification of bacteriorhodopsin (BR), a representative of membrane proteins. In the latter case more useful proved to be "biosynthetic" modification (3) that afforded appropriate analogues for the studies on BR spatial organization with the aid of monoclonal antibodies (mAb) (4), $^{19}F$ NMR and tritium planigraphy (5,6). Thus, with the aid of individual photoactivable neurotoxins it was found that the AchR solubilization affects the topography of its neurotoxin-binding site. Use of Trp(F)-containing BR analogue and $^{19}F$ NMR facilitated the analysis of BR conformation in solution.

AchR binding sites probed with photoactivable neurotoxins

The interaction of neurotoxin II (*Naja naja oxiana*) derivatives, containing the $|^{14}C|$p-azidobenzoyl group ($N_3Bz$) at Lys 26 or Lys 46 (7,8), with the membrane-bound or Triton X-100 solubilized AchR was compared. The efficiency of the UV-induced crosslinking, assessed by DE 81 filter disc assay or HPLC on a Protein Pak 300 SW column in the presence of sodium dodecylsulfate (SDS), showed no significant dependence on the $N_3Bz$ position in the neurotoxin molecule or on the AchR state, solubilized or membrane-bound.

The results of SDS polyacrylamide gel electrophoresis demonstrated that, after crosslinking the Lys 46-derivative to the membrane AchR, almost all radioactivity accounted for by covalent binding was associated with the band of $M_r$ ∿50 K (Fig. 1). Since the neuro-

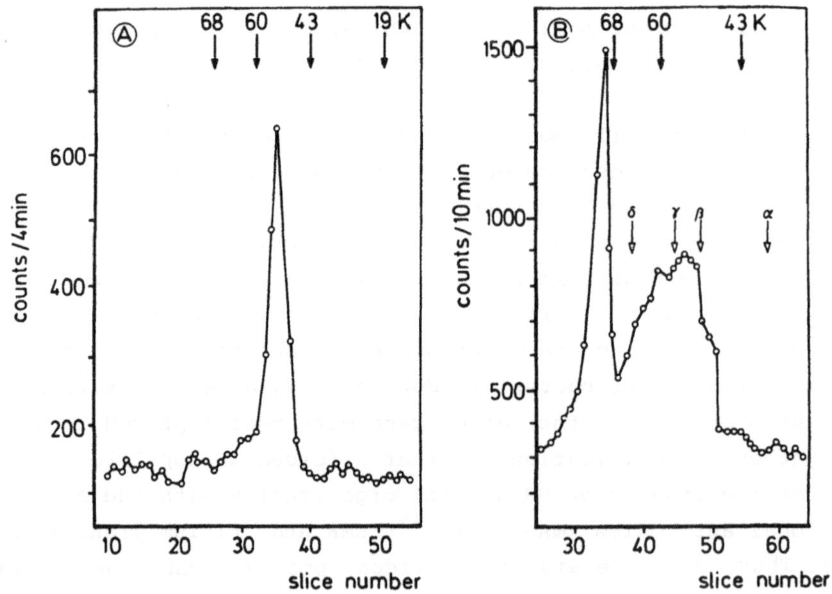


Fig. 1. SDS gel electrophoretic analysis of the $|N_3Bz\text{-}Lys^{46}|$neurotoxin II crosslinking to membrane (A) and solubilized (B) AchR. The arrows indicate the positions of the marker proteins and AchR subunits visualized by Coomassie Blue staining.

toxin derivative has $M_r$ ∿7K, this result points to labeling of the AchR α subunit ($M_r$ ∿40-41 K). Irradiation of the membrane AchR complex with the Lys 26-derivative produced a different radioactivity profile (not shown) with the most pronounced labeling of the γ subunit.

Labeling of the affinity-purified solubilized AchR with either Lys 26- or Lys 46-derivatives resulted in similar radioactivity patterns, the δ subunit being labeled more heavily than α,β or γ.

Although comparison of the neurotoxin binding in terms of the crosslinking efficacy revealed no dissimilarity between the solubilized and membrane-bound AchR, the differences became obvious when labeling of specific subunits was analyzed. Thus, solubilization induces some alterations in the mutual disposition of the bound neurotoxins and AchR subunits. Since the membrane and solubilized AchR share a similar overall structure (9), we apparently detected local conformational changes in the neurotoxin-binding site.

Another type of conformational changes has been disclosed when studying the interaction between AchR in Triton X-100 and the neurotoxin II derivative with the $N_3$Bz group at Lys 25 (10). Irradiation of its AchR complex suppressed subsequent binding of $|^3H|$toxin 3 *Naja naja siamensis*, a long-type neurotoxin, but did not affect binding of $|^3H|$neurotoxin II. Apparently, two molecules of Lys 25-photoactivated derivative in the covalent complex with AchR occupy two "regular" binding sites, whereas photoinduced crosslinks trigger in AchR the conformational changes and create (or uncover) the additional binding sites. These sites (up to 3 per one AchR molecule) can accomodate only short-chain but not the long-chain neurotoxins and are specific: bound radioactive neurotoxin II can be totally displaced by cold neurotoxin II or large excess of acetylcholine.

The neurotoxin II derivative wherein all 6 amino groups (including Lys 25) are trifluoracetylated, shows differring affinities for the two "regular" binding sites of the solubilized AchR (11). When this compound was first added to the AchR followed by $|N_3Bz\text{-}Lys^{15}|$ neurotoxin II, the crosslinking extent appeared twice as low as in the control. If the AchR was preincubated in the dark with the photoactivable neurotoxin and then the latter was displaced by hexa-(trifluoroacetyl)neurotoxin II from one of the two binding sites, subsequent irradiation led to the appearance of the additional binding sites. It seems that one "regular" binding site, that of a higher affinity for hexa(trifluoroacetyl)neurotoxin II, contains a "sensitive locus": interaction with this locus triggers the formation of the additional binding sites. Noteworthy, the nonequivalence of the two "regular" binding sites manifests itself both in the interaction with modified polypeptide neurotoxins and d-tubocurarine (cf. (12)).

The functional role of the additional binding sites is not yet clear. Possibly they are relevant to the low-affinity agonist binding sites reported by Raftery and coworkers (13).

## Bacteriorhodopsin: modification and spatial structure

Chemical modification of integral membrane proteins is more challenging task than modification of such water-soluble proteins as snake venom neurotoxins. Selective labeling of membrane proteins, as a rule, is achieved with novel approaches. For example,a method of BR modification at the sites of limited proteolysis has been worked out at our Institute (14).

Chymotrypsin action generates on the purple membrane surface the free α-amino group of Gly 72 and α-carboxyl of Phe 71 (15). In different conditions papain releases the α-carboxyl of Gly 231 (alone or with the α-amino groups of Ile 4 and Gly 73). The tryptic digestion makes accessible the α-carboxyl of Ser 239. The above-mentioned groupings were modified with the spin-labeling reagents in the BR preparations wherein accessible amino or carboxy groups had been blocked prior to proteolysis. Microenvironment of the spin labels attached at the external and cytoplasmic membrane surfaces was characterized by electron paramagnetic resonance spectroscopy (14).

Photoinduced reduction of the aldimine bond, formed by the retinal and Lys 216, is another example of selective chemical modification giving a fluorescent derivative of BR (see (16) and references therein). In the course of attempts to carry out this reaction in the dark, the $NaBH_4$-induced selective cleavage of the Gly 155-Phe 156 bond was disclosed (16). The resultant large fragments 1-155 and 156-248 were utilized in the studies on BR spatial structure.

Biosynthetic modification seems quite promising for membrane proteins of microbial origin. Using synthetic media containing 5-fluorotryptophan, 3-fluorotyrosine, 3- or 4-fluorophenylalalanine instead of respective aromatic amino acids, the |Trp(F)|-, |Tyr(F)|- and |Phe(F)|BR analogues have been prepared (3). Incorporation of Trp(F) into BR amounted to 95%, while for Tyr(F) and Phe(F) it ranged from 40 to 60%. Fluorinated pigments had the absorption, CD and resonance Raman laser spectra very similar to those of the native BR. Thus fluorination may be considered as nonperturbing modification allowing the study on the role of aromatic amino acid residues. In particular, the data for |Tyr(F)|BR confirmed the effect of tyrosine deprotonation on the rate of the M412 rise, but provided evidence against the direct influence of a tyrosine pK on the chromophore absorption earlier suggested in (17).

Using $^{19}F$ NMR analysis of |Trp(F)|BR, appropriate conditions for studying the BR solution structure were chosen (5). The $^{19}F$ NMR spectrum of |Trp(F)|BR in the $CHCl_3$-$CH_3OH$ (1:1) system with 0.1 M LiCl consists of 8 signals corresponding to 8 Trp(F) residues in the modified BR. A study of the large Trp(F)-containing fragments 1-71, 72-248, 1-155 and 156-248 made possible the signal assignments. In the above-mentioned system of organic solvents, BR was demonstrated to possess the same percentage of regular secondary structure as in Triton X-100 solution and to have an ordered three-dimensional structure apparently similar to that in the membrane.

Fluorinated BR analogues, along with some other modified derivatives and peptide fragments, were used to define the specificity of monoclonal antibodies (mAb) interacting with the exposed determinants on BR. The substitution of Phe for Phe(F) residues resulted in about two-fold decline in the efficiency of the purple membrane interaction with mAbs $A_{14}H_3$ and $H_5E_5$ (Fig. 2), whereas no change

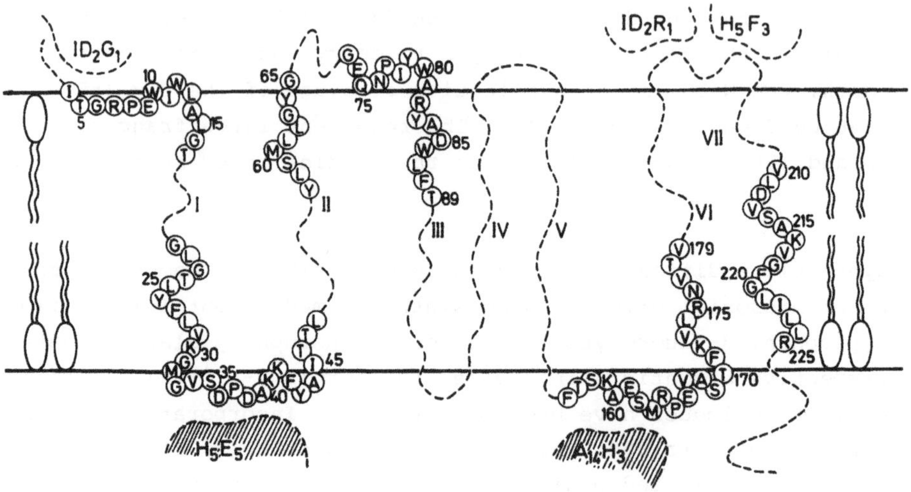


Fig. 2. Bacteriorhodopsin folding according to monoclonal antibody and tritium planigraphy data. Tritium incorporation was determined for the encircled residues.

was observed with the other mAbs. Since the presence of Phe 156 in the $A_{14}H_3$ antigenic determinant has been independently established, these results indicate the involvement of a phenylalanine residue (most probably, Phe 42) in the $H_5E_5$ determinant (4).

A two-stage modification of BR was devised to localize mAbs binding to the extracellular or cytoplasmic membrane surfaces. At first, the fluorescent retinylbacterioopsin had been prepared and then reacted with p-azidobenzylamine in the presence of 1-cyclohexyl-3-(2-morpholinoethyl)carbodiimide metho-p-toluenesulfonate (pH 4.75, final concentration of $CH_3CN$ 12%). Control irradiations ($\lambda_{max}$ 256 nm, 5 min) demonstrated the incorporation of 0.7 mole label/mole BR, that fell to 0.1 mole after cleaving off the C-terminal fragment 232-248 with papain. Thus most of photoactivable labels were attached to the C-terminal tail whose cytoplasmic location has earlier been established (15, 18). If we assume that the remaining labels are evenly distributed between all other carboxyls, then the population of labels on the extracellular surface should be below 5% of the total.

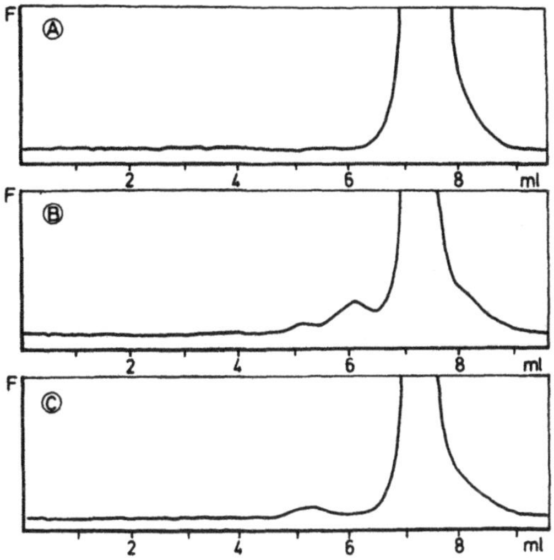


Fig. 3. HPLC separation of monoclonal antibodies covalently bound to photoactivable retinylbacterioopsin. Protein Pak SW 300 column (300 x 7.5 mm), 0.1 M Na-phosphate buffer, pH 6.2, 0.1 % SDS. F - relative fluorescence ($\lambda_{ex}$= 330 nm, $\lambda_{em}$> 480 nm). A - control, B and C - mAb $A_{14}H_3$ and $H_5E_5$ binding, respectively.

The fluorescent photoactivable derivative was incubated with mAbs (0.01 M Na-phosphate buffer pH 7.4, 0.15 M NaCl, 0.05 % Tween 20, 3hr, 20$^oC$) followed by UV-irradiation and denaturation (2 % SDS, 100$^oC$, 3 min). Fig. 3 A refers to the case when the photoactivable BR was UV-irradiated prior to incubation with mAb $H_5E_5$. Similar profiles were obtained after incubating this "photoinactivated" analogue with mAb $A_{14}H_3$, $H_5F_3$, $ID_2G_1$ or with nonspecific mouse antibodies. No fluorescent peak, except that of retinylbacterioopsin, was observed when complexes of the photoactivable BR with mAb $H_5F_3$, $ID_2G_1$ or nonspecific antibodies were subjected to irradiation. However, fluorescent peaks of higher molecular mass than retinylbacterioopsin did appear when mAb $A_{14}H_3$ and $H_5E_5$ were used in the latter protocol. In view of the described control experiments, this finding demonstrates the formation of the covalent crosslinks between the C-terminus and mAbs $A_{14}H_3$ and $H_5E_5$. In turn, it points to the cytoplasmic localization both of these mAbs and their antigenic determinants.

Biosynthetic derivatives with |$^{14}$C|Ile, Tyr, Pro or Phe residues facilitated BR analysis by tritium planigraphy (5, 6). The $^{14}$C-labeled purple membranes were cleaved with $NaBH_4$ or papain and then treated with the thermally activated tritium gas. After removing exchangeable tritium, the peptides 4-65, 73-231 and 156-248 were subjected to Edman degradation, $^{3}$H incorporation being quantified at each step. The presence of $^{14}$C at specified positions made possible the control of the degradation. The cyanogen bromide peptides obtained from the 4-65 and 73-231 fragments were analyzed in a similar manner.

In Fig. 4 one can distinguish the three kinds of radioactivity profiles: $^{3}$H content markedly decreases (A) or increases (B) after a certain residue(s) of the polypeptide chain, or remains at the same level (C). The first case seems to relate to the polypeptide chain entering the membrane from the surface, the second one describes the chain traversing the membrane width and finally emerging on its surface, whereas in the last case one deals with the intramembrane segment.

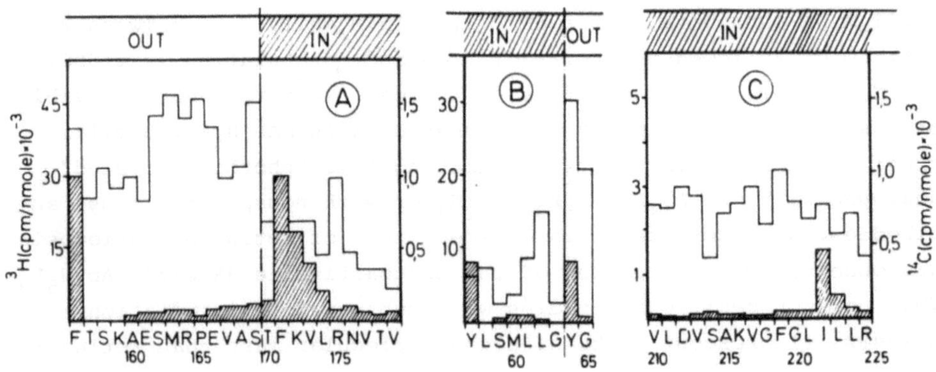


Fig. 4. Edman degradation analysis of tritium incorporation (left-hand ordinates in the plots) into $^{14}$C-labeled (right-hand ordinates, hatced bars) bacteriorhodopsin.

Tritium planigraphy data (see Fig. 2) are in general accord with the earlier models for BR spatial organization (cf.(15)). There are also some interesting features brought to light by this new method: i) helices V and VI are connected by quite a long junction, ii) other interhelical junctions and the N-terminal fragment do not have totally extended and solvent-accessible conformations.

References

1. Ovchinnikov, Yu.A. 1984. Pure and Appl. Chem. 56, 1049-1068.

2. Tsetlin, V.I. 1985. In: Peptides. Structure and Function (C.M.Deber, V.J.Hruby, K.D.Kopple, eds). Pierce chemical company, Rockford, pp. 833-842.

3. Kuryatov, A.B., G.V. Ovechkina, T.N. Alyonycheva, L.P. Minaeva, V.I. Tsetlin. 1984. Bioorgan. Khim. 10, 333-340.

4. Vtyurina, I.Yu., A.B. Kuryatov, A.V. Kiselev, N.I. Khoroshilova, G.V. Ovechkina, N.G. Abdulaev, V.I. Tsetlin, R.G. Vasilov. 1984. Biol. Membrany 1, 1161-1170.

5. Kuryatov, A.B., A.S. Arseniev, T.N. Alyonycheva, L.A. Neiman, V.I. Tsetlin. 1986. In: Retinal proteins (Irkutsk), Abstracts, pp. 76-77.

6. Neiman, L.A., V.S. Smolyakov, A.V. Shishkov. 1985. Radioisotope methods in physicochemical biology. Application of atomic tritium reactions. VINITI, Moscow, pp. 6-208, (in Russian).

7. Pluzhnikov, K.A., A.A. Karelin, Yu.N. Utkin, V.I. Tsetlin, V.T.Ivanov. 1982. Bioorgan. Khim. 8, 905-913.

8. Tsetlin, V.I., K.A. Pluzhnikov, A.A. Karelin, V.T. Ivanov. 1983. In: Toxins as Tools in Neurochemistry (F.Hucho and Yu.A.Ovchinnikov, eds.). Walter de Gruyter, Berlin - N.Y., pp. 159-169.

9. Popot, J.L., J.-P. Changeux. 1984. Physiol. Rev. 64, 1162-1239.

10. Karelin, A.A., K.A. Pluzhnikov, V.I. Tsetlin. 1986. Bioorgan. Khim. 12, 448-456.

11. Tsetlin, V.I., E. Karlsson, A.S. Arseniev, Yu.N. Utkin, A.M.Surin, V.S. Pashkov, K.A. Pluzhnikov, V.T. Ivanov, V.F. Bystrov, Yu.A. Ovchinnikov. 1979. FEBS Letters 106, 47-52.

12. Rousselet, A., G. Faure, J.-C. Boulain, A. Menez. 1984. Eur. J.Biochem. 140, 31-37.

13. Dunn, S.M.J., B.M. Conti-Tronconi, M.A. Raftery. 1983. Proc. Nat. Acad. Sci. USA 22, 2512-2516.

14. Tsetlin, V.I., V.I. Zakis, G.V. Ovechkina, A.B. Kuryatov, T.A. Balashova, A.S. Arseniev, V.N. Maiorov, V.T. Ivanov. 1984. Biol. Membrany 1, 838-857.

15. Ovchinnikov, Yu.A. 1982. FEBS Letters 148, 179-191.

16. Tsetlin, V.I., V.I. Zakis, A.A. Aldashev, A.B. Kuryatov, G.V. Ovechkina, V.L. Shnyrov. 1983. Bioorgan. Khim. 9, 1589-1605.

17. Lemke, H.-D., D. Oesterhelt. 1981. Eur. J. Biochem. 115, 595-604.

18. Gerber, G.E., C.P. Gray, D. Wildenauer, H.G. Khorana. 1977. Proc. Nat. Acad. Sci. USA 74, 5426-5430.

# MONOCLONAL ANTIBODIES AS FUNCTIONAL PROBES OF THE NICOTINIC ACETYLCHOLINE RECEPTOR

Gregor Fels and Alfred Maelicke

Max-Planck-Institut für Ernährungsphysiologie
Rheinlanddamm 201, D-4600 Dortmund, FRG

## Introduction

The nicotinic acetylcholine receptor (AChR) from mammalian muscle and fish electic tissue is an integral signal transducer (1); it contains in its protein moiety binding sites for acetylcholine and its agonists and antagonists (receptor function), the ligand-gated cation channel (response function) and several types of modulator sites (modulator function). Several hundred ligands are known to exist for the AChR, and it therefore may not be obvious why additional ligands such as monoclonal antibodies are desired to probe the receptor's function. However, it is exactly the above noted complex design of the AChR which calls for additional tools in the study of its mechanism of action. The present state of these studies may be illustrated by the fact that at least three basically different models of the receptor's mechanism of action exist (2-4). None of them, however, can satisfactorily explain the full set of electrophysiological and biochemical data available on cholinergic excitation. Among the many unsolved questions are such important ones as (i) how many and which sites must be occupied by transmitter or agonists to avtivate the receptor channel, (ii) is the mutually exclusive binding of cholinergic ligands to the receptor the result of identical sites for these ligands or, instead, the result of allosteric coupling between separate sites for groups of different ligands, (iii) what is the molecular mechanism of desensitisation?

For the purpose of probing questions of this kind, we have tried to obtain by immunological techniques marker molecules which affect the functions of the AChR via other sites or by other mechanisms than the established cholinergic ligands and

Receptors and Ion Channels

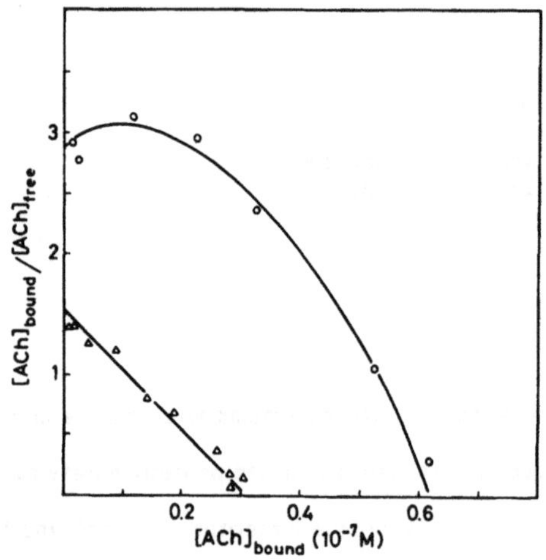


Fig. 1 Scatchard plot of acetycholine binding to the membrane bound AChR from T. marmorata in the absence and presence of antibody WF6.
Experimantal details see (10). Initial concentration of receptor and WF6 were 64 nM and 1000 nM, respectively. In the absence of antibody, acetylcholine binds to two sites per receptor monomer in a positively cooperative fashion. In the presence of saturating concentations of WF6, binding of acetylcholine is to half as many sites and with a single affinity.

modulators. As we show here, this approach may indeed provide new means of unraveling the molecular mechanism of action of the acetylcholine transducer.

The main obstacle to obtaining antibodies against many different surface regions of the same molecule is the limited variation of the common immune response (5,6). Conventional immunization techniques do not lead to many different antibody specificities in immune sera or libraries of monoclonal antibodies directed against the AChR (7). Recently several methods have been developed to overcome this problem (5,6). In addition, we have developed suitable assays to select function-affecting antibodies (8-12). Here we sumarize data mainly obtained with the antibody WF6. We show that (i) this antibody competes with acetylcholine and its agonists but not with low molecular weight antagonists, (ii) the competition with agonists is by allosteric interaction, and (iii) the receptor-integral ion channel is already blocked when one of the two acetylcholine binding sites is allosterically blocked by WF6.

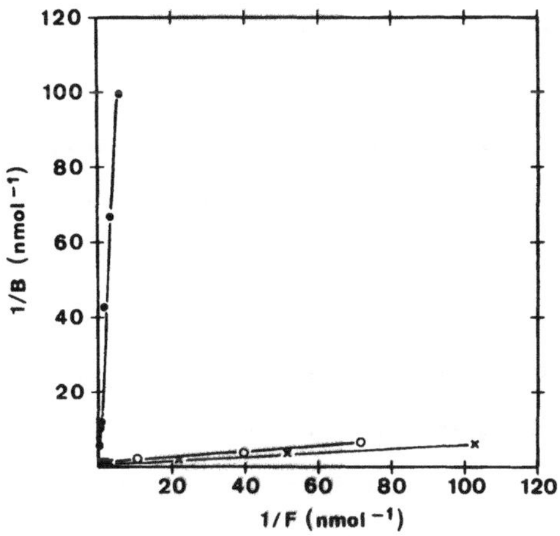


Fig. 2 Competition of WF2 and cholinergic ligands for receptor binding.
Preformed complexes of WF2 (0.2-4.7 nM) and AChR (2 nM) were incubated for 15 min with (x) PBS, (o) hexamethonium (1 mM) and (•) carbamoylcholine (1 mM), respectively. The fraction of bound and free WF2 was determined by a rapid centrifugation assay (equilibrium data: (x) $R_o$=1.2 nmol, $K_D$=64 pmol; (o) $R_o$=1.1 nmol, $K_D$=84 pmol; (•) $R_o$=0.15 nmol, $K_D$=2400 pmol). The data indicate accelerated dissociation of ligand-receptor complexes in the presence of competing cholinergic ligands.

### Interaction of WF6 with the AChR from T. marmorata

Antibody WF6 binds with high affinity and long half life to the receptor ($K_D$=10 pM, $t_{1/2}$=several days) (10). It competes with agonists and α-neurotoxins but not with antagonists (including bismethonium compounds) and local anesthetics for receptor binding. WF6 binds to a single site per receptor monomer (10), thereby blocking all of the sites for α-neurotoxins but only half of the sites for acetylcholine (Fig. 1).

### Interaction of mAb2 with the AChR from T. marmorata

Antibody WF2 also binds with high affinity ($K_D$ =10 pM) and long half life ($t_{1/2}$=several days) to the receptor (12). The antibody competes with agonists, α-neurotoxins and, in contrast to WF6 also with tubocuare for receptor binding while no competition is observed with other antagonists and all bismethonium compounds tested (8,12). Furthermore antibody WF6 completely inhibits binding of WF2 to the receptor while in the reverse experiment WF6 binding is only partially blocked.

Preformed complexes of WF2 and receptor when incubated with high concentration of agonists, dissociate several orders of magnitude faster than is expected from their intrinsic dissociation rate. This effect requires the presence of agonists and is not observed in the presence of antagonists (Fig. 2). For a discussion of accelerated dissociation see the paper by A. Maelicke in this volume.

**Further evidence for allosteric competition between receptor ligands**

The above descibed findings suggest that antibodies WF2 and WF6 (i) do not occupy identical sites and (ii) do not bind directly to the agonist site. The competition between these antibodies and between them and cholinergic ligands must therefore be mediated via allosteric interaction of different binding regions. This allosteric interaction of sites must be bidirectional in the sense that occupation of a ligand or antibody site modulates the binding of other ligands to their sites and vice versa.

To generalize these findings, different groups of ligands appear to induce different conformational changes which therefore allosterically link different surface structures of the AChR. For example, binding of acetylcholine to the AChR induces a conformational change which leads to the disappearance of the epitopes for both antibodies (WF2 and WF6). Consequently, these epitopes form an allosteric network with the acetylcholine binding sites. In contrast, the binding of antagonists (e.g. tubocurare or hexamethonium) results in other conformational changes than those induced by acetylcholine; they affect other (or fewer) epitopes and, therefore, they define other (smaller) allosteric networks of structural regions.

Further evidence for allosteric competition between groups of receptor ligands is provided by cross-competition experiments. As mentioned before, WF6 competes with acetylcholine but not with hexamethonium for receptor binding. As a consequence, the rate of association of WF6 to the receptor is slowed down in the presence of acetylcholine but

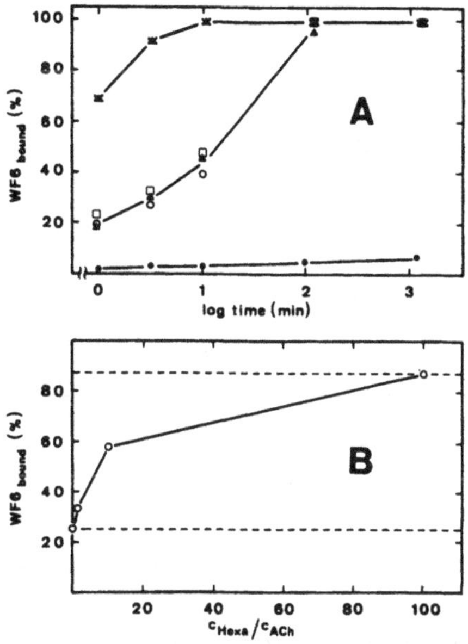


Fig. 3 Effect of hexamethonium on the competition of acetylcholine and WF6 for binding to Torpedo membrane fragments.
(upper) Kinetics of WF6 association in the absence (x) and presence (o) of 0.1 mM acetylcholine. Similar inhibiting effects were observed with NBD-5-acylcholine (▲) and suberyldicholine (□) while the same concentration of hexamethonium (●) had no effect.
(lower) Competition, as determined 3 min after mixing, of WF6 (0.5nM) and acetylcholine (0.1 mM) for receptor binding in the presence of hexamethonium. The dashed lines indicate the levels of WF6 binding in the presence of only hexamethonium (upper line) or acetylcholine (lower line).

not in the presence of hexamethonium (Fig. 3). To test wether these two ligands compete with each other also in the presence of the antibody, mixtures of acetylcholine and hexamethonium were applied in the above kinetic experiment. As shown in Fig. 3, hexamethonium indeed was capable of competing acetylcholine from the receptor thereby preventing the effect of acetylcholine on the association rate of WF6.

In a similar fashion, the accelerated dissociation of WF2-receptor complexes in the presence of acetylcholine is reduced when mixtures of hexamethonium and acetylcholine are applied.

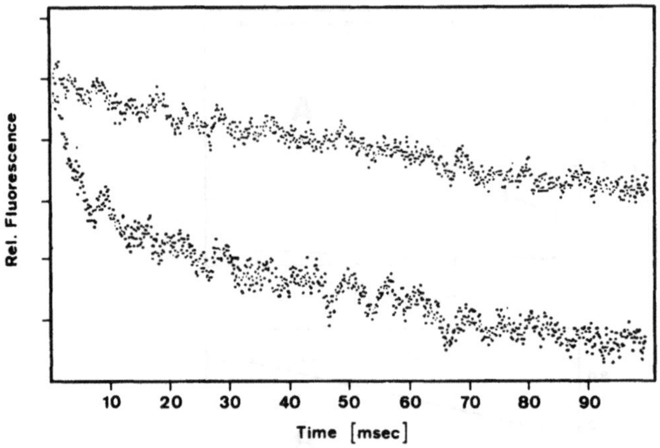


Fig. 4 Effect of WF6 on the kinetics of $Tl^+$ influx into membane vesicles from T. marmorata.
Vesicular membrane fragments (initial concentration of AChR appr. $2*10^{-7}$ M,) were loaded with fluorophore 1,2,6,8-pyrene tetrasulfonate and suspended in 160 mM $NaNO_3$, 10 nM Hepes, pH 7.4. These vesicles were rapidly mixed with equal volumes of a solution containing (lower trace) $10^{-4}$M acetylcholine or (upper trace) $10^{-4}$M acetylcholine and $10^{-6}$M WF6 in 130 mM $NaNO_3$, 30 mM $TlNO_3$, 10 mM Hepes, pH 7.4, and the change in fluorescence was recorded. The upper trace coincides with the control (influx in the absence of acetylcholine). Blockade of half of the acetylcholine binding sites at the AChR by WF6 (Fig. 1) completely abolished the acetylcholine-induced $Tl^+$ influx into the membrane vesicles. Even very high concentrations of acetylcholine sufficient to saturate the suggested additional low affinity site (3,14) did not reactivate the $Tl^+$ influx.

Both effects require the assumption of separate sites for at least two of the three ligands involved. If two can compete with each other by an allosteric mechanism, the same mechanism may also apply for the competition with the third. Thus, it is quite possible that other fully competitive ligands of the AChR also do so by allosteric rather than classical sterical competition.

### Two molecules of acetylcholine are required to gate the receptor channel

Models for channel activation have been suggested (3,14) in which the saturation of one or two low affinity sites, additional and different from the commonly observed two competitive acetylcholine sites of higher affinity (2,4,13) and independent of them, is required for gating. The opposite, namely channel activation by a single acetylcholine molecule has also been suggested (15). Ion flux measurements in the absence and presence of WF6 show that neither of these applies. As shown in Fig. 4, saturating concentations of WF6 (blocking one of the two acetylcholine sites at the receptor (Fig. 1)) fully inhibit the acetylcholine-induced influx of $Tl^{+}$ into sealed AChR-rich menbrane vesicles (9,10). Thus, binding of a single acetylcholine molecule per receptor monomer apparently does not suffive to induce this ion flux. In addition, stopped-flow experiments as shown in Fig. 4 permit to rapidly saturate (within milliseconds) any independent low affinity sites for acetylcholine if they existed. Thus, if Raftery's model (3) were corect, higher concentration of acetylcholine should reinduce $Tl^{+}$ influx even though the second competitive acetylcholine site remains blocked by antibody. This was not observed suggesting that exactly two acetylcholine molecules, not less not more, are required to activate the receptor-integral ion channel.

## Concluding Remarks

Ligand-competitive antibodies have also been obtained by other groups (7,16-18) but have not been used in comparable depth or for the same purposes as in our laboratory. Presently, the major limitation of our library of antibodies is their limited cross-reactivity with receptor preparations other than Torpedo and more suitable for detailed electrophysiological analysis (8). Consequently, their major application presently is in biochemical studies of receptor activation (4,19). In this context, they decisively help to unravel the kinetics of receptor-ligand interactions including such aspects as ordered versus random mechanism (20), preexisting versus ligand-induced active states (21) and the molecular mechanism of desensitisation. With rational procedures for their production available (6) and an initial characterization of some of them performed (8-12), these antibodies may form useful tools for many aspects of AChR studies.

## Acknowledgements

Work from our laboratory is supported by the Deutsche Forschungs-gemeinschaft (SFB 168) and the Fond der Chemischen Industrie.

## References

1. Maelicke, A. 1984. Angew. Chem. Int. Ed. 23, 195.

2. Changeux, J.-P., A. Devillers-Thiery, P. Chemoulli. 1984. Science 225, 1335.

3. Raftery, M.A., S.M.J. Dunn, B. M. Conti-Tronconi, D.S. Middlemas, R.D. Crawford. 1983. Cold Spring Harbor Symp. Quant. Biol. 48, 21.

4. Prinz, H., A. Maelicke. 1983. J. Biol. Chem. 258, 10273.

5. Mathew, W.D., P.H. Patterson. 1983. Cold Spring Harbor Symp. Quant. Biol. 48, 635.

6. Maelicke, A. 1987. Review in preparation.

7. Venter, J.C., C.M. Frazer, J. Lindstrom. 1984. In: Monoclonal and anti-idiotypic antibodies: Probes for receptor structure and function. Receptor Biochemistry and Methology, Vol. 4. Alan R. Liss , Inc. New York, p. 21.

8. Watters, D., A. Maelicke. 1983. Biochemistry 22, 1811.

9. Fels, G., A. Maelicke, D. Schäfer, J.P. Walrond, T.S. Reese. 1985. In: Molecular Basis of Nerve Activity (J.-P. Changeux, F. Hucho, A. Maelicke, E. Neumann, eds.). Walter de Gruyter, Berlin, p.197.

10. Fels, G., R. Plümer-Wilk, M. Schreiber, A. Maelicke. 1986. J. Biol. Chem (in press)

11. Maelicke, A., G. Fels, R. Plümer-Wilk, E.K. Wolff, M. Covarrubias, C. Metfessel. 1986. In: Ion Channels in Neural Membranes. Alan R. Liss, Inc, New York, p. 275.

12. Fels, G., A. Maelicke. 1987, in preparation.

13. Fels, G., E.K. Wolff, A. Maelicke. 1982. Eur. J. Biochem. 127, 31.

14. Pasqaule, E.B., K. Takeyasu, J.B. Udgaonkar, D.J. Cash, M.C. Severski, G.P. Hess. 1983. Biochemistry 22, 5967.

15. Lester, N.A., M.E. Krouse, M.M. Nass, N.H. Wassermann, B.F. Erlanger. 1980. J. Gen. Physiol. 75, 207.

16. Gomez, C., D. Richman. 1983. Proc. Natl. Acad. Sci. USA 80, 4089.

17. James, R., A. Kato, M. Rey, B.W. Fulpius. 1980. FEBS Lett. 120, 145.

18. Moschly-Rosen, C., S. Fuchs. 1981. Biochemistry 20, 5920.

19. Covarrubias, M., H. Prinz, A. Maelicke. 1986. J. Biol. Chem. (in press)

20. Prinz, H., A. Maelicke. 1985. In: Molecular Basis of Nerve Activity (J.-P. Changeux, F. Hucho, A. Maelicke, E. Neumann, eds.). Walter de Gruyter, Berlin, p.437.

21. Maelicke, A., H. Prinz. 1983. In: Modern Cell Biology, Vol 1 (B.H. Satir, ed.). Alan R. Liss, Inc, New York, p.171.

# BINDING OF [$^3$H]-ACETYLCHOLINE TO MEMBRANE-BOUND ACETYLCHOLINE RECEPTOR

Heino Prinz

Max-Planck-Institut für Ernährungsphysiologie
Rheinlanddamm 201, D-4600 Dortmund 1, FRG

## Introduction

The nicotinic acetylcholine receptor is a membrane-bound macromolecule which contains both, the binding sites for acetylcholine and an acetylcholine controlled cation channel (For review see: 1,2). The induced depolarization of the postsynaptic membrane is a transient process which occurs in the time range of milliseconds (3). In order to study the mechanism of cholinergic excitation we therefore have employed fluorescent agonists (4) the binding of which was followed by the corresponding decrease in the spectroscopic signal. For these experiments the acetylcholine receptor was studied in its purified (5,6) and membrane-bound state (7,8). In the case of the membrane-bound receptor, the main part of the association reaction was a slow component which was not detected in the case of the purified receptor protein. This slow component of the association reaction will be the topic of this paper. Its rate constant was sufficiently small (9) to enable us to study it employing [$^3$H]-acetylcholine and a filtration assay.

## Materials and Methods

Membrane fragments were prepared by repeated centrifugation steps (10) from frozen tissue of *Torpedo marmorata*. [$^3$H]-acetylcholine was obtained from Amersham, Braunschweig, W. Germany. Its contamination with non-binding radioactivity (between 9% and 17% of the total radioactivity) was determined for each batch and was considered in data evaluation. Equilibrium binding studies in the presence of an esterase blocker (10) were performed using a Sorvall centrifuge and a SS-34 rotor with adapters for 1.5 ml Beckman tubes. After centrifugation at 48000 g for 1h, the pellets were separated from the supernatant and used for the determination of bound ligand. The concentration of free ligand was determined from radioactivity in the supernatant. Filtration experiments were performed using a Millipore filtration unit XX2702550 and Whatman GF/C filters. The filtration time was less than 2 seconds. The radioactivity in the filtrate was proportional to the free ligand concentration. This was verified by comparison with equilibrium binding data. All experiments were performed at room temperature (20–25 °C) in standard buffer (100 mM NaCl, 4 mM $CaCl_2$, 2 mM $MgCl_2$ and 10 mM PIPES at pH 6.8).

## Results

Fig. 1 shows the association of [$^3$H]-acetylcholine to membrane fragments obtained from *Torpedo marmorata*. For low acetylcholine concentrations (i.e. markedly lower than the concentration of binding sites) the main part of the reaction was so fast that it could not be detected in the filtration experiments. At higher acetylcholine concentrations, i.e. at concentrations near or above the concentration of binding sites, the main part of the reaction had a time constant of less than 0.01 $s^{-1}$. Under these conditions, equilibrium was reached after more than 15 minutes. The observed *decrease* in velocity with increasing ligand concentration is difficult to reconcile with second order association reactions where an *increase* would be expected.

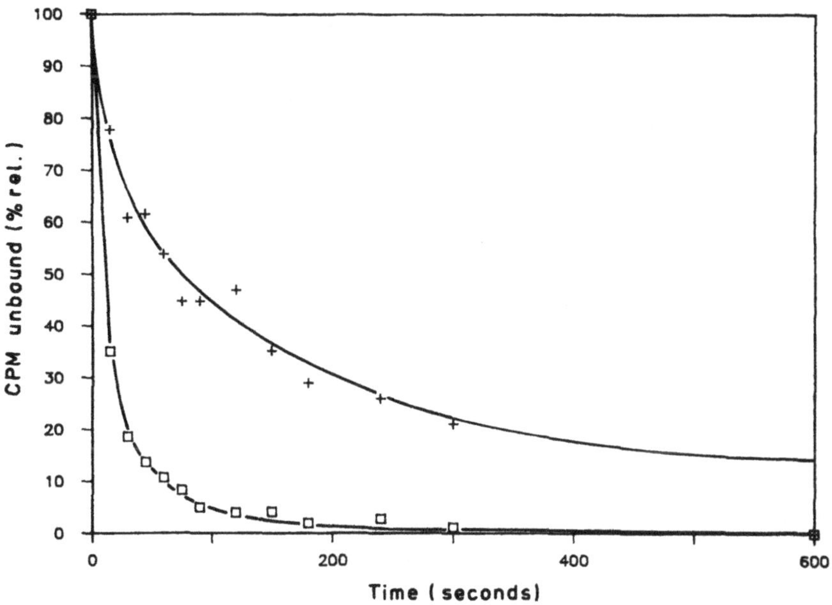


Fig. 1 Association of 13.5 nM and 135 nM [$^3$H]-acetylcholine to membrane fragments of *Torpedo marmorata*. The concentration of [$^3$H]-acetylcholine binding sites was 100 nM as determined from independent equilibrium binding studies. Aliquots of 1 ml were filtered after the indicated times and 100 ul of the filtrate was used to determine the concentration of free ligand. In order to compare the data, the relative concentrations (100% for t=0 and 0% for t = 20 min) are plotted *versus* time. (+): association of 135 nM [$^3$H]-acetylcholine to 100 nM TMF. ([ ]): Association of 13.5 nM [$^3$H]-acetylcholine to 100 nM TMF.

The acetylcholine receptor is known (1,2) to contain at least two classes of binding sites. Assuming that the second binding site is mainly filled at high ligand concentrations, the concentration dependence of the association reaction (fig. 1) shows that the slow component is related to binding of ligands to the second binding site. This may be attributed to intrinsic properties of this site or to properties of the fully occupied receptor: (i) If the association rate for binding to the second site is markedly slower than for the first site, the association reaction at high ligand concentration would show a slow component which would not exist at low ligand concentration. (ii) If a slow conformational change is initiated by the fully saturated receptor, and if this change corresponds to an increase in affinity, it will dominate the binding reaction at high ligand concentrations. In order to discriminate between these alternatives, we studied the association of [$^3$H]-acetylcholine to membrane fragments incubated with other ligands (fig. 2).

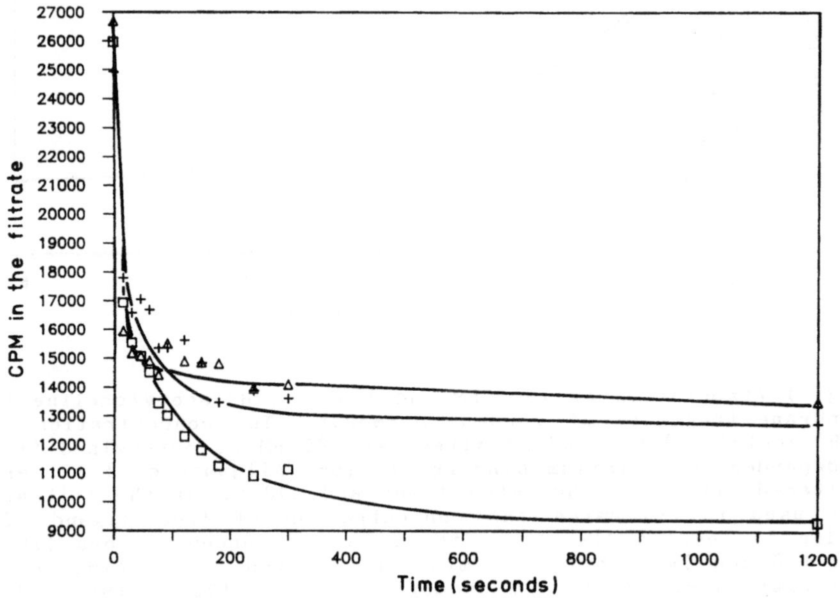


Fig. 2: Association of [$^3$H]-acetylcholine to membrane fragments incubated with cholinergic ligands. Membrane fragments at a concentration of 100 nM [$^3$H]-acetylcholine binding sites were incubated for 30 minutes with cholinergic ligands prior to the addition of 100 nM [$^3$H]-acetylcholine. ([]): Control. (+): Incubation with 300 nM Carbamoylcholine. (Δ): Incubation with 100 nM Tubocurarine.

Fig. 2 shows that the slow component of the association reaction is not a property of the second binding site: If binding to the second site would be intrinsically slow, then only the slow component should be observed if the first site had been occupied with another cholinergic ligand. The experiments gave the opposite results. In all cases where the membrane fragments of *T. marmorata* were incubated with other ligands, the slow component of the reaction was selectively reduced in its amplitude. It should be noted that the slow component decreased only after sufficient incubation times (more than 5 minutes for cholinergic agonists and antagonists).

In order to investigate the influence of membrane structure, the solubilized receptor was compared to the membrane-bound form in rapid kinetic experiments. The association of the fluorescent agonist N-5-C (trimethyl-2-(ω-(7-nitro-4-benzofurazanylamino)-5-alkylcarbonyloxy)ethylammonium chloride) (4) to the purified receptor protein (either from *E. electricus* (6) or *T. marmorata*) was faster than the association to membrane fragments. When these membrane fragments were mixed with detergent (0.01% Tween) the slow component ($k \leq 0.01\ s^{-1}$ for 100 nM binding sites and 100 nM fluorescent ligand) disappeared and the reaction followed the same course as with the purified receptor protein. A complete loss of the slow component in the association reaction was also observed after incubation of the membrane fragments with 10% ethanol or 0.1 mM of the local anesthetic Dibucaine. A partial loss was observed upon increasing the temperature: For membrane fragments of *T. marmorata* at 23.5 °C, the slow component comprised of about 70% of the amplitude of the fluorescence signal. Increasing the temperature to 43.5 °C reduced the relative contribution of the slow component to about 40% .

Filtration experiments with $[^3H]$-acetylcholine showed similar results: The slow component of the association reaction ($k \leq 0.01\ s^{-1}$) disappeared after incubation of the membrane fragments with detergent (0.01% Tween). The same increase in velocity was observed in presence of 10% ethanol or 0.1 mM Dibucaine (fig. 3). Under these conditions, the total amplitude of the association reaction was increased as shown by independent equilibrium binding studies. Detergent, ethanol and Dibucaine increased the affinity of the membrane fragments for $[^3H]$-acetylcholine. The number of binding sites was not changed by any of these treatments.

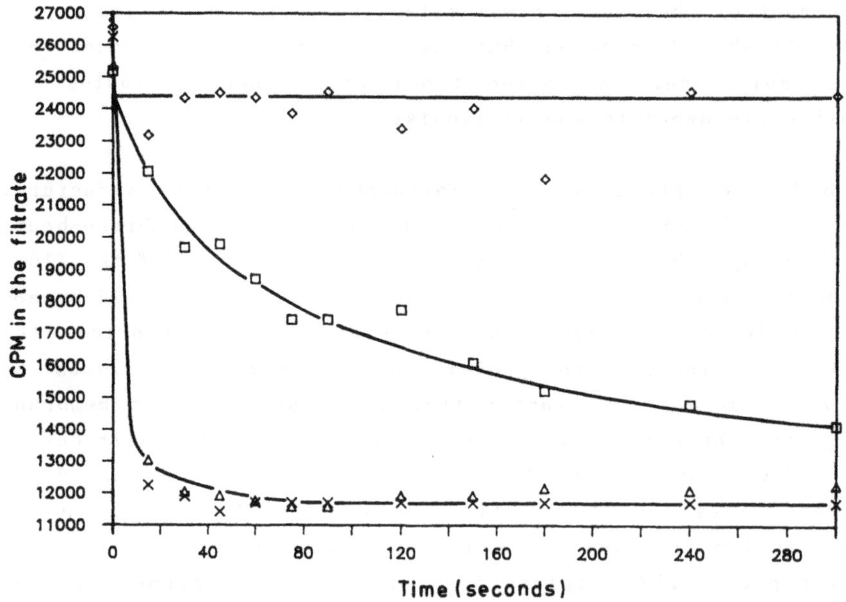


Fig. 3: Association of 135 mM [$^3$H]-Acetylcholine to 100 mM membrane fragments from *T. marmorata*. ([]): Association to untreated membrane fragments. (<>): Membrane fragments incubated for 30 min with 0.1 mM acetylcholine. (Δ): Membrane fragments incubated with 10% ethanol. (X): Membrane fragments incubated with 0.1 mM dibucaine.

## Discussion

Slow components in the association of ligands to membrane-bound acetylcholine receptor have been previously described (8, 11). The reported rate constants were larger than the slow component described here ($k \leq 0.01\ s^{-1}$). Our results show that the amplitude of this slow component is markedly increased at high ligand concentrations and decreased after incubation with other ligands. It cannot be related to activation of the receptor, since the time constant is orders of magnitude slower than can be expected from physiological experiments (12). Since its amplitude increases with ligand concentration, the slow part of the association reaction probably is related to a conformational change observed after saturation of all binding sites at the receptor. For receptor embedded in intact membrane fragments, this part of the reaction is slower than for the solubilized receptor protein. The following molecular mechanism may serve as an explanation:

The membrane matrix functions as a support for membrane proteins. Rapid conformational changes of these macromolecules may be impeded by this matrix, just as rapid movements in a viscous solution. These effects of the surrounding membrane may well have consequences for the function of the cholinergic system. If the observed conformational change is related to desensitization of the receptor, the membrane would slow down this conformational change and thereby stabilize the active state of the receptor protein.

The apparent contradiction, namely that the acetylcholine receptor is known to respond very fast *in vivo* and yet the binding of ligands to the membrane-bound receptor is slower than to the solubilized protein, can be explained by this hypothesis.

Acknowledgement

The technical assistance of Martina Wischnewski is gratefully acknowledged.

References

1. Maelicke, A. 1984.
   Angew.Chem. 96, 193-219.

2. Changeux, J.-P., A. Devillers-Thièry, P. Chemoulli. 1984.
   Science 225, 1335-1345.

3. Sakmann, B., J. Patlak, E. Neher. 1980.
   Nature 286, 71-73.

4. Meyers, H.-W., R. Jürss, H.R. Brenner, G. Fels, H. Prinz, H. Watzke, A. Maelicke. 1983. Eur.J.Biochem 137, 399-404.

5. Prinz, H., A. Maelicke. 1983a. J.Biol.Chem. 258, 10263-10271.

6. Prinz, H., A. Maelicke. 1983b. J.Biol.Chem. 258, 10273-10282.

7. Covarrubias, M., H. Prinz, A. Maelicke. 1984. FEBS Letters 169, 229-233.

8. Covarrubias, M., H. Prinz, H.-W. Meyers, A. Maelicke. 1986. J.Biol.Chem. (in press)

9. Boyd, N.D., J. Cohen. 1980. Biochemistry 19, 5353-5358.

10. Fels, G., E.K. Wolff, A. Maelicke. 1982. Eur.J.Biochem 127, 31-38.

11. Heidmann, T., J.-P. Changeux. 1979. Eur.J.Biochem 94, 255-279; 281-296.

12. Adams, P. R. 1981. J.Membrane.Biol 58, 161-174.

# THE NICOTINIC ACETYLCHOLINE RECEPTOR IS AN ALLOSTERIC PROTEIN; THE SPECIFIC ALLOSTERIC MODEL DOES NOT APPLY TO THE RECEPTOR'S MOLECULAR MECHANISM OF ACTION

Alfred Maelicke

Max-Planck-Institut für Ernährungsphysiologie, D-4600 Dortmund, Federal Republic of Germany

## Introduction

The nicotinic acetylcholine receptor (AChR) is a ligand gated cation channel (1,2) with a considerable number of physiologically distinct "states" (3,4). This paper summarizes results showing that (i) ligand binding induces ligand-specific conformational states of the receptor, and (ii) important functional properties of the receptor are controlled by conformational transitions and/or allosteric interactions between distinct structural domains. There exists increasing evidence, however, that the specific allosteric model (5-7) does not provide a suitable description of the AChR's molecular mechanism of action.

## Results

Conformational transitions and ligand-specific states. - Indirect evidence for conformational transitions in the course of ligand interactions of the AChR is provided by the following electrophysiological and biochemical findings: (i) Single channel recordings show ligand-induced very rapid transitions to and from the open state (16) and to and from sub-states (3,4,9). (ii) The mean open time of AChR-channels depends on the activating ligand applied (10). (iii) From equilibrium binding data, the formation of ligand-receptor complexes is an

Receptors and Ion Channels

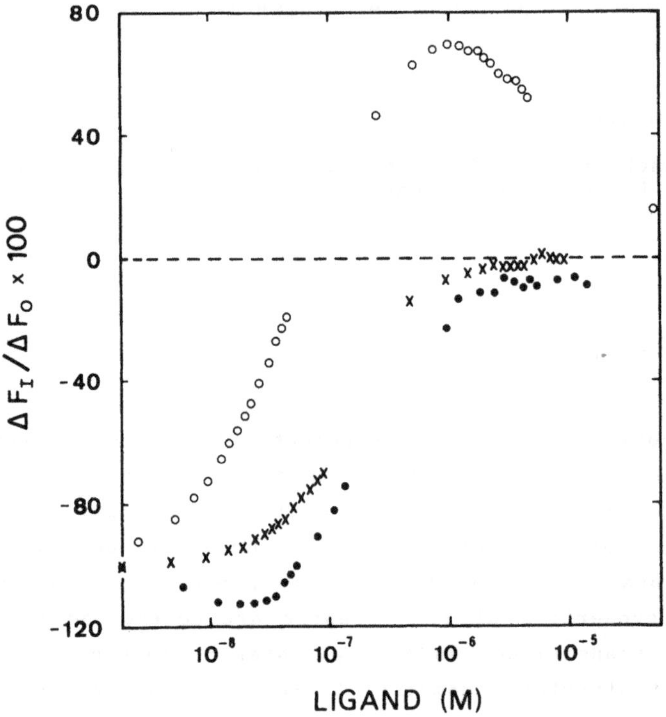


Fig. 1: Fluorescence changes in reaction mixtures of N-5-C and *Torpedo* membrane fragments in the presence of competing ligands.
*Torpedo* membrane fragments (25-40 mM) were incubated with N-5-C (25-40 nM) for 15-20 min followed by stepwise addition (every 8.3 min) of competing ligand. To limit the effect of dilution, two stock solutions were employed for each ligand (low and high concentration range in the figure). Competing ligands acetylcholine (•) suberyldicholine (x), and tubocurarine (o). As was established by experiments with $^3H$-labeled N-5-C, the observed different competition patterns are due to different quantum yields of bound N-5-C in the mixed complexes with competing ligand and receptor. Relative quantum yields of N-5-C in the absence of other receptor ligands for the two classes of binding sites: $Q_1 = 0.50 \pm 0.03$, $Q_2 = 0.75 \pm 0.1$. Quantum yields $Q_3$ in the mixed complexes with acetylcholine, suberyldicholine and tubocurarine were 0.3, 0.5 and 1.4, respectively (15).

entropy-driven reaction (11). (iv) The two binding sites for acetylcholine (and agonists) at the membrane-bound receptor interact positive cooperatively (12,13). Besides suggesting sizable conformational transitions in the course of ligand binding

Table I: Relative quantum yield ($Q_3$) of the fluorescent agonist N-5-C in mixed complexes with competing non-fluorescent ligand and membrane-bound *Torpedo* receptor.

| Ligand | Rel. quantum yield |
|---|---|
| Acetylcholine | 0.3 |
| Carbamoylcholine | 0.2 |
| Suberyldicholine | 0.5 |
| α-Tubocurarine | 1.4 |
| Gallamine | 1.3 |
| Hexamethonium | 1.2 |

The quantum yield of N-5-bound to half saturated receptor in the absence of other ligands is $Q_1 = 0.50 \pm 0.3$. Thus, the agonist suberyldicholine does not change the quantum yield of bound N-5-C while carbamoylcholine and acetylcholine induce different levels of further quenching. In contrast, antagonists increase the fluorescence of bound N-5-C with the resulting $Q_3$ being identical within the limits of experimental error.

and channel gating, these findings indicate that all receptor conformations ("states") are determined by the ligand(s) bound. Furthermore, some of these transitions must be of long range because they affect sites located on separate subunits of the AChR. This applies in particular to the cooperative interaction between agonist sites (12,13) and the modulating effects of local anesthetics on ligand binding (14,15) and channel gating (16).

Direct evidence for ligand-specific conformational states of the AChR is provided by fluorescence binding studies with the acetylcholine analog N-5-C and the membrane-bound *Torpedo* receptor (15). These experiments were performed by initially half-saturating the receptor with N-5-C followed by step-wise addition of non-fluorescent ligand. As shown in Fig. 1, the observed fluorescence competition curves depend on the particular non-fluorescent ligand applied. As shown in detail in the related publication (15), different ligands apparently affect the fluorescence quantum yield of bound N-5-C differently (Table 1). Assuming that the quantum yield of bound N-5-C in these mixed complexes of receptor, fluorescent and non-fluorescent ligand is a suitable parameter to describe the conformational states associated with these complexes, (i) agonists and antagonists induce different conformational states, (ii) antagonists appear to induce the same or very similar states while (iii) the agonist-induced states differ for different agonists.

Modulation of ligand-specific states. - The specific agonist-induced conformations of the AChR are subject to modulation. The best known modulating agents are the non-competitive blockers (e.g. local anesthetics) which bind to sites structurally distinct from the agonist sites (17). The modulating effect of local anesthetics is seen in changed open channel characteristics (16) and binding kinetics (18,19), and in an increase in agonist binding affinity (14,19). Based on these findings, the local anesthetic-modulated states bear resemblance to the desensitized states of the AChR.

As was recently shown by binding and ion flux studies (20) and by direct binding kinetics (25), the membrane environment provides another means of receptor modulation. The close link between receptor conformations and membrane structure is documented by, among others, the following facts: (i) An appropriate membrane fluidity and the presence of specific phospholipids (cholesterol and negatively charged phospholipids) are required for AChR channel gating (20). (ii) Local anesthetics do not bind to the receptor protein in the absence of a lipid environment (11). (iii) The kinetics of ligand binding and ligand-induced state transitions depend very sensitively on the lipid or detergent environment of the AChR (25) with some rate constants varying by orders of magnitude.

Allosteric interactions between separate structural domains. - The cooperative interaction between agonist binding sites, the modulating effect of lipids and local anesthetics on ligand binding and channel gating, and the transition to the open channel state upon agonist binding may all be taken as evidence for allosteric interactions between separate structural domains at the AChR.

A simple model to explain the above observations is to assume that all-or-none effects (such as mutually exclusive binding of competing ligands, and channel opening and closing) are mediated by singular sites whereas modulating effects are caused by allosteric interactions between separate and, possibly, rather distant sites. There exists strong evidence, however, that this clear distinction cannot be made:

(a) Accelerated dissociation of α-neurotoxin-receptor complexes. - Curaremimetic neurotoxins and the agonists and antagonists of acetylcholine are known to bind mutually exclusively to the AChR (1,2). Based on the classical occupational model, this would suggest identical binding sites for these ligands. In contrast, however, the accelerated dissociation of toxin-receptor complexes in the presence of low molecular weight ligands (Fig. 2, (11,22)) suggests the existence of separate binding sites for toxin and small ligands. A separate (or additional) site is required to permit the small ligand to bind to the receptor while the toxin is still bound. The observed increase in the intrinsic rate of toxin dissociation could then result from a ligand-induced conformational transition of the receptor protein leading to the disintegration (e.g. partial collapse of its three-dimensional organization) of the toxin binding site. This would result in a drop in binding affinity and the observed increase in dissociation rate of toxin-receptor complexes. Similarly, toxin binding to the AChR may lead to the partial disappearance of the small ligand binding site(s) which would explain why the phenomenon of accelerated toxin-receptor complex dissociation is observed at a concentration range for the small ligand orders of magnitude higher than the range for mutually exclusive binding. A plausible model for accelerated dissociation is shown in Fig. 2.

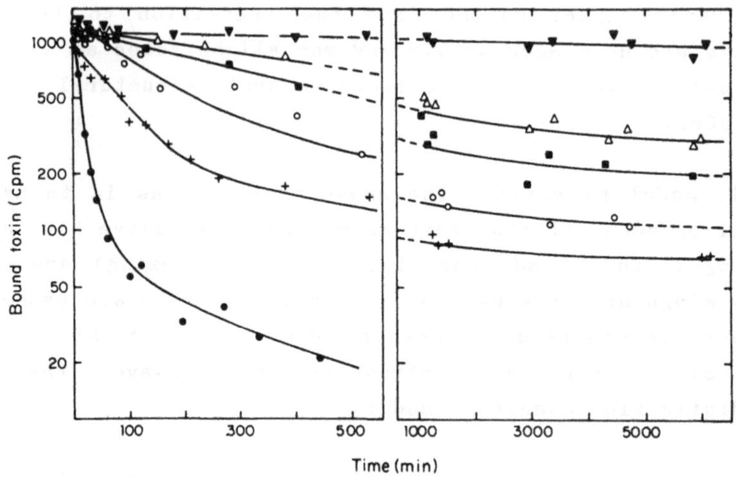
Bound toxin (cpm)
1000
500
200
100
50
20
100
300
500
1000
3000
5000
Time (min)

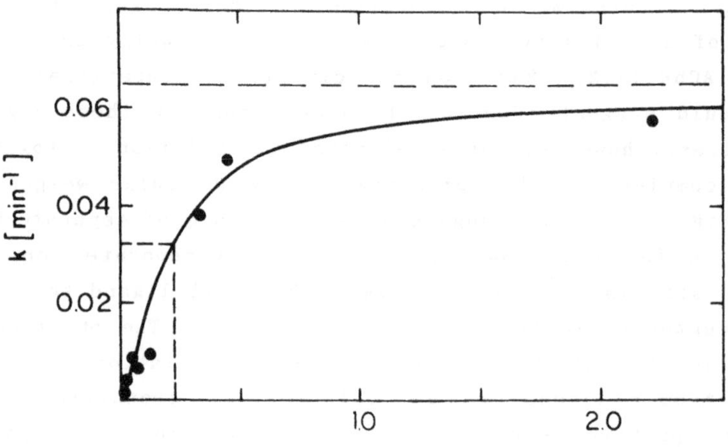
k [min-1]
0.06
0.04
0.02
1.0
2.0

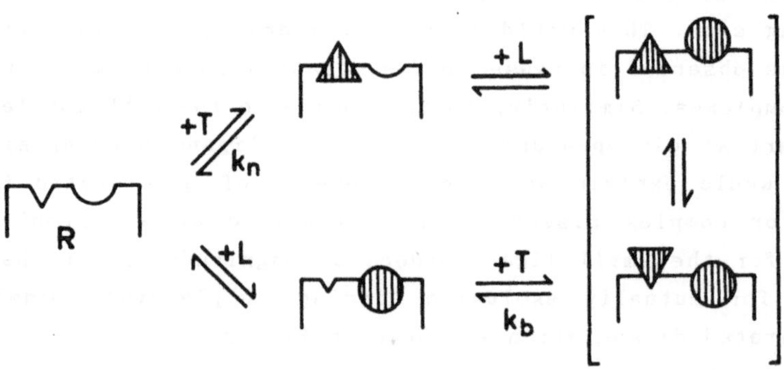
+L
+T
kn
R
+L
+T
kb

Fig. 2: Accelerated dissociation of α-neurotoxin-AChR complexes in the presence of competing ligands.
(a) Dissociation of $^3$H-α-cobratoxin-receptor complexes in the presence of benzoquinonium. After incubation for 20.5 hrs, 500μl of a reaction mixture of $^3$H-toxin and purified AChR from *Electrophorus electricus* were diluted into 50 ml of a benzoquinonium solution in the same buffer, and aliquots of 2.5 ml were removed at the indicated times. They were analyzed for their content of remaining toxin-receptor complexes by filtration through DEAE-filter disks. At the concentrations of toxin and receptor after dilution ($2.9 \times 10^{-10}$M and $8 \times 10^{-10}$M, respectively), spontaneous dissociation of preformed complexes is negligible, and the observed dissociation, therefore, is the result of benzoquinonium binding to the AChR. The applied benzoquinonium concentrations were: (▾), no benzoquinonium, (△), $2 \times 10^{-7}$M, (▪), $6.7 \times 10^{-7}$M, (o), $2 \times 10^{-6}$M, (+) $6.7 \times 10^{-6}$M, and (•), $2.2 \times 10^{-4}$M (11).
(b) Initial rate constants [$min^{-1}$] of toxin-receptor complex dissociation in the presence of benzoquinonium: Original data see (a). $k_{max}$ = 0.065 $min^{-1}$, concentration of benzoquinonium for half maximal rate constant $c1/2 = 2 \times 10^{-5}$M. From these data, the accelerating effect of benzoquinonium is saturable indicating the existence of a low affinity site for this ligand in the presence of bound toxin (11).
(c) A plausible model for accelerated dissociation of toxin-receptor complexes. Receptor interacts with either toxin (▲) or low molecular weight ligand (•) to form the appropriate binary complex. The conformational transition accompanying ligand binding leads to the partial disintegration of the three-dimensional organization of the other ligand's binding site. The result is a large drop in binding affinity for the other ligand. At higher concentrations, however, ternary complexes can be formed.
At the concentration range of mutually exclusive binding, the concentration of ternary complexes is negligible. At higher concentrations, they may become transiently significant thereby leading to accelerated dissociation of the more slowly dissociating ligand.

(b) Competition of the antibody WF6 and cholinergic ligands for receptor binding. - The monoclonal antibody WF6 has been shown to compete with acetylcholine, its agonists and the α-toxins but not with low molecular weight antagonists and local anesthetics for receptor binding (23). This evidence for separate sites at the AChR for groups of cholinergic ligands is further strengthened by the following observations (26): As expected from equilibrium binding experiments (23), acetylcholine and its agonists decrease the rate of WF6 association to the receptor. In contrast, all small antagonists tested do not at all affect the WF6 association kinetics. However, when an antagonist is applied together with acetylcholine, the decrease in WF6 association rate is smaller than in the absence of the antagonist and, at sufficient excess of antagonist over acetylcholine, completely disappears. Obviously, the competition of the antagonist and acetylcholine for receptor binding reduces (and at saturating concentrations eliminate) the competing effect of acetylcholine on WF6 binding. This observation requires to assume that at least one of the three ligands involved (antibody, acetylcholine or antagonist) must bind to site(s) separate from that (those) for the other two ligands. Assuming for argument's sake that the antibody binds to a site separate from that (those) for the small ligands, the competition between acetylcholine and WF6 must then be due to acetylcholine-induced conformational changes leading to the disintegration of the domain (epitope) which is recognized by the antibody. (Similarly, because agonists and WF6 bind mutual exclusively to the receptor, binding of the antibody must also induce a conformational change which leads to the disappearance of the agonist site.) The allosterically induced desintegration of sites may be partial (as in the case of toxin, see above) or complete, depending on the degree of allosteric coupling between the domains involved.

The above reported results suggest that ligands which bind mutual exclusively with each other to the receptor do not necessarily bind to identical sites. Instead, full competition can be the result of ligand-induced conformational transitions causing the partial or complete disappearance of other ligand binding site(s). Conformation coupling between separate structural domains may therefore be of much more importance for the receptor's mechanism of function than was hitherto anticipated.

## Discussion

The findings summarized here suggest a model for the receptor's mechanism of function which is quite different from previously proposed ones (5-7). It assumes that the functionally important states of the AChR all require ligand occupation. Each specific class of ligands (e.g. agonists) induces a specific sequence of conformational transitions of the AChR. These transitions link ligand binding with the discrete functional states observed. The conformational states (and their functional correlates) are subject to ligand-specific variations caused by the particular molecular structure of each individual ligand. As a prerequisite for such properties, the receptor must have a high degree of conformational flexibility and, at the same time, must maintain firm coupling between the domains involved. These structural properties permit a considerable degree of functional complexity: The receptor can individually recognize and respond to ligands, and there exist various levels of functional modulation. As a separate aspect, these properties certainly complicate the elucidation of structure-function relationships of the nicotinic acetylcholine receptor.

The conformational plasticity and the allosteric interactions between distinct domains of the AChR certainly characterize the receptor as an allosteric protein. This is not to say that the specific allosteric model of Monod et al. (24) applies to the mechanism of binding (and channel gating) of the AChR. The application of this model to the AChR (5-7) has several serious drawbacks: (i) The specific allosteric model assumes that the various "states" of the protein also exist in the absence of bound ligand. Consequently, this model cannot easily accommodate the existence of distinct ligand-specific functional states (15) or, if it assumes a related number of preexisting states, looses its advantage of analytical simplicity. (ii) The specific allosteric model predicts a background noise of receptor channel activations. This is because it assumes activating ligands to merely increase the number of activating events without being indispensable for activation (as we suggest). (iii) The specific allosteric model assumes a random mechanism of ligand interaction. We have shown for the *Electrophorus* receptor (27) that ligand interaction is a non-random, strictly ordered process. Other limitations of the specific allosteric model in the analysis of ligand binding to the AChR have been dealt with in separate publications from our laboratory (19,25,27). Thus, from a mechanistic point of view, it is important to make a clear distinction between the general properties of an allosteric protein on the one hand and the specific assumptions and predictions of the Monod model on the other.

(Supported by the Deutsche Forschungsgemeinschaft, SFB 168, and the Fonds der Chemischen Industrie)

References

1. Changeux, J.-P., A. Devillers-Thièry, P. Chenoilli. 1984. Science 225, 1335-1345.

2. Maelicke, A. 1984. Angew.Chem.Int.Ed. 23, 195-221.

3. Colquhoun, D. 1986. In: Structure and Function of the Nicotinic Acetylcholine Receptor (A. Maelicke, ed.) Springer Verlag, Heidelberg.

4. Auerbach, A., F. Sachs. 1983. Biophys. J. 42, 1-10.

5. Changeux, J.-P. 1981. Harvey Lect. 75, 85

6. Karlin, A. 1980. In: The Cell Surface and Neuronal Function (C.W. Cotman, G. Poste and G.L. Nicholson, eds). Elsevier, Amsterdam, pp. 191-229.

7. Conti-Tronconi, B.M., M.A. Raftery. 1982. Ann.Rev.Biochem. 51, 491-527.

8. Neher, E., B. Sakmann, J.H. Steinbach. 1978. Pflüger's Arch. 375, 219-228.

9. Sigworth, F.J. 1985. Biophys.J. 47, 709-720.

10. Colquhoun, D. 1981. In: Drug Receptors and Their Effectors (N.J.M. Birdsall, ed.) MacMillan, London. pp. 107-127.

11. Maelicke, A., B.W. Fulpius, R.P. Klett, E. Reich. 1977. J.Biol.Chem. 252, 4811-4830.

12. Fels, G., E.K. Wolff, A. Maelicke. 1982. Eur.J.Biochem. 127, 31-38.

13. Neubig, R.R., J.B. Cohen. 1979. Biochemistry 18, 5464-5475.

14. Neubig, R.R., E.K. Krodel, N.D. Boyd, J.B. Cohen. 1979. Proc.Natl.Acad.Sci.USA 76, 690-694.

15. Covarrubias, M., H. Prinz, H.-W. Meyers, A. Maelicke. 1986. J.Biol.Chem. (in press)

16. Neher, E., J.H. Steinbach. 1978. J.Physiol. London 277, 153-176.

17. Giraudat, J., C. Montecucco, R. Bisson, J.-P. Changeux. 1986. Proc.Natl.Acad.Sci.USA 83, 2719-2723.

18. Heidmann, T., R. Oswald, J.-P. Changeux. 1983. Biochemistry 22,112-3127.

19. Covarrubias, M., H. Prinz, A. Maelicke. 1984. FEBS Letters 169, 229-233.

20. Fong, T.M., M.G. McNamee. 1986. Biochemistry 25, 830-840.

21. Prinz, H. A. Maelicke (in preparation)

22. Kang, S.S., A. Maelicke. 1980. J.Biol.Chem. 255, 7326-7332.

23. Fels, G., R. Plümer-Wilk, M. Schreiber, A. Maelicke. 1986. J.Biol.Chem. (in press)

24. Monod, J., J. Wyman, J.-P. Changeux. 1965. J.Mol.Biol. 12, 88-118.

25. Prinz, H. 1986. In Nicotinic Acetylcholine Receptor: Structure and Function (A. Maelicke, ed.) Springer Verlag Berlin, pp. 129-146.

26. Maelicke, A., D. Watters, G. Fels. 1986. In Nicotinic Acetylcholine Receptor: Structure and Function (A. Maelicke, ed.) Springer Verlag Berlin, pp. 83-92.

27. Prinz, H., A. Maelicke. 1983. J.Biol.Chem. 258, 10273-10282.

# ORGANIZATION AND FUNCTION OF THE CHOLINERGIC SYNAPSE

V. Witzemann

Abteilung Neurochemie, Max-Planck-Institut für biophysikalische Chemie, Postfach 2841, D-3400 Göttingen

## Introduction

To understand the molecular mechanisms underlying the process of neurochemical transmission, it is essential to establish a correlation between the structural organisation of synapses and the elements functionally involved in the transmission of specific intercellular signals. Besides the characterization of individual molecules, the analysis of differentiation-dependent changes and changes occurring during synapse formation is expected to yield valuable information. The central question is, how can nerve terminals, being responsible for the release of specific transmitters, come into contact with postsynaptic membranes containing the proper receptor molecules.

The electromotor system of Torpedo marmorata provides an ideal source for the purification and characterization of molecules involved in synaptic neurotransmission. The high concentration of synaptic contacts in this purely cholinergic tissue enables one to obtain relatively homogeneous subcellular fractions, such as detached nerve terminals, synaptic vesicles, basal lamina preparations or postsynaptic membranes (1). Embryos of these fish provide in addition an excellent system with which to follow developmental changes (2).

## Development of the electric organ of Torpedo marmorata

The electric organ develops from cylindrical vertically oriented myotubes. At this stage the nicotinic acetylcholine receptor (nAChR) as well as acetylcholinesterase (AChE) are evenly and diffusely distributed over the myotube surface. On morphological differentiat-

Receptors and Ion Channels

ion these cells round up and become horizontally flattened disc shaped cells - the electrocytes. On the ventral surface a basal lamina forms and nAChR and AChE become localized on the ventral membrane. These changes occur without direct neuronal contacts.

The synaptogenic phase is characterized by axons invading the stacks of electrocytes forming synaptic contacts on the ventral side of each cell. During electrocyte differentiation nAChR, AChE and choline acetyltransferase (CAT) are present at low levels. With the formation of synaptic contacts at 50-60 mm embryo length a marked increase of receptor and esterase is seen. CAT-levels show only a moderate increase. AChE and nAChR levels continue to rise until birth. CAT shows a second rising phase at later embryonic stages beginning between 80-90 mm embryo length. This phase coincides with the increase of nerve endings and neuritic coverage of the postsynaptic membranes. The functional maturation of the synapse can be demonstrated by the exponentially increasing electric organ discharge response.

Morphological studies reveal that synthesis of receptor and esterase occurs before neuronal contacts are established. Similarly the formation of the ventral membrane and the localization of these two proteins within this membrane appear not to be controlled by neural factors. The strong increase in nAChR and AChE-levels during synaptogenesis depends however on the formation of synaptic contacts. The results obtained so far by light and electron microscopy, histochemistry and biochemical techniques (2-6) have been confirmed using tissue explants of electric organ at different developmental stages. There it has been shown that electrocyte differentiation occurs in vitro as in vivo despite the absence of any neural tissue, and that differentiated embryonic electrocytes can be maintained in vitro for periods of up to 3 weeks (7). Biochemically it is shown that the complex changes in AChE forms occurring during electrocyte differentiation (8) are also observed in vitro and are not under neural control. Furthermore the results suggest that the increased AChE and nAChR accumulation after the formation of synaptic contacts may be triggered by an external, possible neural factor (9). Further studies will have to concentrate on the identification of such putative neural factors. By analysing the developmentally regulated changes in the expression of AChE molecular forms and the synthesis of AChR (9) it is confirmed that the explanted cells differentiate not only morphologically but also biochemically. Tissue explants therefore provide a useful system for the study of nAChR and AChE synthesis and their dependence on neuronal regulation. A schematic representation of some of the events occurring during the embryological development of Torpedo marmorata is given in Fig. 1.

## The postsynaptic membrane during synaptogenesis

The adult electric organ is an ideal source for the isolation of postsynaptic membranes. Reorienting sucrose gradient centrifugation (10) results in a membrane fraction highly enriched in nAChR-protein, which is separated from lighter membranes due to its high protein content. Using embryonic electric organs significant differences in the enrichment of nAChR in this membrane fragment fraction are observed. From adult organs the majority of the nAChR-molecules are recovered together with these "heavy" membranes. Using embryonic tissue from 80 mm embryonic stages - by this time the nAChR content has already reached about 80% of adult levels - 5 to 10 times less toxin binding sites are found to co-sediment with the "heavy" membrane fraction and the majority is found in the "lighter" membranes at the top of the gradient. Analysis of the "heavy" nAChR-enriched membranes on SDS-polyacrylamide gels reveals significant changes in polypeptide composition indicating that during the functional maturation of the postsynaptic membrane distinct changes lead to the structural stabilization of this membrane. The most prominent differens occurs with regard to actin and the 43 K polypeptides. These have been implicated in stabilizing the receptor arrangements in the postsynaptic membrane. Fig. 1b shows that with development actin, initially a prominent component of the embryonic membranes, decreases, whereas the 43 K polypeptides become increasingly enriched together with the nAChR polypeptides.

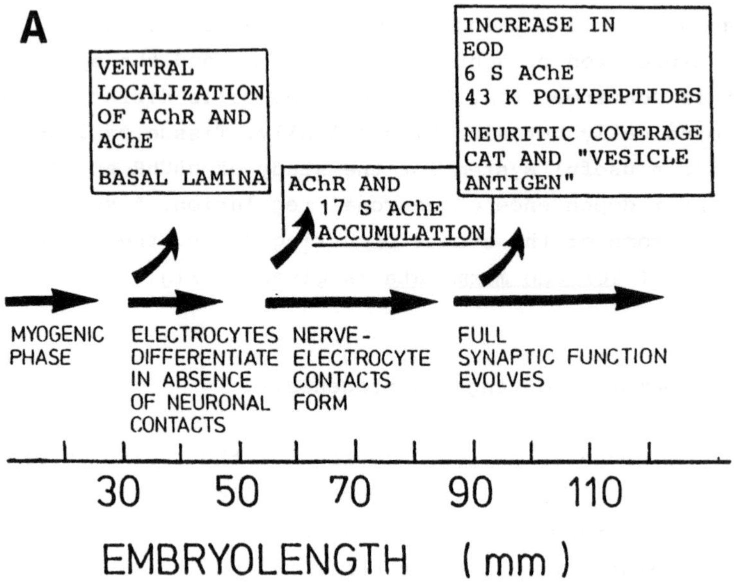


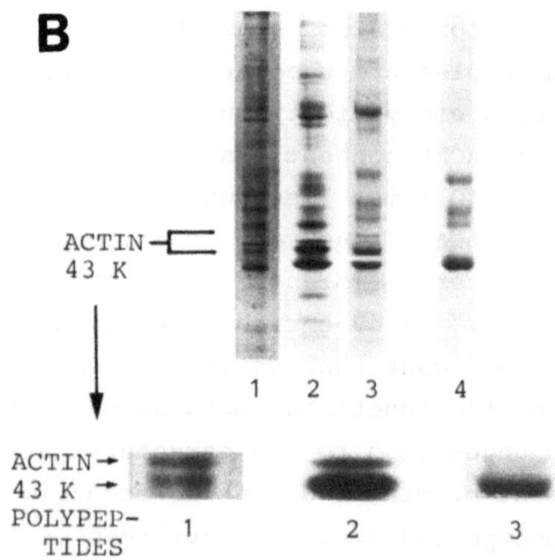


Fig. 1:

A) A schematic representation of events occuring during the embryological development of Torpedo marmorata. EOD, electric organ discharge, a measure of functional maturation.

B) SDS-Polyacrylamide gel electrophoresis of membrane fragments isolated from electric organs at different stages of development. (1) 93 mm, (2) 111 mm, (3) adult, (4) purified AChR-subunits. The membranes from adult electric organ are highly enriched in AChR- and 43 K polypeptides. The AChR content of embryonic membranes is reduced and comparing the contents of actin and 43 K polypeptides a characteristic shift is observed: Actin decreases, whereas the 43 K polypeptides show a marked increase, reflecting probably developmentally regulated changes in the organization of the postsynaptic membrane. The changing amounts of actin and 43 K polypeptides can be clearly seen in the enlarged section at the bottom of Fig. 1B.

Cytoskeleton and extracellular matrix

Control of transmembrane protein distribution undoubtedly involves cytoskeletal elements. Analysis of nAChR-enriched membrane fragments shows that both actin and desmin-like polypeptides like the 43 K polypeptides are associated in a peripheral manner with these membranes (11,12). The desmin-like polypeptides occur like actin in large amounts in the electric organ. Their presence in the nAChR-containing membrane fragments could therefore be the result of non-specific association. Immunohistochemically they are shown to extend throughout the electrocytes where they probably represent part of the intracellular framework necessary to maintain the unusual structure of the electrocytes. A gel overlay assay has been used to test whether any of the polypeptides present in receptor-enriched membranes could interact with actin. None of the receptor subunits binds actin. However the 43 K polypeptides appear to be able to bind actin with high affinity under these conditions. This finding suggests that these polypeptides may act as a link between the membrane-bound nAChR and cytoskeletal structures (12). Further studies are however needed to prove such an interaction in vivo. The possible role of the postsynaptic cytoskeleton in nAChR organization has been recently reviewed (13).

Components present in the extracellular matrix of the synaptic region have been implied in organizing postsynaptic structures (14). A major core constituent of synaptic vesicles has been characterized as a heparan sulphate proteoglycan (15). This highly antigenic molecule is synthesized in the cell bodies of the electromotor neurons and axonally transported to the nerve terminals. Specific antibodies have shown that this proteoglycan is released together with the neurotransmitter from synaptic vesicles and deposited in the extracellular matrix (16). The same antigen can be detected on the nAChR-enriched membrane fragments (17). Immunochemical analysis of extracts from electric lobe and electric organ during development confirms the vesicular origin: The antigen is synthesized in lobe tissue at early embryonic stages. In the electric organ on the other hand it can be detected only when electrocytes begin to differentiate, i.e. when axons start to invade the electric organ.

During the functional maturation of the electromotor system the antigen increases strongly in both tissues, but it becomes more abundant in the electric organ than in electric lobe tissue, supporting the view that it is deposited in the extracellular matrix. This vesicular heparan sulphate proteoglycan may be a component involved in specifying the correct intercellular interaction between neurons and their electric organ target (17).

## Functional properties of the acetylcholine receptor

An important question is to what extent is nAChR function dependent on the components of the local environment. What is, for example, the molecular basis for the observed differences between junctional and extrajunctional nAChR of mammalian muscle? Are the different nAChR populations modulated by soluble factors, post-translational modifications, cytoskeletal elements or components of the extracellular matrix? Recombinant DNA techniques recently resulted in the discovery of a novel nAChR subunit of the calf muscle nAChR (18). Besides α, β, γ and δ subunits, a fifth subunit exists, the so-called ε-subunit. The different forms of the nAChR observed during muscle development apparently arise from different combinations of the subunits (19). In Torpedo marmorata only one type of nAChR has been found (5). One approach to analysing receptor function is to isolate poly $A^+$ mRNA and inject it into Xenopus oocytes. The conductance and gating properties of nAChR channels expressed by the oocytes, can then be determined (20). RNA from adult and embryonic electric organs (between 80-110 mm embryo length) exhibits no significant differences (unpublished observations). It may be that at that stage of development only one class of nAChR exists in Torpedo. Earlier embryonic stages (especially before innervation of the electric organ) should be analysed before a final conclusion can be drawn. On the other hand the results may suggest that species-specific mechanisms may underlie the developmental regulation of nAChR molecules and these may differ considerably between the specialized electric organ of Torpedo marmorata and the neuromuscular junction of mammals.

References


1. Whittaker, V.P. 1977. Naturwissenschaften 64, 606-611.
2. Krenz, W.-D., Tashiro, T., Wächtler, K., Whittaker, V.P., Witzemann, V. 1980. Neuroscience 5, 617-624.
3. Fox, G.Q., Richardson, G.P. 1978. J. Comp. Neurol. 185, 293-315.
4. Fox, G.Q., Richardson, G.P. 1979. J. Comp. Neurol. 224, 337-343.
5. Witzemann, V., Richardson, G.P., Boustead, C. 1983. Neuroscience 8, 333-349.
6. Witzemann, V., Schmid, D., Boustead, C. 1983. Eur. J. Biochem. 131, 235-245.
7. Richardson, G.P., Krenz, W.-D., Kirk, C., Fox, G.Q. 1981. Neuroscience 6, 1181-1200.
8. Witzemann, V., Boustead, C. 1982. J. Neurochem. 39, 747-755.
9. Richardson, G.P., Witzemann, V. 1986. Neuroscience 17, 1287-1296.
10. Elliot, J., Dunn, S.M.J., Blanchard, S.G., Raftery, M.A. 1979. Proc. Natl. Acad. Sci. USA 76, 2576-2579.
11. Walker, J.H., Boustead, C.M., Witzemann, V., Shaw, G., Weber, K., Osborn, M. 1985. Eur. J. Cell Biol. 38, 123-133.
12. Walker, J.H., Boustead, C.M., Witzemann, V. 1984. EMBO J. 3, 2287-2290.
13. Froehner, S.C. 1986. TINS 9, 37-41.
14. Carlson, S.S., Caroni, P., Kelly, R.B. 1986. J. Cell Biol. 103, 509-520.
15. Stadler, H., Dowe, G.H.C. 1982. EMBO J. 1, 1381-1384.
16. Kiene, M.-L., Stadler, H. (submitted)
17. Stadler, H., Witzemann, V. (in preparation)
18. Takai, T., Noda, M., Mishina, M., Shimizu, S., Furutani, Y., Kayano, T., Ikeda, T., Kubo, R., Takahashi, H., Takahashi, T., Kuno, M., Numa, S. 1985. Nature 316, 761-764.
19. Mishina, M., Takai, T., Imoto, K., Noda, M., Takahashi, T., Numa, S., Methfessel, C., Sakmann, B. 1986. Nature 321, 406-411.
20. Methfessel, C., Witzemann, V., Sakmann, B., Takahashi, T., Mishina, M., Numa, S. 1986. Pflüger's Arch. (in press)

# DIRECTED MODIFICATION OF THE BRAIN CHOLINERGIC SYSTEM

Yu.G.Plyashkevich, I.V.Victorov, I.G.Dementieva, V.P.Demushkin
Laboratories of neurochemistry and functional synaptology, All-Union Center of Mental Health of AMS USSR, Moscow, USSR

## Introduction

Cholinergic systems comprise an essential part of the total number of organism regulatory systems. Certain pathophysiological and clinical phenomena such as visual reception disoders, hypokinesia, Parkinson's disease, senile dementia of Alzheimer's type, and other mental diseases are connected with their disfunction (1,2). Studies on directed chemical modification play a vital role in the investigation of cholinergic systems. Directed modification is used in vitro for the study of the molecular structural features of cholinergic receptors (preferably neuro-muscular) (3,4,5), while in vivo investigations are aimed to the modification of the cholinergic systems in the whole brain ( mostly to the systems involved in acetylcholine and choline utilisation (6,7)).
The overwhelming majority of the reagents used can interact not only with cholinergic systems, therefore investigation of these systems, brain-specific in particular, demands development of the novel approaches. The main goal of the present investigation was to synthetize the affinity reagents and to assess the perspectives of their use for the study of the cholinergic brain systems in vitro and in vivo.

## Results and discussion

Using the information concerning nicotinic and muscarinic acetylcholine receptor (AChR) binding site structures, formulated on the basis of analysis of cholinergic ligands structural pecularities (8) the synthesis of two classes of compounds for directed modification of cholinergic receptors was accomplished.

Receptors and Ion Channels

Such radioactive and nonradioactive derivatives as N-methylazidocytisine (1), p-azidophenacyl cytisine (2), (p-azidophenacyl)quinuclidinyl benzilate (3), p-azidophenacyl atropine (4), p-azidophenyl choline ether, which were used for photoaffinity modification of AChRs, belong to the first group (See tab.1).

Table 1. Reagents for directed modification of AChR's

| Reagent | Kd | |
|---|---|---|
| | mAChR | nAChR |
| 1. N-methylazidocytisine | - | 600 nM |
| 2. p-azidophenacyl cytisine | - | 800 nM |
| 3. p-azidophenacylquinuclidinyl benzilate | 0.8 nM | - |
| 4. p-azidophenacyl atropine | 9 nM | - |
| 5. p-azidophenyl choline ether | 120 uM | 200 uM |
| 6. cyanoesther of choline | 1300 uM | 500 uM |
| 7. 2-methylenecyclohexanedione trimetyl ammonium iodide | - | 20 uM |
| 8. epoxypropyltrimethyl ammonium chloride | 2.2 nM | - |

The affinities of the reagents were estimated according to inhibition of $^{3}$H-atropine and $^{3}$H-quinuclidinil benzilate (QNB) specific binding with membrane-bound muscarinic receptor from N.caudatus of bovine and rat brain and binding of $^{14}$C-tubocurarine and newly synthesized by us $^{3}$H-methylcytisine with membrane-bound nicotinic receptor from optical ganglia of squid (B.magister) (9,10). Radioactive ligand binding parameters $K_d$ and $B_{max}$ were estimated on the basis of the data about specific receptor binding depending on added ligand concentration with the aid of our own programm "Ligand" which was realised by microcomputer "Labtam" (CCP/M-86 operation system, Australia).
Both specificity and products of modification were determined by the incorporation of the radiolabel into the receptor preparations

after modification with reagent in presence or absence of ligand as a protector ($10^{-5}$ M nicotine or $10^{-5}$ M platifiline for membrane-bound nAChR and mAChR respectively) and estimation of molecular weight by liquid chromatography and SDS-PAG-electrophoresis. Table 1 demonstrates that in terms of the competitive inhibition data the strongest interactions were observed between receptor and compound 1 to 4 and 8. The most effective affinity modification of membrane-bound receptor was obtained with compounds number 1 and 3, which were synthesized as $^3$H-derivatives. Introduction of arylazido groups into reagents as evidenced by the activity binding in the dark practically did not tell upon their affinity to receptor and $B_{max}$.

Gel-filtration of the products of chemical modification of nicotinic receptor by reagent 1 after its solubilisation in 1% Triton X-100 revealed molecular weight of receptor component modified appared to be 400 kD. Destruction of the protein-protein interaction by organic solvent systems on the basis of 2-chloroethanol yielded molecular weight of components modified to be equal 40-80 kD. Similar results have been obtained after SDS-PAG electrophoretic analysis (See Fig.1) which demonstrated that molecular weights of ganglionar and neuro-muscular nicotinic receptor were the same. The modified component with molecular weight of 40 kD hasn't been retained by Concanavalin A-Sepharose. This distinguishes it from similar subunit of neuro-muscular nAChR.

Since N-methylcytisine is more reactive towards nAChR from ganglia one may suppose reagent 1 to be more specific towards not only ganglionar receptors but also to other types of nicotinic receptors of CNS. However this assumption should not be considered as a finally proved.

After specific modification of muscarinic receptor by $^3$H-reagent 3 and its solubilisation in 2% sodium cholate and Sepharose CL-6B gel-filtration radioactivity was observed mainly in fraction which corresponded to molecular weight of about 400 kD, one half of these fractions by weight being represented by phospholipids. We have shown earlier (11) that N.caudatus preparation from bovine brain contained two subpopulations of receptors B1 and B2 which were similar to M2 and M1 subpopulations by their properties. Comparison of dose/response dependence between photoactivated

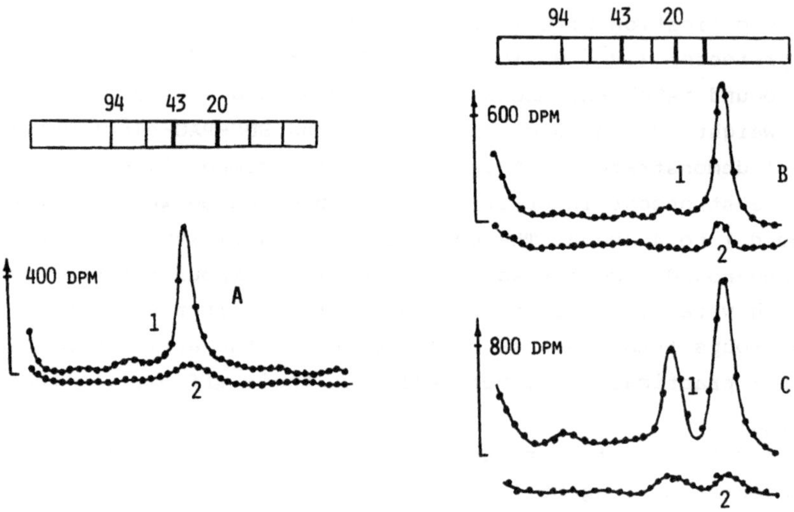


Fig.1. PAG scanes modified components of AChRs. Modification nAChR by compound 1 - (A); modification mAChR by <10 nM - (B) and >50 nM - (C) compound 3 at absence of protectors - (curve 1), at presence of protectors - (curve 2).

reagent concentration and muscarinic receptor modification degree showed, that population B1 was modified by $^3$H-reagent 2 about 50 times as rapid as population B2 was. At a low reagent concentration (<10 nM) subpopulation B1 was modified preferentially while at concentrations above 50 nM both population were modified. Molecular weights of receptor components B1 and B2 subpopulations were found to be 12.5 and 25 kD respectively (see Fig.1).
It should be noted that component with molecular weight of 12.5 kD in the composition of muscarinic receptor was found ealier (12,13). Special experiments have shown that under standard conditions of fixation in aqueous mixture of isopropanol and acetic acid this component can quite easily be lost from the PAG plate. The 25 kD-component of muscarinic receptor has also been detected after chemical modification by benzylyl choline mustard (14).
Components with higher molecular weights (80 kD) were observed after modification of brain mACHR with QNB azido-derivatives, which containes azido-group in phenyl ring of benzylic acid (15). Since maximal distance between azido-groups of reagent 3 and azido-QNB may range up to 15 angstroms it can not be excluded that

these reagents modify different components of mACHR.
Existence of two modifiable components and constant ratio between their content was found independently whether the modification was carrid out immediately after animal sacrifice or after storage of brain membranes for 4 hr at +4 $^{o}$C or 4 months at - 20 $^{o}$C. Besides we found that both light and heavy synaptosomes contained both B1 and B2 subpopulations and their quantitive ratio remains the same in membrane fractions from the N.caudatus of bovine and rat brains.
The low molecular wight synthetic derivatives, having structural elements, providing the affinity to cholinergic receptors and carring groups able to modify functional groups of proteins which may be used for modification of AChR in vivo can be placed to the second group of compounds. They are cyano-esther of choline - 6, 2-metylcyclohexanedione thrimetylammonium iodide - 7 and epoxypropyl trimethylammonium chloride - 8. The most selective ligand of this serie proved to be compound 8. Dissosiation constant of the complex of this compound with mAChR determined according to inhibition of specific binding of $^{3}$H-QNB was 2.2 nM. Incubation of mAChR membrane preparations in presense of 10 uM compound 8 during 1 hr under physiological pH haven't been resulted in irreversible inhibition of receptor activity. However, intraventricular injection of this compound caused prolonged (5-6 days after injection) alterations of stereotypical behaviour of animals, this fact urged us to investigate the neurotoxic activity of compound 8 in more details.
Data obtained on fractions of isolated neuronal membranes gave a reason for the experiments dealing with the investigation of neurotoxicity of synthetised compound on animals. Investigated compounds in Simms' balaced salt solution were injected according to stereotaxic coordinates into the left lateral ventricle of the brain of anasthetized (chloral hydrate 350 mg/kg) adult Wistar rats of both sexes. 1-9 days after injection the brains of the experimental and control animals were fixed and embeded in paraffin. 12-15 micron sections were stained with cresyl violet according to the method of Nissl.
The study of histological preparations showed that intraventricular injection of 2.5-250 umol epoxypropyl trimethylammonium chloride led to the total dose-dependent lysis of neurons and glial

cells in subcortical structures of the brain located near the left lateral ventricle (septum, striatum, thalamus, hippocumpus ect.) and accompanied by degeneration of the neurones in the cortex. As a rule exepiremental animals werecharacterized by general suppression, decreased reaction to the light and sound irritatements, increased sensitivity to tacktile stimulations, and forced pose, hind limbs paralysis, forced circular movements. Most of the animals died on the 1st - 2nd days of experiment. The intraventricular injection of 10-25 nmol of compound 8 caused the destructive and distrophic alterations of neurons in the cortical and subcortical strustures of the brain (oedema and shrinkage, tigrolysis and in some cases caryolysis). In this group of experimental animals definite behavioural and neurogical disturbances weren't observed during the experiment lasting 2-3 days. Some of the effects are demonstrated in fig.2 .

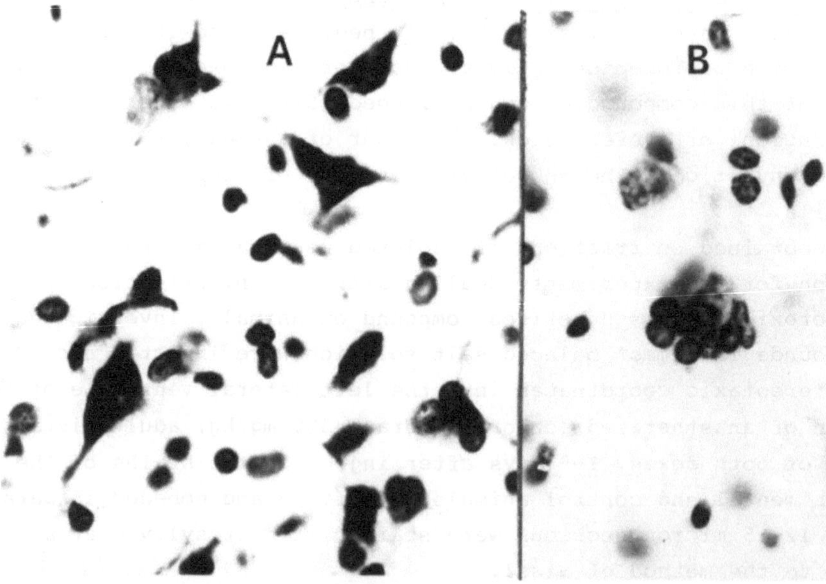


Fig.2. Degenerative changes of neurones 5th days after the intaventricular injection of 25 nmol of epoxypropyl trimetylammonium chloride in the frontal cortex (A). Neuronal degeneration and neurophagia in the striatum (B).

Intraventricular injection of allyl trimethylammonium (one of the probable precursor of epoxypropyl trymetylammonium) in dose of 2.5 umol hasn't caused massivve distructions in the local subcortical structures of the brain similar to that observed after the injection of the same dose of epoxypropyltrimethyl ammonium, but was accompanied by degeneration of some populations of neurons in the cortex and striatum, in the cholinergic structures of forebrain and in the substancia nigra. The data obtained in these experiments showed the certain similarities in the character and localization of neuronal degeneration after intraventricular injections of 10-25 nmol compound 8 and allyl trimetylammonium iodide. The definite neurological disturbances in the animals of these experimental groups weren't observed. However, the instrumental investigations of the animal behaviour on the 3rd, 6th and 9th days after the intraventricular injection of compound 8 allowed us to notice some decrease in total motional activity of rats which were more distinctly pronounced on the 6th day of the experiment.
Thus, a number of low molecular weight ligands for chemical modification of brain AChR was synthetized and used in this study. Compounds 1 and 3 proved to be useful tools for labelling of n- and mAChR component in vitro. Epoxypropyl and allyl trimethylammonium were shown to posess a neurotoxic activity and could be used in the study of brain receptor systems in vivo and as well as some other neurocytotoxic agents ( kainic acid, ibotenic acid etc.) might be served as a tool in experimental neuroanatomy for investigation of neurochemically specific neuronal systems of the brain.

References


1. Denisenko P.P. 1980. The role of cholinergic mechanisms in regulatory prosesses (Godolina E.A.,ed.). Meditsina, Moscow, p.292.
2. Norberg A., Winblad B. 1986. Abstracts of the Sixth ESN General Meeting , Prague, 1-6 september, 325.
3. Popot J.,-L.,Changeux J.-P. 1984. Physiol.Rev.,64, p.1163.
4. Demushkin V.P., Zotov V.M., Plyashkevich Yu.G. 1982. Vestnik AMN USSR 1,15.
5. Plyashkevich Yu.G., Demushkin V.P. 1985. Biochimia 50, 1167.

6. Mantion C.R., Zigmond M.J., Fisher A., Hanin I. 1983 J.Neurochem. 41, 251.

7. Walsh T.J., Tilson H.A., DeHaven D.L., Malmnan R.B., Fisher A., Hanin I. 1984. Brain Res. 321, 31.

8. Demushkin V.P., Kotelevtsev U.V., Plyashkevich Yu.G., Khramtsov N.V. 1982. Mol.Biologia USSR 16, 190.

9. Demushkin V.P., Khramtsov N.V. 1981. Biochimia USSR 46, 674.

10. Demushkin V.P., Kotelevtsev U.V. 1980. Biochimia USSR 45, 1773.

11. Plyashkevich Yu.G., Demushkin V.P. 1986. Abstracts of the Sixth ESN General Meeting, Prague, 1-6 september, 148.

12. Peterson G.L., Herron G.S., Yamaki M., Fullerton D.S., Schimerlink M.I. 1984. Proc.Natl.Acad.Sci. USA 81, 4993.

13. Hoda K., Hoda T. 1985. J.Biol.Chem. 260, 7927.

14. Rues K.-P., Lieflander M. 1979. Biochem.Biophys.Res.Commun. 88, 627.

15. Amitai G., Avissar S., Balderman D., Sokolovsky M. 1982. Proc.Natl.Acad.Sci.USA 79, 243.

# MOLECULAR MECHANISMS OF CHANNEL BLOCKADE IN NEURONAL NICOTINIC ACETYLCHOLINE RECEPTOR

V.I. Skok, A.A. Selyanko, V.A. Derkach

Bogomoletz Institute of Physiology, Kiev-24

V.E. Gmiro

Institute of Experimental Medicine, Leningrad П -22

## Introduction

It was found recently that some simple bis-quaternary ammonium compounds (BAC), selective ganglion-blocking agents, blocked open ionic channels in nicotinic acetylcholine receptors (AChRs) of autonomic ganglion neurones rather than their channel-gating sites. This mechanism was inferred from the observation that BAC decreased in voltage-dependent manner a time constant, $\tau_s$, of decay of excitatory postsynaptic current (EPSC) recorded from a neurone of autonomic ganglion (1,2). The aim of present work was to investigate i) which kinetic component in single AChR channel activity corresponds to $\tau_s$, and ii) whether this kinetic component can be changed by BAC similarly to $\tau_s$.

## Methods

Single-channel currents were recorded using patch-clamp method in its cell-attached mode (3) from the neurones of rat superior cervical gang-

Receptors and Ion Channels

lion treated by collagenase to clean the cell surface. The experiments were performed at 24° C in Tris-buffered Krebs solution. The AChRs were activated by $3.10^{-5}$M ACh and blocked by $3.10^{-5}$M heptamethonium ($C_7$) added to Krebs solution in patch pipette. $C_7$ was used because the $C_7$-induced channel-blocking effect was more voltage-sensitive than in other BACs. (8). This allowed to test whether the blockade of AChRs observed was produced by $C_7$ simply by changing membrane potential in the membrane patch. Single-channel currents were recorded at about -110 mV membrane potential level, at a frequency band width of 0-3.5 kHz, digitalized at 20 kHz and analysed with the SM-3 computer. Pulses and interpulse intervals shorter than 150 µs were ignored. Mean values of current pulse durations (channel open time) and of the inter pulse intervals (channel closed time) were measured as time constants of their exponential distributions (4).

## Results

Fig. 1,A and Fig. 2,A show examples of single AChR channel activity recorded from different patches of rat superior cervical ganglion neurones when no blocking agent was present in the patch pipette. Single current pulses and bursts of pulses occured in stochastic manner, their mean amplitude corresponded to mean channel conductance 20.0 ± 0.2 pS. Sometimes larger currents that corresponded to about 50 pS channel conductance were seen (not shown in Fig. 1 and Fig. 2); large currents were not further analysed. The analysis of complex distributions of interpulse intervals yielded four components of interpulse intervals, or channel closed times, with their mean values 0.15 ± 0.02 ms, 1.78 ± 0.38 ms, 80.2 ± 23.3 ms and 1083 ± 292 ms (n=4). Assuming the shortest component, $\tau_c$, corresponded to inter pulse intervals within the burst, the mean burst duration was estimated by ignoring all interpulse intervals shorter than 4 x 0.15 ms (this should include 98 % of an exponentially distributed population of events with a mean 0.15 ms). Using this procedure, two components of current durations, or channel open time, were obtained, with their mean values 0.32 ± 0.06 ms and 8.54 ± 1.22 ms. The former value corresponded to durations of separate single opening while the latter one corresponded to duration of a burst of openings ($\tau_b$). Each single opening within a burst, as an average, was 2.6 ± 0.1 ms long ($\tau_o$). The measured duration of each single opening within a burst was apparently overestimated due to the fact that the inter pulse intervals shorter than 150 $\mu$s remained unresolved. The corrected value of $\tau_o$ (for correction methods see 5) was 1.3 ± 0.2 ms. Thus, there were 6 single openings within the burst, as an average.

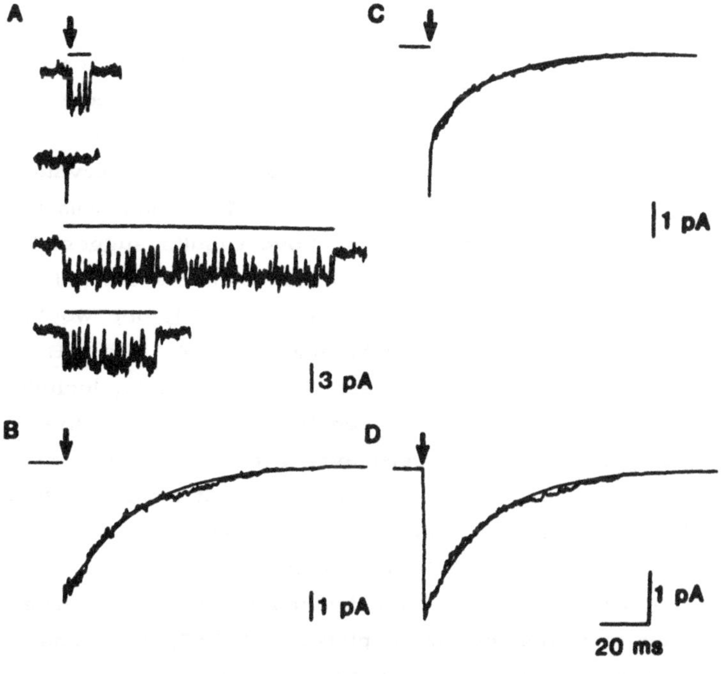


Fig. 1.

Reconstruction of synaptic current by averaging of single-channel currents recorded from cell-attached patch. A: Examples of single-channel currents recorded from the same patch at -110 mV calculated membrane potential and identified as single events (indicated by bar above each record), when short intervals (shorter than 4 x $\tau_c$) were ignored. B,C and D show reconstructed synaptic currents obtained by synchronous averaging of 106 "true" bursts (containing two and more current pulses) (B), or by synchronous averaging of 59 single-pulse events together with the "true" bursts (C), or by non-synchronous averaging of both single-pulse currents and bursts (D), some of which are shown in A. In D delays introduced for single events varied according to the Gaussian distribution, with $\sigma$ = 0.3 ms. The reconstructed currents were fitted by single exponential curves in B and D (time constants 29.5 and 25.6 ms, respectively) or by the sum of two exponential curves in C (time constants 0.5 and 28.2 ms). In contrast to other records, the records shown in Fig. 1 were obtained in bicarbonate buffered solution (25 mM $NaHCO_3$ and 118 mM NaCl, instead of 10 mM Tris-HCl and 133 mM NaCl).

The time constant, $\tau_s$, of the EPSC decay in rat superior cervical ganglion, if measured at a temperature (23°C) and membrane potential ( -110 mV) similar to those used in the present work, is 13,9 ± 0.6 ms (n= 4) (Derkach, Selyanko and Skok, unpublished observation). This value of $\tau_s$ is close to $\tau_b$ rather than to $\tau_o$ found from the analysis of single AChR channel activity. The above results suggest that by averaging "true" synchronously started bursts of current pulses recorded from single AChR channel (as shown in Fig. 1,A), one would obtain a current with a time course similar to that of EPSC. Fig. 1,B shows that such current indeed can be obtained. When all events, including separate single current pulses (which can be considered as the bursts containing only one opening) were averaged, the current exhibited a double-exponential decay with a slow component similar to that in EPSC and a fast component which had no counterpart in EPSC (Fig. 1,C). However, rising phase in EPSC is usually S-shaped (6) indicating that there are delays in activation of individual channels by nerve-released ACh. In order to model the rising phase of EPSC, we introduced delays for single events according to a Gaussian distribution. By changing the variance in this distribution, we found that the curve changed from double-exponential to single-exponential at $\sigma$ = 0.3 ms (Fig. 1,D). It thus can be concluded from the above results that activation of AChR resulting from single preganglionic volley results in the appearence of a burst which, as an average, consists of about 6 single openings.

One thus could expect that BAC which shorten $\tau_s$ should also shorten the burst duration, $\tau_b$. In order to test this suggestion, the effect of

$C_7$ on single AChR channel activity was studied in four membrane patches of the rat superior cervical ganglion neurones. The results are illustrated by Fig. 2 and Table 1. It was found that $C_7$ shortened both $\tau_b$ and $\tau_o$ without affecting mean amplitude of the current flowing through single AChR channel and mean interpulse interval within the burst, $\tau_c$.

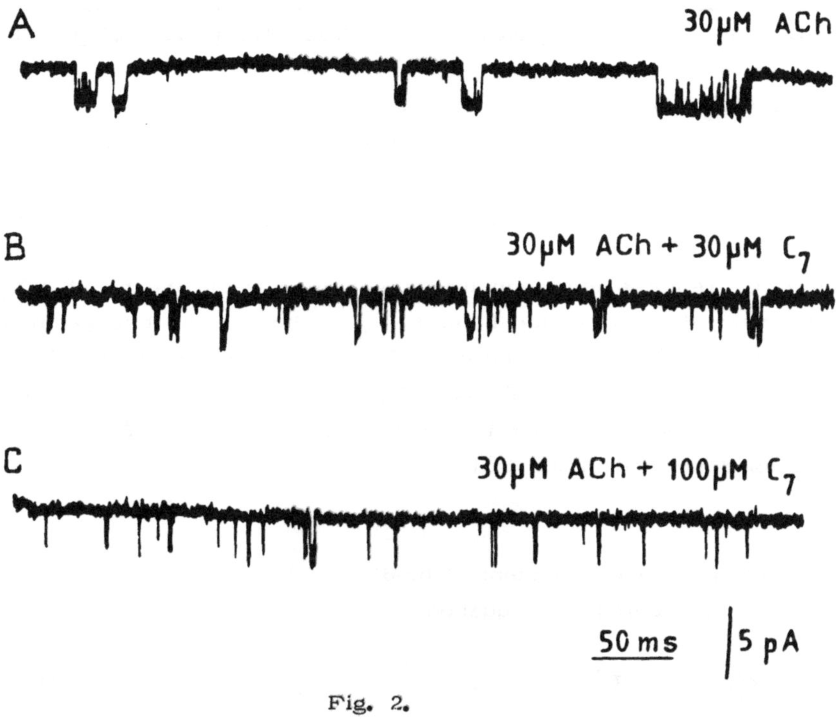


Fig. 2.

Single channel currents recorded with a pipette that contained ACh only (30 µM) or ACh and $C_7$ (30 µM or 100µM). Records were obtained from three different patches, A, B and C.

The effects observed are in agreement with a model in which $C_7$ blocks open channel of AChR (7):

$$AR \underset{\alpha}{\overset{\beta}{\rightleftharpoons}} AR^* + B \underset{k^*_{-B}}{\overset{k^*_{+B}[B]}{\rightleftharpoons}} AR^*B, \qquad (1)$$

where AR, AR* and AR*B are closed-channel state, open-channel state and blocked-open-channel state of the agonist-receptor complex,

B is a blocking agent in concentration [B], and $\alpha$, $\beta$, $k^*_{+B}$ and $k^*_{-B}$ are rate constants. It can be shown (see 4) that $\tau_o = \alpha^{-1}$ and $\tau_b = n(\tau_o + \tau_c) + \tau_o$; n is a number of closings in burst.

| Pipette solution contained | i (pA) | $\tau_c$ (ms) | $\tau_o$ (ms) | $\tau_b$ (ms) |
|---|---|---|---|---|
| ACh (30 $\mu$M) (n = 4) | 2.2 ± 0.01 | 0.15 ± 0.02 | 1.3 ± 0.2 | 8.5 ± 1.22 |
| ACh (30 $\mu$M) and $C_7$ (30 $\mu$M) (n = 4) | 2.0 ± 0.07 | 0.12 ± 0.02 | 0.4 ± 0.1 | 1.5 ± 0.13 |

Table 1. $C_7$ reduces the mean time spent open within the burst ($\tau_o$) and the mean duration of the burst ($\tau_b$). There is no change in the time spent closed within the burst ($\tau_c$) or in the current amplitude (i). Note that the values of $\tau_c$ and $\tau_b$ were estimated from the inter-pulse intervals and burst duration distributions, whereas $\tau_o$ was calculated as described in the text.

The "true" mean rate constant of binding of B to open channel, $k^*_{+B}$, can be calculated from the equation

$$k^*_{+B} = [(\tau'_o)^{-1} - (\tau_o)^{-1}] \times [B]^{-1} \qquad (2)$$

where $\tau'_o$ is mean duration of single channel opening in the presence of $C_7$. The $k^*_{+B}$ thus found was $64.8 \times 10^6 M^{-1}s^{-1}$. When $\tau_b$ and $\tau'_b$ (mean burst duration in the presence of $C_7$) are used instead of $\tau_o$ and $\tau'_o$, the eq.2 gives the mean "apparent" value of $k^*_{+B}$ equal to $17.6 \times 10^6 M^{-1}s^{-1}$. The latter value is not much different from that found when $\tau_s$ and $\tau'_s$ (the EPSC decay time constant in the presence of $C_7$) were used instead of $\tau_o$ and $\tau'_o$, correspondingly, in eq. 2, provided that membrane potential is −110 mV and that $k^*_{+B} \gg k^*_{-B}$ (7). That the latter condition is fulfilled is evidenced by the fact that the EPSC decay in presence of $C_7$ remains single exponential. Thus, the results obtained in this work are consistent with the suggestion that $C_7$ blocks open channel of AChR.

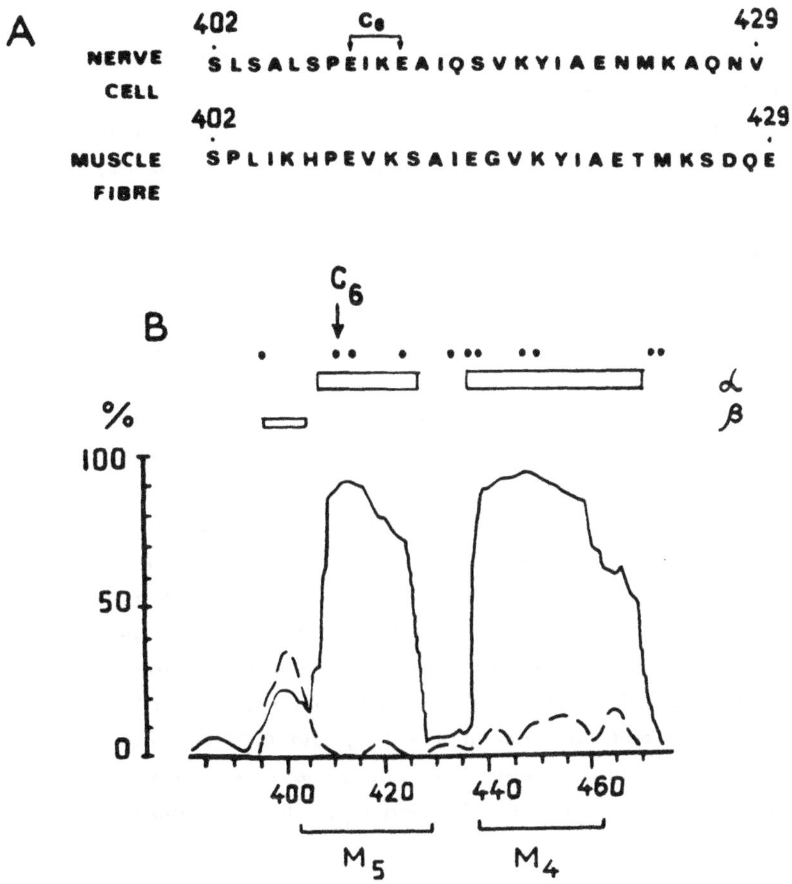


Fig. 3.

Amino acid sequence and predicted secondary structure of $M_5$ portion of neural AChR α-subunit. A. The amino acid sequence is shown in one-letter code. The tentative binding site for $C_6$ is pointed by arrows. For comparison, the amino acid sequence of muscle AChR α-subunit is shown in bottom line. B. Numbers of amino residues (abscissa) and probabilities of α-helix (smooth line) and β-structure (broken line) (ordinate). Dark spots indicate negatively charged residues. Broad and narrow rectangles indicate most probable α-helix and β-structure, correspondingly. $M_4$ and $M_5$ portions are shown (11).

Hexamethonium ($C_6$) and pentamethonium ($C_5$) are most potent among simmetrical BACs both in their open channel-blocking and ganglion-blocking activities (see 8). A question arises whether a site can be identified in the channel-forming portion of the AChR protein that might selectively bind $C_5$ and $C_6$. It was suggested that the ionic channel in nicotinic AChR of fish electric organ was lined by $M_5$ (or L) portions yielded by each of five subunits of the AChR molecule (9, 10). A protein encoded by clone PCA48 of cDNA obtained from rat phaeochromocytoma cell line PC12 was thought to be similar to $\alpha$-subunit of AChR in sympathetic ganglion neurones (11). The $M_5$ portion of this protein contained three glutamate residues with their negatively charged carboxyl groups that might bind cationic groups of BAC. One of glutamates, E-412, is absent in the homologous portion of $\alpha$-subunit from muscle AChR (Fig. 3,A), which, in contrast to ganglionic AChR, is insensitive to a channel-blocking influence of $C_5$ and $C_6$ (12). Using a method of theoretical prediction of protein secondary structure (13), we confirmed the earlier results (see 11) that the $M_5$ portion is an amphipatic $\alpha$-helix (Fig. 3,B). A distance between two glutamate residues E-409 and E-412 (Fig. 3,A) is about 0.7-0.8 nm, assuming the helix possesses conventional parameters (diameter = 0.96 nm, 3.6 residues per turn and helical pitch = 0.54 nm). This distance is very close to the intercharged distances in $C_5$ and $C_6$ molecules in their most stable conformations, which are 0.75 nm and 0.88 nm at $\varepsilon = 3.1$, and 0.75 nm and 0.81 nm at $\varepsilon = 81$, correspondingly (see 14). Thus, the site E-409 - E-412 is one of possible binding sites for $C_5$ and $C_6$, selective channel blockers of neural AChR.

## References

1. Selyanko, A.A., V.A. Derkach, V.I. Skok. 1981. Adv. Physiol. Sci. 4, 329.

2. Skok, V.I. 1986. Neuroscience 17, 1.

3. Hamill, O.P., A. Marty, E. Neher, B. Sakmann, F.G. Sigworth. 1981. Pflügers Arch. 391, 85.

4. Derkach, V.A., R.A. North, A.A. Selyanko, V.I. Skok. J. Physiol. ( in press)

5. Colquhoun, D., B. Sakmann. 1985. J. Physiol. 369, 501.

6. Gage, P.W. 1976. Physiol. Rev. 56. 177.

7. Adams, P.R. 1976. J. Physiol. 260, 531.

8. Skok, V.I., A.A. Selyanko, V.A. Derkach, V.E. Gmiro. 1984. Neurophysiology 16, 46.

9. Guy, H.R. 1984. Biophys. J. 45, 249.

10. Finer-Moore, J., R.M. Stroud. 1984. Proc. natn. Acad. Sci, U.S.A. 81, 155.

11. Boulter , J., K. Evans, D. Goldman, G. Mar tin, D. Treco, S. Heinemann, J. Patrick. 1986. Nature 119, 368.

12. Rang, H.P., R.J. Rylett. 1984. Br. J. Pharmac. 81, 519.

13. Ptitsyn, O.B., A.V. Finkelstein. 1983. Biopolymers. 22. 15.

14. Skok, V.I. 1985. Biomembranes 2, 245.

# PROPERTIES OF THE HIGH AFFINITY CHOLINE CARRIER AND ACETYLCHOLINE RECEPTORS IN THE NERVOUS SYSTEM OF INSECTS

H. Breer, M. Knipper, D. Benke, W. Hanke
Fachbereich Biologie/Chemie, Universität Osnabrück, FRG

## Introduction

Communication between neurons which is mediated by specific compounds and which occurs at specialized structures, the synapses, is a fundamental process in neuronal function. Although in the nervous system of vertebrates and several invertebrates many transmitters compounds and the enzymes which metabolize them has been characterized, the detailed evaluation of the molecular elements and microphysiological processes is still a most challenging problem in neurobiology.
Acetylcholine (ACh) was the first substance to be recognized as chemical transmitter, but our knowledge on functions and molecular mechanisms of neurons and synapses that utilize ACh as transmitter, cholinergic neurons, is still limited and mainly based on the wealth of information obtained by studying the electrophysiology of the vertebrate neuromuscular junction and by exploring the biochemical properties of preparations from electric tissue; in each case synapses between neurons and muscle, resp. muscle-derived, cells.
The nervous system of arthropods was found to be high cholinergic innervated (12) with acetylcholine concentrations two orders of magnitude higher than in the vertebrate brain. One of the reasons for the high concentration of cholinergic synapses in the ganglia of arthropods is probably the different neurochemical innervation pattern in these species: the efferent neurons were found to be glutaminergic, whereas all identified afferent pathways appeared to be cholinergic. Thus, the nervous tissue of arthropods may be a suitable source for studying molecular aspects of neuronal cholinergic synapses.

Receptors and Ion Channels

High affinity choline transport.

One distinct possibility for regulating the production of acetylcholine in cholinergic terminals, where the capacity to synthesize the transmitter considerably exceeds the normal requirement, is the supply of choline. The use of synaptosomes in rapid tracer flux studies have evaluated the existence of a sodium-dependent, high affinity uptake system for choline (22), and in subsequent approaches evidences have been accumulated demonstrating that the high affinity choline carriers are apparently unique to cholinergic nerve terminals and the choline accumulation via this high affinity pathway is obviously the rate-limiting, regulatory step for the synthesis of acetylcholine (17); this process is thus of particular importance for cholinergic synapses.
Synaptosomal preparations from locust were found to accumulate exogenous choline in a high affinity carrier-mediated process and convert most of it to acetylcholine (3). The choline transport is known to be essentially dependent on $Na^{+}$-ions and blocked by hemicholinium-3, but the principles how this process is energized and regulated is still poorly understood; this is partly due to the fact that an adequate interpretation of transport data has always been complicated by intracellular metabolic activities and sequesteration in intact nerve endings. More recently there has been significant progress in exploring synaptosomal transport processes following a shift from the complex synaptosomes to membrane vesicles obtained after osmotic lysis of synaptosomes. Such "synaptosomal ghosts" have proven to be very useful for studying neurotranmitter transport in isolation from other processes; but unfortunately it was found that the transport activity for choline was lost following osmotic lysis in mammalian preparations (15,18). Synaptosomal ghosts derived from the highly cholinergic insect nervous tissue, however, loaded with $K^{+}$ ions and suspended in NaCl, were capable to accumulate choline via a high affinity, carrier-mediated process (Fig. 1) indicating that the accumulation of choline was energized by ion gradients only and showing that ATP and ATPases are not directly involved (4,9). Manipulations of the ion compositions in the intra- and extravesicular medium have revealed that the $Na^{+}$ -gradient must be considered as the main driving force for choline accumulation and that choline is possibly translocated as a complex of

2 $Na^+$ : 1 $Cl^-$ : 1 choline. This points to an electrogenic process; i.e. net charges cross the membrane and the membrane potential should affect choline transport. In fact, we found that valinomycin, which increases the membrane potential enhanced the transport rate, whereas CCCP reduced choline accumulation (5). The results favour the view that the high affinity uptake of choline is catalyzed by thightly coupled $Na^+$/Ch symporters energized by electrochemical gradients.

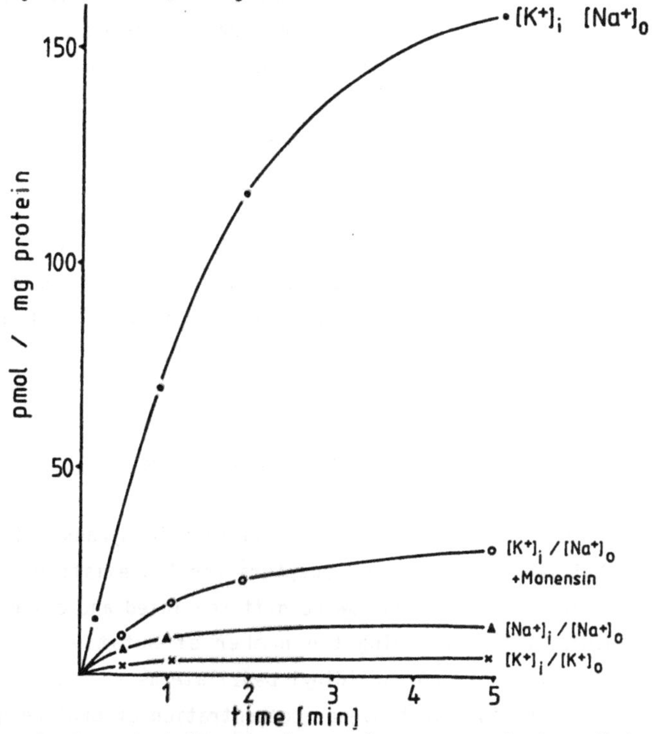


Fig.1 Accumulation of choline by locust "synaptosomal ghosts" in the presence of different ion concentrations. Choline is only transported in the presence of an appropriate sodium

Studies on the efflux of choline from preloaded membrane vesicles have indicated the bidirectionality of the transport and that the carrier is symmetrical with respect to the membrane; thus the vectoral translocation under physiological conditions is caused by ion gradients and electrical potential across the membrane (8); this view is further supported by transactivating effects of choline, i.e. the rates of translocation de-

pends (within limits) on the concentration of choline on the opposite side of the membrane. Apparently, the carrier mediates transport in both directions and its binding site translocates faster when it is loaded with choline. The transport is however apparently inhibited by compounds, like acetylcholine, that bind to the carrier but cannot be transported; the physiological significance of this phenomenon for regulating acetylcholine synthesis and concentration in the terminal is unclear yet.
Recent observations indicate that ATP may be considered as a modulator, as an inhibitor of choline carrier. Extracellular ATP was found to inhibit uptake of choline in synaptosomes in submillimolar concentrations.
This finding is of particular interest, since ATP might be released together with acetylcholine from cholinergic synapses of insects (7), as has already been shown for other cholinergic nerve terminals (24). This view is further supported by the observation that the transport of GABA was not affected by nucleotides. Experiments using various nucleosides and nucleotides as well as ATP-analogues suggest that the effect of ATP may be mediated by a kinase reaction (16).

## Receptors for acetylcholine in insect nervous tissue

From the earliest days of research on cholinerigic synapses it has been recognized that two categories of receptors for ACh exist: nicotinic and muscarinic receptors, which can now be differentiated and estimated using specific ligands. When monitoring the number of putative ACh-recptors using -bungarotoxin and quinuclidinyl benzilate as specific ligands, it was found that there is a much higher concentration of cholinergic receptors in insects than in vertebrates and furthermore the relative level for the two different binding sites was reversed (Fig.2): predominantly muscarinic receptors in the vertebrate brain, very high concentration of putative nicotinic receptors in insect ganglia.
The preponderance of nicotinic binding sites and convincing physiological evidences indicate that in insect these sites are functional acetylcholine receptors (20). In view of the enormous progress in identifying the peripheral AChR in vertebrates (11) it was of particular interest to explore the molecular properties of the insect AChR.

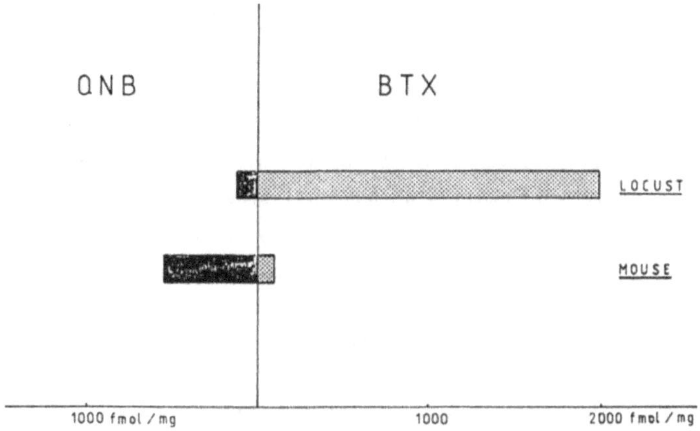


Fig. 2 Concentration of α-bungarotoxin and quinuclidinyl benzilate binding sites in the locust ganglia and mouse brain.

Acetylcholine receptors, as probed by α-toxin binding, have been solubilized from locust neuronal membrane preparations and subjected to an affinity chromatography purification procedure. The toxin binding sites was found to be a high molecular weight glycoprotein, with a sedimentation coefficient of about 10S; a value similar to that found for the vertebrate receptor. In analysis on polyacrylamid-microelectrophoresis under nondenaturing conditions the purified protein gave a single band corresponding to about $M_r$ 300,000, which confirms the 10S value; under denaturing conditions in a SDS-gel, the same protein migrated again as a single band now at a position corresponding to $M_r$ 65,000 (10). This result suggest, that the native receptor apparently represents an oligomer of 4-5 identical or very similar polypeptides and would thus significantly differ from the vertebrate receptor. But before drawing such a conclusion it was necessary to evaluate whether the isolated toxin binding protein represents in fact an acetylcholine receptor.

In a first approach immunohistochemical techniques have been used for a topochemical localization. Monospecific antisera against the affinity purified protein were used to incubate cryostate sections from insect ganglia; the antigenic sites were visualized by the peroxidase-antiperoxidase technique. In the head and thoracic ganglia of various insect

species very distinct areas of the neuropil were found to be labelled; zones which are known to be rich in neuronal connections and several of which are supposed to have many cholinergic synapses. No labelling was found over the fibers, the peripheral sheets and cell-layers. Thus, the appearance of the antigenic sites in immunocytochemial preparations would be consistent with a location at neuronal synapses.
In a second approach the crossreactivity with monoclonal antibodies against the Torpedo receptor was analysed. In Western blots it could be demonstrated that a few antibodies out of a monoclonal libarary (21), significantly crossreacted with the insect receptor polypeptides, pointing to some molecular relatedness of the two receptor types. The immunological approaches thus provide further evidences that the purified protein is in fact a constituent of the insect neuronal receptor.
The ultimate proof, however, that the isolated protein represents the functional AChR and not only the ligand binding component can only be achieved by reconstituting the protein in artificial lipid membranes, e.g. planar lipid bilayer. To approach this goal, the purified insect receptor protein has been incorporated into liposomes and these proteoliposomes subsequently fused into planar lipid bilayer; the conductance of this bilayer was then analyzed under voltage clamp conditions and at high time resolution, which allows to resolve single channel events.

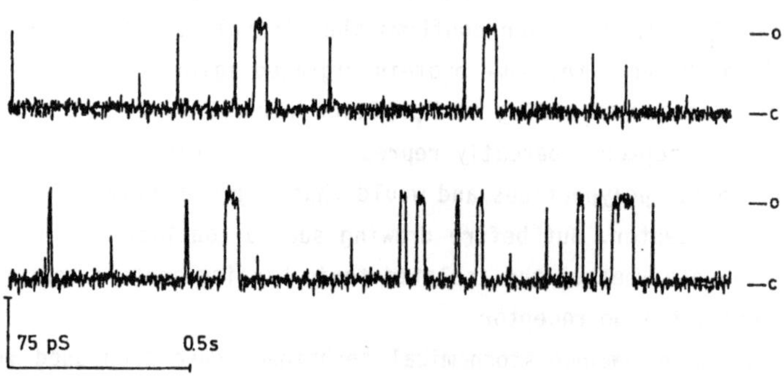


Fig. 3 Fluctuation of an agonist activated AChR-channel isolated from locust neuronal membranes and reconstituted in planar lipid bilayer.

Without agonists in the aqueous solution no conductance was observed, however the addition of agonists induced the appearance of specific channel fluctuations; single channels, selectively permeable for cations, which display a conductance of about 75pS and a mean life time of a few milliseconds were recorded (13,14). Thus for the first time a neuronal ACh-controlled ion channel, a functional AChR from nerve cells, has been reconstituted.

The molecular organisation of the neuronal AChR from insect, which is apparently quite different from the peripheral vertebrate receptor, is of some interest in view of the receptor evolution, since it has been suggested the 4 genes encoding the subunits of the vertebrate receptor must have been originated from a common ancestral gene via duplication (19). Whether the insect receptor can be considered as a prototype of such an ancient form is unclear and can only be decided on the basis of a completely deciphered primary structure. As a first approach the purified protein was subjected to gas-phase microsequencing. Unfortunately the amino terminus of the polypeptide was found to be blocked, however, a short stretch of amino acid sequence from a fragment of the receptor could be identified (23); an almost identical sequence is present in all identified vertebrate $\alpha$-subunits. The complete primary structure, however, can only be explored using recombinant DNA and the approaches of molecular genetics.

In order to evaluate whether receptor specific mRNA can be isolated from insect nervous tissue, polyA$^+$-RNA preparation from young locusts were microinjected into Xenopus oocytes, which are known to express vertebrate mRNA, perform all posttranslational modification and even incorporate receptor protein into plasma membrane (1). After several days $\alpha$-bungarotoxin binding activity could be detected, depending linearly on the amount of applied RNA, and binding sites were found in the surface membrane of the oocytes, indicating that AChR molecules were inserted into the membrane. Immunoprecipitation of receptor polypeptides synthesized in the presence of radiolabelled amino acids, followed by electrophoresis and autoradiography, revealed that obviously a homogenous population of polypeptides was isolated, indicating that the <u>in ovo</u> synthesized receptor proteins have a similar size as the native subunits. In ion flux studies it was subsequently verified that the oocytes have expressed ACh-gated ion channels, functional AChR. When oocytes, previously injected with insect mRNA were treated with cholinergic agonists, a significant influx of $^{86}Rb^{+}$ isotops was induced, which could be blocked by $d$-tubocurarine (6). These results thus indicate, that Xenopus oocytes do express insect mRNA and that the polyA$^{+}$-RNA preparations from nervous tissue of young locusts do contain receptor-specific mRNAs and may be used as template to produce the appropriate complementary DNA, a first step towards a molecular analysis of the insect neuronal ACh-receptors.

## Conclusion

The application of powerful new approaches to neuronal preparations from invertebrates not only can contribute to unravel the molecular architecture of the arthropod nervous system but may also significantly contribute to explore molecular details of chemical signalling between nerve cells. Comparative studies on molecular neurobiology of invertebrates may gain new information concerning the evolution and phylogenetic development of biochemical processes and molecular elements involved in synaptic transmission. More detailed knowledge of synaptic elements in the nervous system of insects is also considered as an essential prerequisite for analyzing the mode of action of chemicals that may considered as putative insecticides, and furthermore to detect critical sites in the nervous system of insects, which might represent new targets for insecticides.

## Acknowledgements

The authors express their graditude to G. Hinz and U. Mädler for skilful technical assistance and to G. Moehrke for preparing the manuscript. The experimental studies were supported by the Deutsche Forschungsgemeinschaft.

## References

1. Barnard, E.A., Beeson, D., Bilbe, G., Brown, D.A., Constanti, A., Houamed, K., Smart T.G. 1984. J. Recept. Res. 4, 681.
2. Breer, H. 1981. Neurochem. Int. 3, 155-163.

3. Breer, H. 1982. J. Neurobiol. 13, 107-117.

4. Breer, H. 1983. FEBS Lett. 153, 345-348.

5. Breer, H. 1986. In: Neuropharmacology and Neurobiology (N.G. Ford, P.N.R. Usherwood, R.C. Ray, G.G. Lunt, eds.) Ellis Horwood Books, pp. 384-413.

6. Breer, H., Benke, D. 1986. Molecular Brain Research -in press-

7. Breer, H., Knipper, M. 1984. Insect. Biochem. 14, 337-344.

8. Breer, H., Knipper, M. 1985. Cellul. Molec. Neurobiol. 5, 285-296.

9. Breer, H., Lueken, W. 1983. Neurochem. Int. 5, 713-720.

10. Breer, H., Kleene, R., Hinz, G. 1985. J. Neuroscience 5, 3386-3392.

11. McCarty, M.P., Earnest, J.P., Young, E.F. Choe, S., Stroud, R.M. 1986. Ann. Rev. Neurosci. 9, 383-413.

12. Florey, E. 1963. Can. J. Biochem. Physiol. 41, 2619-2626.

13. Hanke, W., Breer, H. 1986a. Nature 321, 171-174.

14. Hanke, W., Breer, H. 1986b. J. Gen. Physiol.

15. Kanner, B.I. 1983. Biochim. Biophysi. Acta 726, 293-316.

16. Knipper, M., Breer, H. 1986. Neurosci. Lett. - in press-

17. Kuhar, M.J. Murrin, L.C. 1978. J. Neurochem. 30, 15-21.

18. Meyer, E.M. Cooper, J.R. 1983. J. Neurosci. 3, 987-994.

19. Raftery, M., Hunkapiller, M.W., Strader, C.D., Hood, L.E. 1980. Science 208, 1454-1457.

20. Sattelle, D.B., Harrow, I.D., Hue, B., Pelhate, M., Gepner, J., Hall, L.M. 1983. J. exp. Biol. 107, 473-489.

21. Watters, D., Maelicke, A. 1983. Biochemistry 22, 331

22. Yamamura, H.I., Snyder, S.H. 1973. J. Neurochem. 21, 1355-1374.

23. Zenssen, Hinz, G., Beyreuther, K., Breer, H. 1986.

24. Zimmermann, H. 1982. In: Neurotransmitter Vesicles (R.L. Klein, H. Lagercrantz, H. Zimmermann, eds.) London, Academic Press, pp. 305-359.

# I Receptors

## b) Other Receptors

EFFECT OF SULFHYDRYL REAGENTS ON ANTAGONIST BINDING WITH MUSCARINIC RECEPTORS

J. Järv, A. Rinken
Department of Organic Chemistry, Tartu State University
Tartu, Estonian SSR

## Introduction

Chemical modification of thiol and disulfide groups of muscarinic receptor has been widely used for investigation into the structure and properties of the receptor binding sites. Many investigators have studied the influence of sulfhydryl reagents on agonist binding with muscarinic receptor. Less attention has been paid to the alteration of the antagonist binding properties of the receptor, although radiolabelled potent antagonists (e.g. L-[$^3$H]quinuclidinyl benzilate, [$^3$H]QNB) are widely used as reporter ligands in experiments with agonists (1 - 4). It has been reported in several papers that modification of the receptor protein with N-ethylmaleimide (3-9), 5,5'-dithiobis(2-nitrobenzoate) (5, 10, 11) and dithiotreitol (2, 5) has no effect on [$^3$H]QNB binding. According to other papers (10, 12-14), however, these reagents and p-chloromercuribenzoate (5, 10, 13-15) have been found to influence [$^3$H]QNB binding. As the effects described in the latter papers seem to be dependent upon the reaction time and the reagent concentration, kinetic analysis of the modification process is necessary for meaningful discussion of these phenomena. In the present paper this aspect of chemical modification of the receptor protein with several thiol and disulfide reagents has been studied in the case of membrane-bound and solubilized muscarinic receptors from rat cerebral cortex. Digitonin was used for receptor solubilization (16). The number of the receptor binding sites was determined by the specific binding of [$^3$H]QNB, measured by the common filtration assay in the case of membranes (17) or by the gel-filtration assay in the case of the solubilized receptor (16). Simultaneous experiments were made with the receptor-[$^3$H]QNB complex, where the radioligand

Receptors and Ion Channels

had been bound with the receptor before its chemical modification.

Mercaptication with p-chloromercuribenzoate

Incubation of the membrane-bound muscarinic receptor in 20-500 μM solution of p-chloromercuribenzoate led to a decrease in the number of the [$^{3}$H]QNB binding sites. Complete inactivation of the receptor can be achieved if sufficiently high concentrations of the reagent were used. The semilogarithmic plots of the specific [$^{3}$H]-QNB binding vs. incubation time yield straight lines (Fig 1), which point to the pseudo-first order kinetics of this process and allow the calculation of the rate constants $k_{obs}$. The linear dependence of $k_{obs}$ upon the reagent concentration gives the apparent second-order rate constant $k_{II}$ = 25 ± 5 $M^{-1}s^{-1}$ (Fig 2) for the modification process. Similar kinetic regularities were found in the

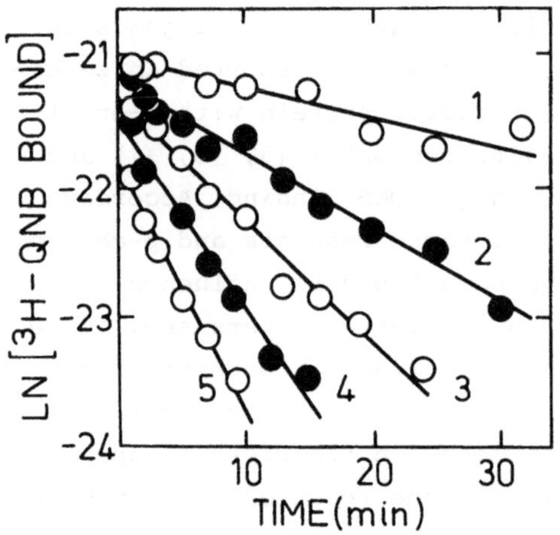


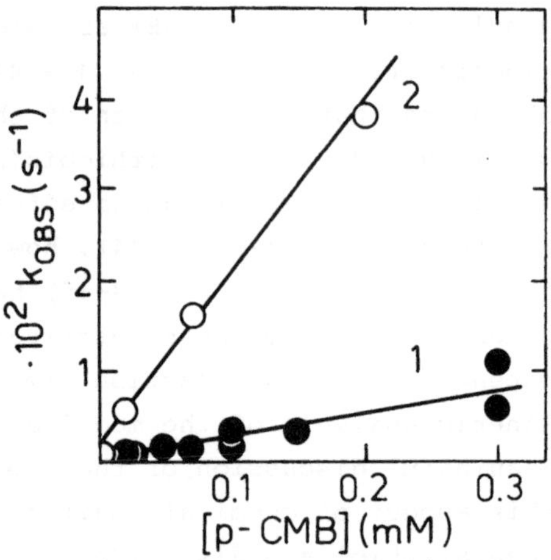


Figure 1 (left). The effect of p-chloromercuribenzoate on the specific binding of [$^{3}$H]QNB with muscarinic receptor. Membranes from rat cerebral cortex were incubated with 1- 0.03 mM, 2- 0.07 mM, 3- 0.15 mM, 4- 0.3 mM, 5- 0.5 mM p-chloromercuribenzoate during the time indicated (0.05 mM K-phosphate buffer pH = 7.4, 25°C). After that [$^{3}$H]QNB was added to the reaction mixture (5 nM) and the bound radioligand was determined after 15 min incubation by the filtration method. The non-specific binding of [$^{3}$H]QNB was measured in the presence of 100 μM atropine.

Figure 2 (right). Inactivation of the membrane-bound and solubilized muscarinic receptors from rat cerebral cortex by p-chloromercuribenzoate (p-CMB) in 0.05 M K-phosphate buffer pH = 7.4, 25°C.

case of the solubilized receptor for which $k_{II}$ = 190 ± 10 $M^{-1}s^{-1}$ was calculated. The addition of p-chloromercuribenzoate to the incubation medium containing the receptor-[$^3$H]QNB complex, has no measurable effect on its stability. The latter conclusion is also valid for the solubilized receptor-[$^3$H]QNB complex. The results obtained clearly show that a single SH-group governs the specific binding of [$^3$H]QNB with the receptor. However, there should be remarkable hindrances to the accessibility to this group by p-chloromercuribenzoate as the inactivation velocity of the receptor is approximately $10^6$ times smaller than the mercuration rate of such model SH-compounds as glutathione and 2-mercaptoethanol ($k_{II}$ = = $6 \cdot 10^6$ $M^{-1}s^{-1}$) (18). The acceleration of the inactivation in the case of the solubilized receptor in comparison with the membrane-bound receptor can be explained by the destruction of the structure-stabilizing lipid environment of the receptor protein.

Thiol-disulfide exchange with 5,5'-dithiobis(2-nitrobenzoate)

0.1 - 5 mM solutions of 5,5'-dithiobis(2-nitrobenzoate) also caused measurable decrease in the concentration of the [$^3$H]QNB binding sites. This reaction is much slower than the inactivation of muscarinic receptor by p-chloromercuribenzoate and can be characterized by the rate constant $k_{II}$ = (5.0 ± 0.4) $10^{-3}$ $M^{-1}s^{-1}$. As the reaction of 5,5'-dithiobis(2-nitrobenzoate) with model SH-compounds is much faster (19), the slowness of the receptor modification can also be explained by steric factors. The results obtained give evidence of the existence of an important SH-group in the antagonist binding site of the muscarinic receptor. On the other hand, 5,5'-dithiobis(2-nitrobenzoate) has no measurable effect on the stability of the receptor-[$^3$H]QNB complex, pointing to the importance of the thiol group only on the step of [$^3$H]QNB binding.
The application of 5,5'-dithiobis(2-nitrobenzoate) also allowed us to estimate the total number of sulfhydryl groups in brain membranes available for modification under the experimental conditions used (20). The titration of these SH-groups gave 0.25 µmole/mg protein, which exceeds more than $10^6$-fold the number of the receptor sites determined by using [$^3$H]QNB.

The influence of the alkylating reagent N-ethylmaleimide

The treatment of brain membranes with 0.1 - 10 mM N-ethylmaleimide led to a remarkable modification of the receptor binding properties as shown in Fig 3.

In summary, the effects observed were the following. Firstly, a rapid and dose-dependent decrease in the concentration of the receptor sites, which bound [$^3$H]QNB during a short incubation time (10 - 15 min), could be observed. This process of receptor modification is too fast to be kinetically studied by means of the common receptor assay system.

Secondly, slow [$^3$H]QNB binding with brain membranes could be followed after the N-ethylmaleimide treatment. The observed rate constant for this reaction did not depend on N-ethylmaleimide concentration in the incubation mixture and its value was approximately 500-fold smaller than the corresponding value for [$^3$H]QNB binding with the native membrane-bound receptor (21).

Thirdly, the slow binding reaction was not complete and clearly pointed to the dose-dependent inhibition of the receptor sites.

These data can be explained by two alternative reaction schemes. The first possible model assumes the simultaneous existence of al-

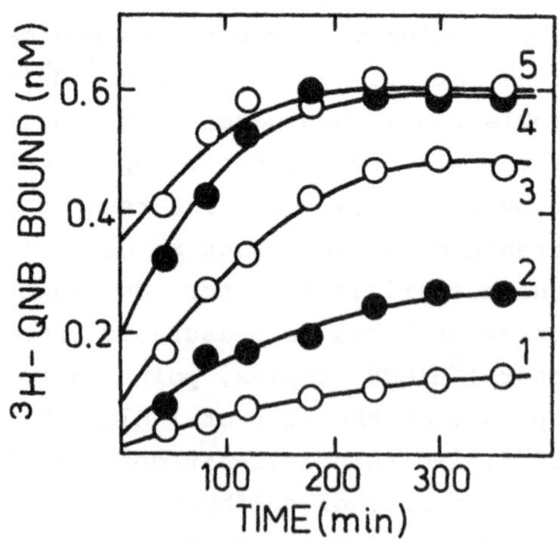


Figure 3. Binding of [$^3$H]QNB (5 nM) to membrane-bound muscarinic receptor from rat cerebral cortex, treated with 1 - 11,5 mM; 2 - 2.9 mM, 3 - 0.7 mM; 4 - 0.2 mM; 5 - 0.04 mM N-ethylmaleimide. The treatment was carried out for 60 min at 25°C in 0.05 M K-phosphate buffer pH = 7.4.

kylation of SH-group and reversible binding of N-ethylmaleimide with the receptor protein. The latter complex should possess a very slow dissociation rate. The second possible model involves consecutive modification of two different SH-groups. The alkylation of one of these groups slows down the $[^3H]$QNB binding rate, while the modification of the second SH-group leads to a complete loss of $[^3H]$QNB binding with the receptor.

## Disulfide reducing with dithiothreitol

The loss of $[^3H]$QNB binding sites occurred in 0.02 - 0.4 M dithiothreitol solutions in the concentration-dependent manner that allowed the estimation of the second-order rate constants. For membrane-bound and solubilized receptors the $k_{II}$ values were close, $(1.2 \pm 0.1)10^{-3}\ M^{-1}s^{-1}$ and $(1.0 \pm 0.2)10^{-3}\ M^{-1}s^{-1}$, respectively. A similar conclusion could be drawn in the case of the membrane--bound and solubilized receptor-$[^3H]$QNB complex, for which $k_{II} = (1.3 \pm 0.1)10^{-4}\ M^{-1}s^{-1}$ and $(2.3 \pm 0.3)10^{-4}\ M^{-1}s^{-1}$, respectively. Besides that, the degradation rate of the free receptor and the receptor-$[^3H]$QNB complex differ only 10-20-fold in the case of both membrane-bound and solubilized receptors. This difference is remarkably smaller than the effects found in the case of the sulfhydryl reagents studied above. Quite similar inactivation velocity of the free receptor and receptor-ligand complex as well as of the membrane-bound and solubilized receptors points to the fact that the attack of dithiothreitol on the crucial disulfide bond is not hindered by the membrane environment or the bound ligand.

## Discussion

Chemical modification of sulfhydryl groups on brain membranes leads to the inhibition of antagonist binding with the muscarinic receptor. A complete loss of the receptor binding sites can be achieved if sufficiently high reagent concentrations are used. In the case of p-chloromercuribenzoate and 5,5'-dithiobis(2-nitrobenzoate) the inhibition process follows the first-order reaction course, indicating that the modification of only one sulfhydryl

group by these reagents is crucial for the loss of the receptor activity. As the receptor-antagonist complex is insensitive to treatment with sulfhydryl reagents, the crucial SH-group seems to govern the binding properties of the receptor and is probably located in the appropriate binding site. If only a partial loss of the antagonist binding sites is observed in the modification experiments, either an insufficient amount of the sulfhydryl reagent has been used or the modification reaction has not been followed up to the end. A large excess of the reagent should be used in such experiments, for the total number of the SH-groups available for modification in the membranes considerably exceeds the number of the receptor sites. Therefore, the data on a partial change in the receptor activity resulting from the modification of the sulfhydryl groups can hardly be regarded as sufficient reason for biochemical differentiation of the receptor subtypes as done in (13, 15).
Besides the sulfhydryl groups some disulfide bonds also seem to play an important role in the stabilization of muscarinic receptor, as treatment with dithiothreitol leads to the inactivation of both membrane-bound and solubilized receptor preparations. But differently from sulfhydryl reagents dithiothreitol quite effectively also decomposes the receptor-antagonist complex. This means that the receptor-bound ligand does not protect the protein effectively enough against reduction of the disulfide group. Consequently, these groups do not seem to be related to the ligand binding site of muscarinic receptor.
It should be realized that besides the the loss of binding sites the chemical modification of sulfhydryl groups can also change the antagonist binding properties of muscarinic receptor. It has been found in the present study that the treatment of the receptor with N-ethylmaleimide can decrease the $[^3H]$QNB binding rate approximately 500-fold. A more thorough kinetic analysis of antagonist binding with the modified receptor is necessary to better understand the mechanism and the structural background of this phenomenon.
In summary, the kinetic study of the chemical modification of sulfhydryl and disulfide groups has revealed their participation in antagonist binding with the muscarinic receptor. The same groups can also be expected to play some role in agonist binding with the receptor. However, at the present stage of kinetic studies with antagonists, it seems to be rather difficult to obtain meaningful

data about the influence of sulfhydryl and disulfide reagents on the agonist binding as long as radiolabelled antagonists are used as reporter ligands in such common displacement experiments.

References


1. McMahon, K.K., M.M. Hosey. 1983. Biochem.Biophys.Res.Commun. 111, 41 - 46.

2. Wei, J.-W., P.V. Sulakhe. 1980. Naunyn-Schmiedeberg's Arch. Pharmacol. 314, 51 - 59.

3. Harden, T.K., A.G. Scheer, M.M. Smith. 1982. Mol.Pharmacol. 21, 570 - 580.

4. Aronstam, R.S., G.O. Carrier. 1982. Br.J.Pharmacol. 77, 89 - 95.

5. Aronstam, R.S., L.G. Abood, W. Hoss. 1978. Mol.Pharmacol. 14, 575 - 586.

6. Aronstam, R.S., W. Hoss, L.G. Abood. 1977. Eur.J.Pharmacol. 46, 279 - 282.

7. Nukada, T., T.Haga, A.Ichiyama. 1983. Mol.Pharmacol. 24, 374 - - 379.

8. Korn, S.J., M.W.Martin, T.K. Harden. 1983. J.Pharmacol.Exp. Ther. 224, 118 - 126.

9. Martin, M.W., T. Evans, T.K. Harden. 1985. Biochem.J. 229, 539 - 544.

10. Carson, S. 1980. FEBS Lett. 109, 81 - 84.

11. Uchida, S., K. Matsumoto, K. Takeyasu, H. Higuchi, H. Yoshida. 1982. Life Sci. 31, 201 - 209.

12. Dennison, R.L., D.A. Wenger, R.S.Aronstam. 1985. Res.Commun. Chem.Pathol.Pharmacol. 47, 465 - 468.

13. Hedlund, B., T. Bartfai. 1979. Mol.Pharmacol. 15, 531 - 544.

14. Hurko, O. 1978. Arch.Biochem.Biophys. 190, 434 - 445.

15. Birdsall, N.J.M., A.S.V. Burgen, E.C. Hulme, E.H.F. Wong. 1983. Br.J.Pharmacol. 80, 187 - 196.

16. Rinken A.A., Ü.L. Langel, J.L. Järv. 1984. Biol.Membrany. 1, 341 - 348.

17. Langel, Ü.L., A.A. Rinken, L.J. Tähepôld, J.L. Järv. 1982. Neirokhimia. 1, 343 - 351.

18. Hasinoff, B.B., N.B. Madsen, O. Avramovic-Zikic. 1971. Can.J. Biochem. 49, 742 - 751.

19. Ellmann, G.L. 1959. Arch.Biochem.Biophys. 82, 70 - 77.

20. Habeeb, A.F.S.A. 1972. Methods Enzymol. 25, 457 - 464.

21. Sillard, R.G., J.L. Järv, T. Bartfai. 1985. Biol.Membrany. 2, 426 - 432.

# BIOCHEMISTRY AND MOLECULAR BIOLOGY OF RECEPTORS AND ION CHANNELS IN THE CENTRAL NERVOUS SYSTEM (CNS)

Heinrich Betz, Bertram Schmitt, Cord-Michael Becker, Gabriele Grenningloh, Axel Rienitz, Petra Knaus, Irm Hermans-Borgmeyer, Dieter Zopf, Patrick Schloß, Erich Sawruk, Eckart Gundelfinger and Hubert Rehm.

ZMBH, Zentrum für Molekulare Biologie der Universität Heidelberg, Im Neuenheimer Feld 282, 6900 Heidelberg, FRG

Chemosensitivity and electrical excitability are the key properties of nerve cells upon which information processing in the brain is based. The proteins providing these capacities are neurotransmitter receptors and ion channels located in the neuronal plasma membrane. Since some years, our group has focussed on the pharmacological and structural characterization of CNS receptors and ion channels. Here, we summarize results recently obtained in our laboratory.

## The membrane receptor for the presynaptic neurotoxin ß-bungarotoxin: a subtype of nerve terminal $K^+$ channels?

ß-Bungarotoxin (ß-Btx) is a presynaptically active protein neurotoxin with phospholipase A2 activity. At the neuromuscular junction, ß-Btx blocks neurotransmitter release in a complex triphasic fashion (1). Upon prolonged incubation, ß-Btx is cytotoxic. In the CNS of the developing chick embryo, cholinergic and GABA-ergic neurons are destroyed by ß-Btx (2, 3).

A high-affinity ß-Btx binding site was identified in chick brain membranes using radioligand-binding methods (4).

Receptors and Ion Channels

Photoaffinity cross-linking of the same membrane preparation in the presence of $^{125}$I-ß-Btx allowed the identification of a toxin-binding polypeptide of Mr 95.000 (5). This peptide is thought to be a subunit of the ß-Btx binding protein complex. Sucrose gradient centrifugation and gel filtration of the detergent-solubilized ß-Btx binding protein revealed a total Mr of about 430.000 for the native toxin binding site (6). The ß-bungarotoxin receptor thus can be concluded to be a large membrane protein containing several polypeptide subunits.

What may be the physiological role of the ß-Btx binding protein? A first hint came from solubilization experiments which showed that $K^+$ ions have to be present in the detergent buffer if the solubilized ß-Btx binding protein is to be held in a native, i.e. toxin-binding, conformation (6). Furthermore, protease inhibitor homologues from Dendroaspis venom (i.e. dendrotoxin, toxin I) were found to inhibit $^{125}$I-ß-Btx binding to CNS membranes (6, 7). These protease inhibitor homologues have recently been shown to block A-type $K^+$ currents in hippocampus slice preparations (8). The ß-Btx binding protein thus can now be tentatively classified as a subtype of neuronal $K^+$ channel. Current experiments in our laboratory aim on its isolation by affinity chromatography and further elucidation of its molecular structure.

## Protein structure of the glycine receptor from mammalian spinal cord

The amino acid glycine is a major inhibitory neurotransmitter in the CNS of vertebrates and many invertebrates (9). At the postsynaptic membrane, glycine produces an increase in chloride conductance, i.e. it hyperpolarizes the target neuron. This inhibitory action of glycine is selectively antagonized by strychnine, an alkaloid we have found to be a potent tool for analyzing and purifying the postsynaptic glycine receptor protein.

After solubilization in non-ionic or ionic detergents, the glycine receptor behaves as a strychnine-binding membrane protein exhibiting an apparent Mr of 250.000 (10-12). By UV-induced incorporation of $[^3H]$-strychnine, the antagonist binding subunit of the glycine receptor was identified as a polypeptide of Mr 48.000 (13, 14). Two additional polypeptides (Mr 58.000 and 93.000, respectively) were revealed by SDS-polyacrylamide gel electrophoresis of rat, pig and mouse glycine receptor preparations obtained after affinity chromatography on aminostrychnine-agarose (11, 12, 15). Photoaffinity labelling experiments showed that the Mr 48.000 and, to a lesser extent, the Mr 58.000 polypeptides participate in the formation of the ligand binding site(s) of the glycine receptor (12). The physiological function of the Mr 93.000 polypeptide is unknown. Immunocytochemical (16, 17) and biochemical (18) data revealed the Mr 93.000 polypeptide as a peripheral membrane protein associated with cytoplasmic domains of the "postsynaptic glycine receptor complex". This polypeptide therefore has been implicated in specialized functions, e.g. anchoring of the receptor in the postsynaptic membrane and/or transmembrane signalling (18, 19). Also, preliminary data on the ontogenesis of glycine receptor polypeptides during spinal cord development indicate that the Mr 93.000 polypeptide is regulated independently from the Mr 48.000 and 58.000 polypeptides (C.-M. Becker, unpublished).

The production of monoclonal antibodies against the rat glycine receptor (20) as well as partial amino acid sequence determinations of the Mr 48.000 polypeptide (collaboration with K. Beyreuther, Köln) provide the basis for a molecular biology approach to the glycine receptor. The isolation and DNA sequence determination of putative glycine receptor subunit clones isolated from cDNA libraries established in bacteriophages $\lambda$gt10 and $\lambda$gt11 are under current investigation in our laboratory (G. Grenningloh and A. Rienitz, unpublished).

## Characterization of the cDNA and gene of a putative nicotinic acetylcholine receptor protein of the Drosophila CNS

The nicotinic acetylcholine receptor of the vertebrate neuromuscular junction and of the related fish electric organ has been extensively characterized and shown to be a pentameric protein of the subunit stoichiometry $\alpha_2\beta\gamma\delta$ (21). Acetylcholine receptors of nicotinic pharmacology are also present in the CNS of vertebrates and invertebrates. Due to their low abundance, their characterization is, however, much less advanced.

Ligand binding studies have shown that insects contain comparatively high numbers of neuronal nicotinic acetylcholine receptors (22). Using DNA probes of the *Torpedo* acetylcholine receptor $\gamma$-subunit, we have isolated cDNA clones encoding a putative CNS acetylcholine receptor protein of *Drosophila* (ARD protein). The predicted mature ARD polypeptide has a calculated Mr of 57.430 and possesses extensive amino acid sequence homology with vertebrate nicotinic acetylcholine receptor subunits (23). Briefly, the *Drosophila* protein has four hydrophobic segments long enough to form transmembrane $\alpha$-helices and one amphipathic region which might form an additional charged transmembrane $\alpha$-helix. Also, two cystein residues found in all vertebrate acetylcholine receptor subunits as well as a potential cyclic AMP-dependent protein kinase phosporylation site have been conserved in the ARD protein. On the other hand, two consecutive cysteins proposed to be involved in acetylcholine binding to receptor $\alpha$-chains (24) are not present in the ARD polypeptide; we therefore tentatively classify it as a non-$\alpha$ type receptor subunit.

The ARD protein exhibits the highest degree of homology with a recently analyzed putative neuronal acetylcholine receptor $\alpha$-subunit isolated from the pheochromocytoma cell line PC 12 (25). Northern blot analysis showed that the expression of ARD mRNA is highly regulated during development. A strongly hybridizing poly(A)$^+$ RNA species of about 3.2 kb is detected in late embryos and in pupae, i.e. at developmental stages when the embryonic and adult nervous systems differentiate (23).

Considering that acetylcholine is present in the CNS, but not at the neuromuscular junction of insects, these results strongly suggest that the ARD protein is indeed a neuron-specific gene product.

In an attempt to define the genetic elements responsible for the differentiation- and tissue-specific expression of the ARD mRNA we have begun to analyze the structure of the ARD gene (26). The currently available data show that its organization is similar to that of vertebrate acetylcholine receptor subunit genes. However, the ARD gene has only some of the introns present in vertebrate $\alpha$- and $\gamma$-subunit genes (27, 28). Southern blot analysis of Drosophila genomic DNA using ARD cDNA as a probe indicates that more than one ARD-related gene is present in the Drosophila genome. Whether this (these) other ARD-related gene(s) correspond(s) to other subunits of the Drosophila neuronal nicotinic acetylcholine receptor, or whether they constitute developmentally regulated isoforms of the ARD protein, remains to be established.

## Acknowledgments

This work was supported by the Bundesministerium für Forschung und Technologie, the Deutsche Forschungsgemeinschaft and the Fonds der Chemischen Industrie. We thank C. Schröder, H. Krischke and C. Udri for expert technical assistence and J. Rami for help during the preparation of this manuscript.

## References

1. Abe, T., S. Alema, R. Miledi. 1977. Eur. J. Biochem. 80, 1.
2. Hirokawa, N. 1978. J. Comp. Neurol. 180, 449.
3. Rehm, H., T. Schäfer, H. Betz. 1982. Brain Res. 250, 309.

4. Rehm, H., H. Betz. 1982. J. Biol. Chem. 257, 10015.

5. Rehm, H., H. Betz. 1983. EMBO J. 7, 1119.

6. Rehm, H., H. Betz. 1984. J. Biol. Chem. 259, 6865.

7. Othman, I.B., J.W. Spokes, J.O. Dolly. 1982. Eur. J. Biochem. 128, 267.

8. Halliwell, J.V., I.B. Othman, A. Pelchen-Matthews, J.O. Dolly. 1986. Proc. Natl. Acad. Sci. USA 83, 493.

9. Aprison, M.H., E.C. Daly. 1978. Adv. Neurochem. 3, 203.

10. Pfeiffer, F., H. Betz. 1981. Brain Res. 226, 273.

11. Pfeiffer, F., D. Graham, H. Betz. 1982. J. Biol. Chem. 257, 9389.

12. Graham, D., F. Peiffer, R. Simler, H. Betz. 1985. Biochemistry 24, 990.

13. Graham, D., F. Pfeiffer, H. Betz. 1981. Biochem. Biophys. Res. Commun. 102, 1330.

14. Graham, D., F. Peiffer, H. Betz. 1983. Eur. J. Biochem. 131, 519.

15. Becker, C.-M., I. Hermans-Borgmeyer, B. Schmitt, H. Betz. 1986. J. Neurosci. 6, 1358.

16. Triller, A., F. Cluzeaud, F. Pfeiffer, H. Betz, H. Korn. 1985. J. Cell. Biol. 101, 683.

17. Altschuler, R.A.,H. Betz, M.H. Parakkal, K.A. Reeks, R.J. Wenthold. 1986. Brain Res. 369, 316.

18. Schmitt, B., P. Knaus, C.-M. Becker, H. Betz. 1986. Biochemistry, in press.

19. Betz, H., B. Schmitt, C.-M. Becker, G. Grenningloh, A. Rienitz. 1986. Biochim. Soc. Transactions, in press.

20. Pfeiffer, F.,R. Simler, G. Grenningloh, H. Betz. 1984. Proc. Natl. Acad. Sci. USA 81, 7224.

21. Stroud, R.M., J. Finer-Moore. 1985. Ann. Rev. Cell Biol. 1, 317.

22. Dudai, Y. (1978) Biochem. Biophys. Acta 539, 505.

23. Hermans-Borgmeyer, I., D. Zopf, R.-P. Ryseck, B. Hovemann, H. Betz, E.D. Gundelfinger. 1986. EMBO J. 5, 1503.

24. Mishina, M., T. Tobimatsu, K. Imoto, K. Tankana, Y. Fujita, K. Fukuda, M. Kurasaki, H. Takahishi, Y. Morimoto, T. Hirose, S. Inayama, T. Takahishi, M. Kuno, S. Numa. 1985. Nature 313, 364.

25. Boulter, J., K. Evans, D. Goldman, G. Martin, D. Treco, S. Heinemann, J. Patrick. 1986. Nature 319, 368.

26. Gundelfinger, E.D., I. Hermans-Borgmeyer, D. Zopf, E. Sawruk, H. Betz. 1986. in: The Acetylcholine Receptor (Maelicke, A., ed.) Springer, Heidelberg-New York, in press.

27. Nef, P., A. Mauron, R. Stader, C. Alliod, M. Ballivet. 1984. Proc. Natl. Acad. Sci. USA 81, 7975.

28. Shibahara, S., T. Kubo, H.J. Pershi, H. Takahashi, M. Noda, S. Numa. 1985. Eur. J. Biochem. 146, 15.

# RECONSTITUTION OF GLUTAMATE RECEPTORS INTO PLANAR BILAYERS

B.A.Tashmukhamedov, E.M. Makhmudova, I. Kazakov, A.G.Khafizov, T.M. Lim

Institute of Physiology, Academy of Sciences of the Uzbek SSR, Tashkent, USSR

Early it has been shown that *Argiopa lobata* spider venom blocks irreversibly the locust glutamatergic synapses (1). Using the toxic fraction of this venom as a ligand for affinity chromatography makes possible the isolation of membrane glycoproteins from the crab, crayfish and cockroach neuromuscular junctions, as well as from rat brain. These glycoproteins induce glutamate-sensitive conductance of bilayer lipid membranes BLM (2-4). Blocking of the induced conductance by diethyl glutamate or by the venom toxic fraction, as well as the conductance enhancement after concanavalin A addition allow us to consider the obtained membrane components as glutamate receptors. The membrane fractions isolated by this affinity chromatography method from rat liver failed to induce glutamate-sensitive conductance in BLM.

Column chromatography was used for further purification of the membrane-active fractions. After gel chromatography of the membrane-active fraction from crab neuromuscular junctions on Sephadex G200 we obtained two protein fractions of high and low molecular weight, 240 and 13 kD respectively (Fig. 1). Each of them could induce glutamate-sensitive conductance in BLM.

Alternatively, the total fraction of the crab neuromuscular junction membrane-active components was subjected to gel filtration on Sephadex G15, followed by Sephadex G10 chromatography resulting in four main protein fractions.

The N-terminal analysis according to Hartley and Gray (5) was used to check the purity of obtained preparations. The three first fractions had the same N-terminal residues (Ile, Val, Leu) in spite of

Receptors and Ion Channels

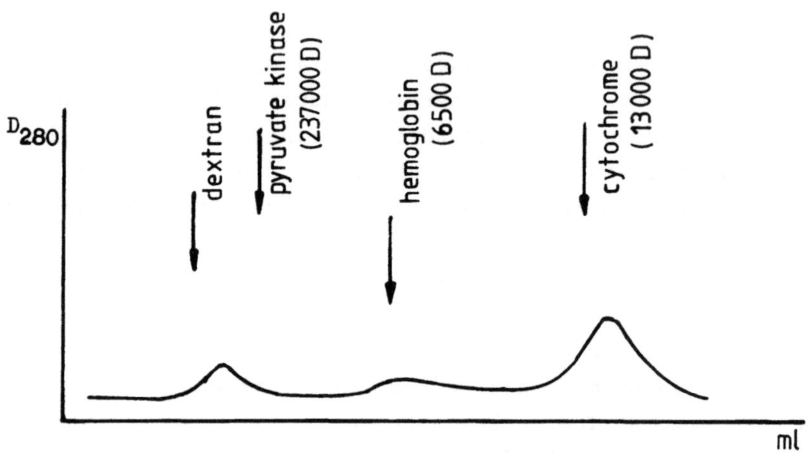


Fig. 1. Sephadex G-200 chromatography of the membrane-active components from crab neuromuscular junctions.

different chromatographic mobility. The fourth fraction was found to be enriched with aminosugar and histidine.

Fractions I-III induce the conductance in BLM in Na-containing solution only after addition of glutamate; in some cases the presence of concanavalin A was required. Fraction IV, without any additives, increases the condactance of BLM in the Na-containing solution by more than 2 to 3 orders of magnitude.

Electrophoretic separation of the isolated fraction in 10% polyacrylamide gel in the presence of SDS and dithiothreitol revealed three bands with the average molecular masses of 14, 30, and 60 kD. Sometimes the band of ∿8 kD was also observed. The ratio of the obtained molecular masses point to the possibility of aggregate formation. Since the first three fractions have the same N-termini, these fractions may correspond to different degrees of aggregation. On the other hand the existence of different types of glutamate receptors isolated by affinity chromatography cannot be ruled out.

In our experiments we measured the potential induced in BLM in the presence of a 10-fold $Na^+$-concentration gradient. The membrane glycoproteins from rat brain, crab, cockroach and crayfish neuromuscular junctions were used. We observed changes in the value and sign of potential with time. The same potential changes were observed during measurement of biionic potentials (30 mM NaCl, 30 mM KCl) (Fig. 2).

Since the total protein factions, not subjected to Sephadex chromatography, were employed in these experiments, one may suggest that at first one type of receptors ("depolarizing receptors") are incorporated followed by another type ("hyperpolarizing receptors") with the concomitant change of the $Na^+$ for $Cl^-$ conductivity. However, further comparative pharmacological and ion-selectivity analysis of every protein band obtained after electrophoresis is required to show that the different species of receptors were obtained.

A single-channel registration method allowed us to study the action of $Ca^{2+}$ and $Mg^{2+}$ ions on current fluctuations of rat brain receptor protein modified BLM. As it is shown in Fig. 3, $Ca^{2+}$ ($10^{-5}$M) causes a decrease in the channel amplitude and an increase in the average life-time of single-opening events. $Mg^{2+}$ ions ($10^{-5}$ M) cause a transient decrease in the current fluctuations amplitude (Fig. 4). Prolonged opening events of channels observed in Fig. 4 were explained by the presence of concanavalin A. Fig. 5(B) shows the increase in the average channel life-time of opening events induced by receptor fractions from crayfish neuromuscular junctions after concanavalin A application. The amplitudes registered in the present case correspond to 60-350 pS. Noteworthy, the glutamate channel conductance of $23.5 \pm 7$ pS was carlier measured by the voltage-clamp method on crayfish muscle fibers (6). As noted in (4), the average life-time of single opening events in our reconstituted system was longer than that reported for intact post-

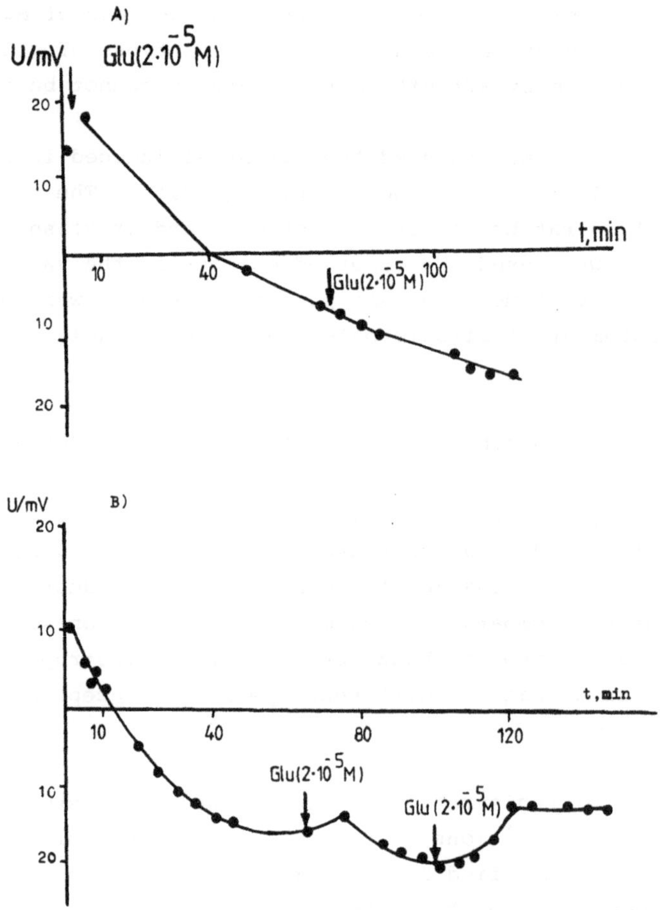


Fig. 2. Time-course of the changes of potential induced in BLM. The membrane - active glycoprotein from rat brain was added to both sides of BLM. A) The potential was measured as it developed across bilayer due to the presence of 10-fold NaCl gradient. B) Biionic potential was measured as it developed across the bilayer due to the presence of 30 mM $Na^+$ ions on one side of BLM and 30 mM $K^+$ ions on the other side.

synaptic membrane. When comparing quantitatively the reconstituted glutamate receptor system with the intact membrane current patterns, the difference in species used and in the experimental condition should be taken into account. These differences include ion concentration, lipid composition of cell and artificial membrane, the presence of solvent in BLM, etc.

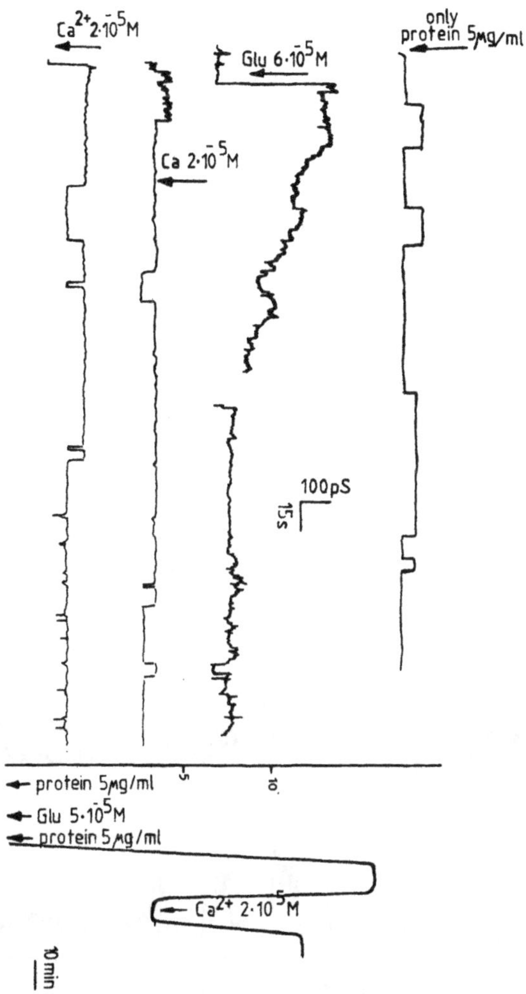


Fig. 3. Effects of $Ca^{2+}$ on current fluctuations induced in BLM by membrane active glycoprotein fraction from rat brain.

The glutamate-binding protein (GBP) has been isolated from rat brain synaptic plasma membranes. Glutamic acid and concanavalin A were used as ligands for affinity chromatography (7-9). The molecular mass of this protein, based on amino acid and carbohydrate analyses was found to be 14300 (8). It should be noted that our membrane components show some properties similar to those of the above mentioned protein. We also found that heating of protein samples for

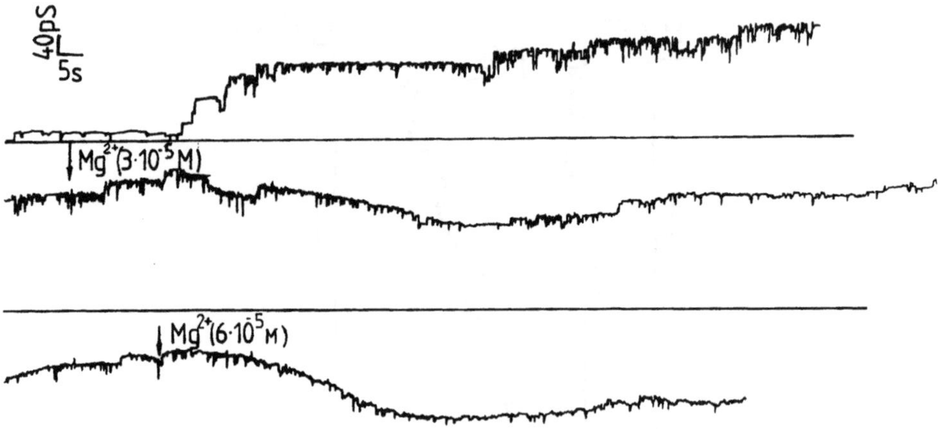


Fig. 4. Effects of $Mg^{2+}$ ions on current fluctuations induced in BLM by membrane active glycoprotein fraction from rat brain.

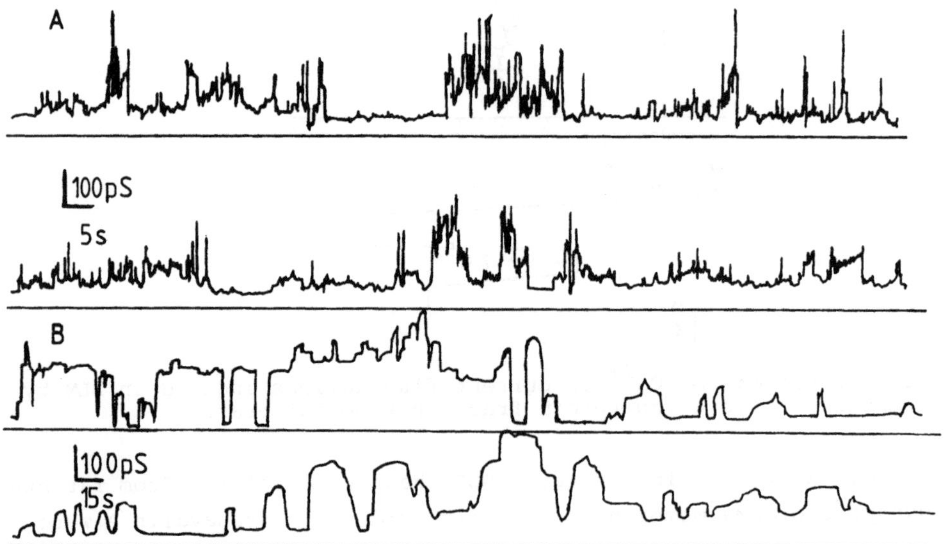


Fig. 5. A) Current fluctuations of crayfish receptor-protein (10 μg/ml) modified BLM in the presence of glutamate ($10^{-5}$M). B) Concanavalin A ($10^{-6}$M) effects on the induced current fluctuations.

2 or 3 min at 100° C in the presence of SDS and dithiothreitol caused progressively greater degrees of aggregate formation and incomplete penetration into polyacrylamide gels. At 10 % acrylamide concentration, the larger fraction of protein remained as an aggregate at the start. However, N-terminal residues of our membrane glycoproteins, isolated from crab neuromuscular synapses, differ from the N-terminal residue of rat brain GBP identified as tyrosine (8).

The molecular mass, assessed by gel filtration on Sephadex G200 of a total glycoprotein fraction isolated by affinity chromatography from crab neuromuscular synapses, is in aggrement with the data of Bardsley and Roberts (10). By radiation inactivation method they estimated the molecular mass of high affinity binding sites for glutamate in brain synaptic membrane as $263 \pm 34$ kD and $75 \pm 15$ kD in the presence and absence of glutamate, respectively.

Radioactive mediator binding method, which is very useful in membrane receptor investigations, allows one to distinguish two different glutamate binding sites in the rat brain synaptic membranes: one type is $Cl^-$-dependent and another is $Cl^-$-independent. It has been revealed that $Ca^{2+}$-ions enhance $Cl^-$-dependent binding and have no influence on the $Cl^-$-independent sites (11). The $Ca^{2+}$ effects on the parameters of current fluctuations induced by the rat brain membrane glycoprotein fraction are in agreement with the model of Lewis and Slewents (12). They assumed that $Na^+$, $K^+$, and $Ca^{2+}$ ions compete at a binding site in the pore of the ion channel of acetylcholine receptor at the frog end-plate membrane. The occupation of this site by $Ca^{2+}$ ions would prevent the passage of $Na^+$ or $K^+$ ions, thus reducing the conductance, and would keep the channel in the open conformation (12). It may be supposed that it is the causative factor which increases integral BLM conductance by $Ca^{2+}$ ions in the case of the glutamate receptor (Fig. 3). It should be noted that the $Ca^{2+}$ effects on the induced conductivity strongly depend on concentration of these ions.

The action of $Mg^{2+}$ ions, as well as other putative amino acid antagonists, has been studied on central neurons in culture by the intracellular recording method (13). This investigation demonstrated that one glutamic acid receptor is coupled to mechanism of excitation resulting from an increase in the input conductance, while second distinct receptor mediates its effects by means of an apparent decrease in the input conductance. The decrease in the input conductance was more sensitive to $Mg^{2+}$ ions than the increase. In our experiments $Mg^{2+}$ ions failed to suppress the conductance, at least at the employed concentrations.

Further purification of receptor molecules and their subunits, investigation of their properties in model systems that better mimick biological membranes will shed light on the function mechanisms of receptors in the excitable membranes.

References


1. Tashmukhamedov,B.A., P.B. Usmanov, I. Kazakov, D. Kalikulov, L.Ya. Yukelson, B.U. Atakusiev. 1983. In: Toxin as Tools in Neurochemistry (F. Hucho, Yu.A. Ovchinnikov, eds.). Walter de Gruyter. Berlin, New York, p. 311-323.

2. Tashmukhamedov, B.A., E.M.Makhmudova, P.B. Usmanov, I. Kazakov. 1983. Uzb. Biol. J. 12, 57-58.

3. Tashmukhamedov B.A., E.M. Makhmudova, P.B. Usmanov, I. Kazakov, B.U.Atakuziev. 1984. DAN SSSR 276, 977-979.

4. Tashmukhamedov, B.A., E.M. Makhmudova, P.B. Usmanov, I. Kazakov. 1985. Gen. Physiol. Biophys. 4, 625-630.

5. Gray, W.R., B.S. Hartley. 1975. In: Molecular Biology, Biochemistry and Biophysics. 8. Protein Sequence Determination. Springer-Verlag Berlin, Heidelberg, New York, p.42-54.

6. Slettmeier H., W. Finger, J. Dudel. 1983. Pflugers Arch. 397, 20-24.

7. Michaelis E.K. 1975. Biochem. Biophys. Res. Commun. 65, 1004-1012.

8. Michaelis, E.K., M.L. Michaelis, T.M. Stormann, W.L. Chittenden, R.D. Grubbs. J. Neurochem. 40, 1742-1753.

9. Dambinova, S.A., V.I. Besedin, M.N.Demina. 1984. Biokhimiya 49, 67-74.

10. Bardsley, M.E., P.J. Roberts. 1985. Biochem. Biophys. Res. Commun. 126, 227-232.

11. Mena, E.E., S.R. Whittenmore, D.T. Monagham, C.W. Cotman. 1984. Life Sciences. 35, 2427-2433.

12. Lewis, C.A., C.F. Stevens. 1979. In: Membrane Transport Processes (Stevens C.F., Tsien R.W. eds.). Raven Press New York, p. 133-151.

13. McDonald, T.F., I.M. Wojtowicz. 1981. Can. J. Physiol. and Pharmacol. 60, 283-296.

# PHARMACOLOGICAL PROPERTIES OF AMINO ACID RECEPTORS IN ISOLATED HIPPOCAMPAL NEURONS

O.A. Krishtal, N.I. Kiskin, E.M. Kljuchko, A.Ya. Tsyndrenko
A.A. Bogomoletz Institute of Physiology, Ukrainian Academy of Science, Kiev, USSR

## Introduction

There is a strong evidence that certain amino acids, including $\gamma$-aminobutyric acid, glycine and glutamate, play a role of neurotransmitters in the mammalian central nervous system (CNS), particularly in the hippocampus (1,2). Glutamate and/or aspartate are supposed to be responsible for the transmission of excitation. Postsynaptic receptors sensitive to these excitatory amino acids and other structurally related compounds are subdivided into three major classes on the basis of their susceptibility to the action of agonists and blockade by specific antagonists (3,4,5): 1) NMDA receptors with D-$\alpha$-aminoadipate (D$\alpha$AA) and 2-amino-5-phosphonovalerate (APV) as most potent antagonists, antagonized also by $Mg^{2+}$ ions (6), 2) quisqualate (QA) receptors, preferentially blocked by glutamic acid diethylester (GDEE), 3) kainate (KA) receptors which form separate class because no selective antagonist to the excitatory action of KA is known at present time. The major part of electrophysiological evidence concerning the excitatory amino acid receptors was obtained by using ionophoretic or pressure application of substances on the CNS neurons <u>in situ</u> and in some cases to the cultured neurons. The validity of obtained information largely depends, however, on certain limitations and restrictions of ionophoretic techniques, such as unknown amount of applied substances and their non-uniform distribution over the cell surface, difficulties in preventing the

Receptors and Ion Channels

leakage of substances from the pipettes, dilution by external fluid, etc. These restrictions do not permit to quantify adequately the drug-receptor interactions and to visualize their kinetics. Moreover, complex nature of multicellular preparation with numerous metabolic processes occuring in it, including amino acid uptake, and with complicated network of pre- and postsynaptic amino acid-sensitive sites of action is a considerable and sometimes principal obstacle in the electrophysiological study of amino acid receptors. In order to circumvent these difficulties we have applied the `concentration clamp` method combined with voltage clamp to the study of excitatory amino acid receptors in isolated internally perfused neurons of rat hippocampus.

Methods

To obtain the isolated cells we incubated the slices of rat hippocampus for 60 min at 37 °C in the permanently oxygenated (95% $O_2$ and 5% $CO_2$) saline containing (in mM): NaCl 152, KCl 5, $NaHCO_3$ 26, EGTA 1, $CaCl_2$ 1, glucose 10 with 0.2% pronase E and 0.1% collagenase IV. Then the enzymes were completely washed out in the same saline with addition of bovine serum (10%). The treated cells were mechanically dissociated with coarse-tipped glass pipette. Micropipettes for the whole-cell voltage clamp and intracellular perfusion (tip opening diameter 2-4 µm) were prepared from soft glass by the two-stage pooling procedure (7) and filled with a mixture of KF 100 mM and Tris-Cl 30 mM (pH 7.2). External solution contained (in mM): NaCl 152, $CaCl_2$ 2.6, $MgCl_2$ 1.1, HEPES-NaOH 10 (pH 7.4). The micropipette with perfused cell was placed into the opening of V-shaped glass tube so that it could be transferred into different bathes with various test salines. The application of the saline occured when electromagnetic valve connected the tube with the source of negative hydrostatic pressure. The technique of `concentration clamp` allowed to perform a complete change of external solution near the cell (and/or a step-wise application of a given substance) within 10-20 ms (8).

## Results

All pyramidal neurons examined (total number 120) were electrically excitable, demonstrating both inward sodium and outward potassium voltage-operated currents. Most of the neurons (95%) were sensitive to L-glutamate (L-Glu). Application of L-Glu in the concentrations $2\times10^{-5}$-$2\times10^{-2}$ M resulted in transient inward current which rapidly faded in the presence of agonist, demonstrating profound desensitization to 5-10% of the initial peak value. The kinetics of desensitization was independent of L-Glu concentration and holding voltage with the time constants of exponential current decline ranging from 20 to 80 msec.

The neurons sensitive to L-Glu also responded with inward currents to the applications of L-Glu analogues- QA, KA, both D- and L-homocysteate (HC) and willardiine (1-(2-amino-2-carboxyethyl)uracil). Responses to all these agonists were reversibly depressed in sodium-free Tris-substituted saline and were not detected in those few cells which did not respond to L-Glu. Similar to L-Glu pattern of desensitization was observed with applications of all agonists except KA. The latter substance produced steady-state plateau-like inward currents with no sign of the desensitization. Fig. 1 demonstrates linear current-voltage relationships for the responses to L-Glu, KA and QA, and the reversion of currents at positive holding voltages. Identical reversal potentials of these responses indicated that ionic permeability changes which mediate excitatory action of L-Glu, KA and QA were very similar and corresponded to potassium and sodium permeability ratio $P_{K+}/P_{Na+}= 0.6$. Similar results were obtained with D- and L-HC.

The dose-response relationships measured for the peak va-

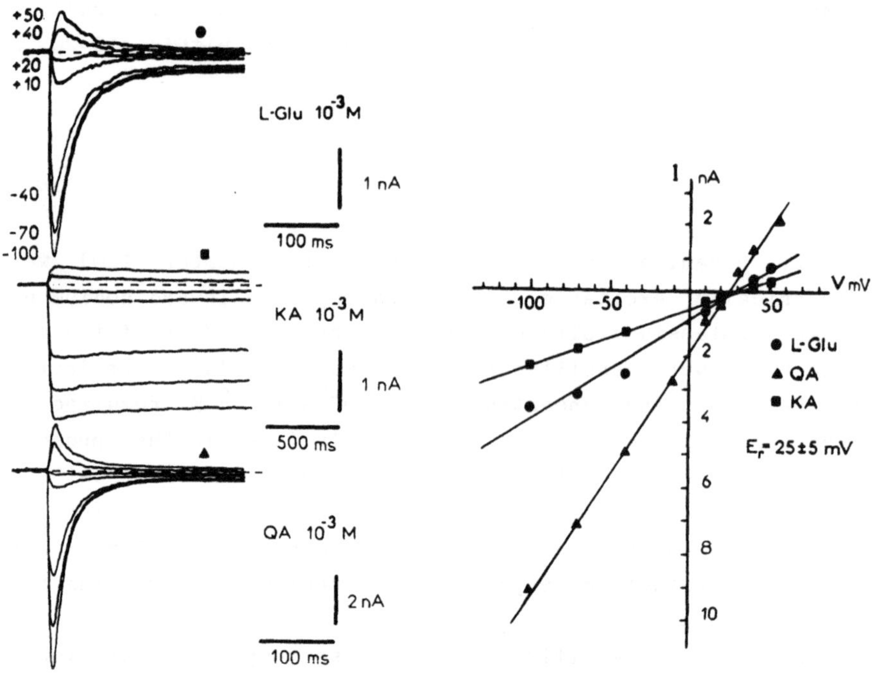


FIG. 1. Voltage dependences for the responses elicited by L-Glu, KA and QA at concentration 1 mM for each agonist. Corresponding holding voltages are indicated near the L-Glu curves. Right, corresponding current-voltage curves for the peaks of current. Lines are drawn to obtain the best fit using the least-squares method.

lues of current showed no considerable deviations from single-site binding isotherm for all the agonists tested (see also (9)). `Functional` $K_d$ values for the tested agonists are demonstrated in Table 1. These data indicate that QA is so far most potent agonist. The response to L-HC had a similar concentration dependence to that of D-isomer. When the measurements were made in the same cell, maximal (saturating) response to QA was the same as to L-Glu or sligthly larger, while maximal responses to KA and HC (both isomers) were smaller

Table 1. Relative Potencies of L-Glu Agonists on Isolated Hippocampal Neurons

| | QA | KA | L-Glu | D-HC |
|---|---|---|---|---|
| $K_d$ value (M) | $9.3\times10^{-5}$ | $5.0\times10^{-4}$ | $1.1\times10^{-3}$ | $4.2\times10^{-3}$ |
| Hill coefficient | 0.89 | 1.02 | 0.95 | 1.04 |

(20-40% of L-Glu response). QA analogue willardiine, when tested in the concentration of 5 mM, produced very small inward current (near 10% of L-Glu response).

The ability of agonists to produce profound and nearly complete desensitization of target receptors was used in our experiments for the purpose of determining whether these agonists activate the same system of membrane receptors or different ones. We measured the concentration dependences of the steady-state desensitization produced by L-Glu and QA. It was found that the responses to L-Glu and QA demonstrated complete and reversible cross-desensitization, i.e. L-Glu desensitized QA response just in the same manner as L-Glu response itself, with identical concentration dependence, and vice versa (9). Since application of KA caused rapid activation of the steady-state current, we could see the effect of desensitization produced by L-Glu or QA on KA response: the amplitude of initial step-wise activation of KA-induced current was strongly affected in a concentration-dependent manner by preincubation in L-Glu or QA. The concentration dependences of the steady-state desensitization produced by L-Glu and QA also showed one-to-one agonist-receptor interactions with apparent $K_d$ values of $9.8\times10^{-6}$ M and $2.7\times10^{-7}$ M, respectively.

Fig. 2A represents the cross-desensitization experiments with L-HC. In high concentrations (up to 5 mM) this weak agonist was also capable of producing nearly complete desensitization of L-Glu response (Fig. $2A_a$). The response to KA was affected by L-HC in the similar manner as by L-Glu (Fig. $2A_b$): rapid phase of its activation was almost completely supressed. Note also relatively fast (100 ms) removal of the desensitiza-

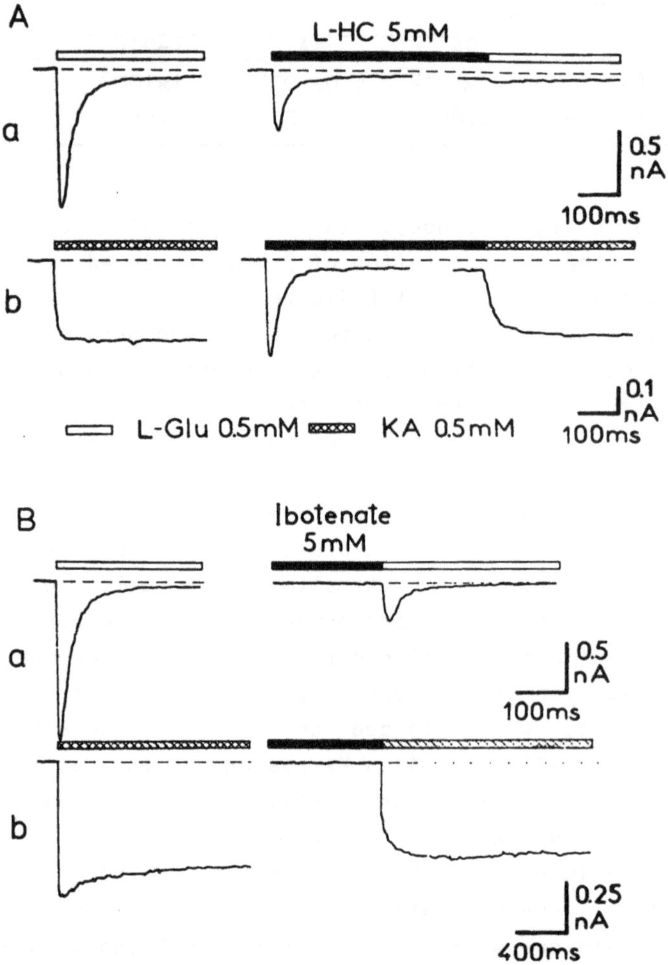


FIG. 2. Desensitization of responses to 0.5 mM L-Glu (a) and 0.5 mM KA (b) produced by preincubation in 5mM L-HC (A) and 5mM ibotenate (B). Desensitizing agonists were applied for 30 s.

tion. In the experiments with L- (or D-) HC applied on the background of desensitization caused by L-Glu it was found that HC-activated responses were affected by L-Glu in the same manner as the response to L-Glu itself (not shown). These results clearly indicate that both forms of HC activate the same system of membrane receptors which also interacts with L-Glu, KA and QA.

Naturally occuring carboxylated muscimole analogue, ibotenic acid, was reported to be a potent excitant of the mammalian CNS neurons (10,11), interacting preferentially with NMDA receptors. Though NMDA- and/or aspartate-activated receptors were not found in isolated hippocampal pyramidal neurons, as reported earlier (9), we tried this conformationally restricted Glu analogue in order to clarify structure-activity requirements for the agonist-receptor interactions (Fig. 2B). It turned out that ibotenate, in the concentration range up to 5 mM, did not elicit any measurable response, but was nearly equipotent in producing the desensitization of L-Glu (Fig. $2B_a$) and KA (Fig. $2B_b$) responses. We cannot, however, exclude a possibility that ibotenate may have very weak excitatory effect when tested at much higher concentrations.

There is a number of potent and selective antagonists known to supress excitatory action of L-Glu and its analogues at different preparations. DαAA and APV are considered as selective and 2-amino-4-phosphonobutyric acid (APB) as less selective antagonists of responses mediated via activation of NMDA receptors, and γ-D-glutamylglycine (γDGG), cis-2,3-piperidine dicarboxylic acid (PDA) and GDEE as antagonists of responses mediated via QA receptors and, to a lesser extent, KA receptors (3,4,5). All antagonists mentioned were tested on isolated hippocampal neurons in order to determine their relative potencies. It was found that, in contrast to the observations on hippocampal slices (12), NMDA, both isomers of aspartate, D-Glu and quinolinic acid were completely incapable of producing any permeability changes when applied to isolated hippocampal neurons, both in normal and $Mg^{2+}$-free solutions (6), but occured to be the antagonists of responses elicited by L-Glu or KA on this preparation. The inhibition data are summarized in Table 2. They qualitatively demonstrate that no

Table 2. Inhibition of Responses to L-Glu and KA by Antagonists

| Antagonist | Concentration | Test response | % Inhibition |
|---|---|---|---|
| DαAA | 1 mM | KA 0.5 mM | 65 |
| γDGG | 1 mM | KA 0.5 mM | 49 |
| APV | 5 mM | KA 1 mM | 35 |
| APB | 8 mM | KA 1 mM | 57 |
| PDA | 2 mM | KA 1 mM | 41 |
| GDEE | 5 mM | L-Glu 0.5 mM | 23 |
| NMDA | 5 mM | KA 1 mM | 62 |
| L-aspartate | 5 mM | KA 1 mM | 42 |
| D-aspartate | 5 mM | KA 1 mM | 62 |
| Quinolinate | 8 mM | KA 1 mM | 36 |
| D-Glu | 5 mM | KA 1 mM | 51 |

specific antagonist can be suggested at present for the responses to L-Glu and KA on isolated neurons. All the tested antagonists have similar weak potency in millimolar concentrations, with DαAA, γDGG and PDA only slightly stronger than the others (see also (12)).

## Discussion

Our data indicate that the isolated pyramidal neurons of rat hippocampus are sensitive to L-Glu and its analogues, QA, KA, L- and D-HC, willardiine but not to NMDA and aspartate. Inward ionic currents elicited by a step-wise application of these substances, except KA, showed profound desensitization, a property which has not been described earlier for these responses, at least in the voltage-clamp conditions. The permeability changes which mediate drug-activated currents were identical for all the agonists tested and included the increases in permeabilities to $Na^+$ and $K^+$ with poor discrimination between these cations. The cross-desensitization procedure for these agonists showed (see also (9)) that all drug-activated responses could be completely and reversibly cross-desensitized. This implies that all the agonists mentioned activate the same system of membrane `non-NMDA` receptors and none of them can activate some different receptors that could be detected in this preparation. These data also make questionable the existence of separate classes of KA and QA receptors. Recent reports on isolated retinal cells give a support to the latter idea (13,14), as well as the binding studies which have demonstrated the displacement of KA binding by L-Glu, but not by L-aspartate or NMDA (4,5,15) and the absence of NMDA binding to the membranes.

Quantitative data demonstrated that `non-NMDA` receptors could be desensitized by each agonist (except KA) with similar time courses and at much lower agonist concentrations than those required for the activation of response (compare $K_d$ values for activation and desensitization of L-Glu or QA responses). It may be supposed that two different receptor sites are involved in the agonist action, one being responsible for the receptor activation, and the other- for its desensitization. The ability of KA to activate receptors without desensitization as well as the ability of ibotenate to elicit desensitization without activation give additional support to this suggestion.

The presented data can also clear up some `structure-activity` considerations proposed earlier (4,5) for the action of excitatory amino acids. The structure of all agonists which activate isolated hippocampal neurons (see above), according to known minimal and maximal distances between carboxylic and amino groups (4), correspond to the structure of L-Glu in almost completely `extended` conformation. The data with conformationally restricted L-Glu analogues, KA and ibotenate, form a basis for this suggestion. NMDA and aspartate molecules, which cannot `extend` to such `long` distances between $\alpha$- and $\omega$-carboxylic groups, were inactive at this site of action.

Data obtained with antagonists also point out that the `extended` structure is necessary for antagonistic action, though all known antagonists demonstrate very low specificity. It should be noted that both optical isomers of HC were similarly active in producing inward currents in this experiments. This can be due to the substitution of $\omega$-carboxylic group in HC molecule with more acidic sulphonic group of larger molecular dimensions which makes it possible for the `extended` forms of both isomers to fit the three-point L-Glu receptor template.

Acknowledgements

We are grateful to Dr. B.S. Drach for the willardiine synthesis and to Dr. N. Akaike for his generous gift of antagonist drugs.

References

1. Storm-Mathissen, J. 1977. Progr. in Neurobiol. 8, 119-181.

2. Cotman, C.W., A. Foster, T. Lanthorn. 1981. In: Glutamate as a Neurotransmitter (G. DiChiara and G.L. Gessa, eds.). Raven Press, New York, pp. 1-27.

3. Watkins, J.C., R.H. Evans. 1981. Ann. Rev. Pharmacol. Toxicol. 21, 165-204.

4. McLennan, H. 1981. In: Glutamate as a Neurotransmitter (G. DiChiara and G.L. Gessa, eds.). Raven Press, New York, pp. 253-262.

5. McLennan, H. 1983. Progr. in Neurobiol. 20, 251-271.

6. Nowak, L., P. Bregestovski, P. Asher, A. Herbet, A. Prochiantz. 1984. Nature 307, 462-465.

7. Hamill, O.P., A. Marty, E. Neher, B. Sakmann, F.J. Sigworth. 1981. Pflügers Arch. 391, 85-100.

8. Krishtal, O.A., S.M. Marchenko, V.I. Pidoplichko. 1983. Neurosci. Lett. 35, 41-45.

9. Kiskin, N.I., O.A. Krishtal, A.Ya. Tsyndrenko. 1986. Neurosci. Lett. 63, 225-230.

10. Krogsgaard-Larsen, P., T. Honorè, J.J. Hansen, D.R. Curtis, D. Lodge. 1981. In: Glutamate as a Neurotransmitter (G. DiChiara and G.L. Gessa, eds.). Raven Press, New York, pp. 285-294.

11. Nistri. A., J.F. MacDonald, J.L. Barker. 1981. In: Glutamate as a Neurotransmitter (G. DiChiara and G.L. Gessa, eds.). Raven Press, New York, pp. 245-252.

12. Collingridge, G.L., S.J. Kehl, H. McLennan. 1983. J. Physiol. 334, 19-31.

13. Ariel, M., E.M. Lasater, S.C. Mangel, J.E. Dowling. 1984. Brain Res. 295, 179-183.

14. Ishida, A.T., J. Neyton. 1985. Proc. Natl. Acad. Sci. USA 82, 1837-1841.

15. Roberts, P.J., N.A. Sharif. 1981. In: Glutamate as a Neurotransmitter (G. DiChiara and G.L. Gessa, eds.). Raven Press, New York, pp. 295-305.

# II Ion Channels

# cAMP-ACTIVATED IONIC CHANNELS IN THE NERVE CELL MEMBRANE

P.G. Kostyuk, N.I. Kononenko, A.D. Shcherbatko
Department of General Physiology of the Nervous System,
A.A. Bogomoletz Institute of Physiology, Academy of Sciences of the Ukrainian SSR, Kiev 252601

## Introduction

A hypothesis about participation of the cyclase system of a nerve cell in mediating the effect of different biologically active substances (neurotransmitters and neurohormones) on the properties of the neuronal surface membrane is highly attractive nowadays (1). It is suggested that a neurotransmitter by activating adenylate cyclase of the cell increases the cAMP level in the cytoplasm. Then cAMP activates protein kinases which, in turn, bring about phosphorylation of the corresponding membrane proteins forming ionic channels of the cell membrane. In fact, microinjection of cAMP into giant mollusc neurons (2) resulted in depolarization of the surface membrane and generation of action potentials. We report here the effects of iontophoretic injection of cAMP into the Helix neurons on the properties of their surface membrane.

## Results

Iontophoretic cAMP injection into different identified snail neurons evoked depolarization of the membrane. If the neuron did not possess its own activity, cAMP injection led to generation of spikes (Fig. 1a). Injection of cAMP into spontaneously active neurons produced either an increase in the frequency of spike generation (Fig. 1b) or a change in the pattern of spontaneous discharges (Fig. 1c). Analogous results were also obtained by other authors (3,4).

To elucidate ionic mechanisms responsible for depolarization of the membrane induced by cAMP injection, we performed the experiments with membrane potential clamp. As it was expected, in this case intracellular cAMP injection leads to generation of an inward current

Receptors and Ion Channels

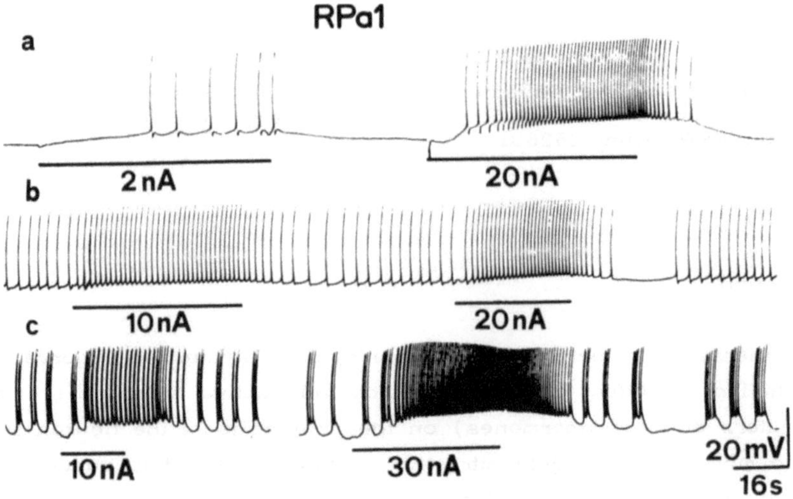


Fig. 1. Effect of cAMP injection on electrical activity of RPa1 bursting neuron. Bar in this and subsequent figures indicates the time of injection and numbers = injection current.

(cAMP-current), which continued to rise some time after the end of injection and having reached its maximal value restored to its initial level (Fig. 2).

Prolongation of cAMP injection increased the amplitude of cAMP-current; strengthening of injection current increased the rate of rise and, correspondingly, the amplitude of cAMP-current.

Further experiments showed that drugs influencing one or another enzyme of the adenylate cyclase system of the cell affect accordingly the cAMP-current. For example, theophylline, an inhibitor of phosphodiesterase, upon its external application caused an increase in the amplitude of the cAMP-current, whereas imidazole, an activator of phosphodiesterase, produced its decrease.

Intracellular injection of papaverine, another inhibitor of phosphodiesterase of cyclic nucleotides, largely increased the amplitude of the cAMP-current. The effect of intracellular injection of theophylline was removed in several dozens of minutes. The most dramatic changes in the cAMP-current have been produced by tolbutamide, a known inhibitor of cAMP-dependent protein kinase (5). It almost completely and reversibly blocked the cAMP-current. A noticeable inhibitory effect on the cAMP-current was exerted by lowering of temperature. The apparent activation energy

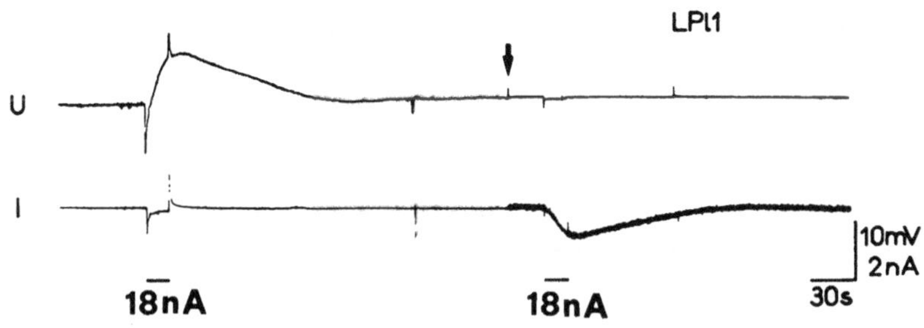


Fig. 2. Changes in membrane potential and transmembrane current induced by iontophoretic cAMP injection. Upper record - membrane potential; lower record - membrane current. At arrow membrane potential was clamped. Holding potential -61 mV.

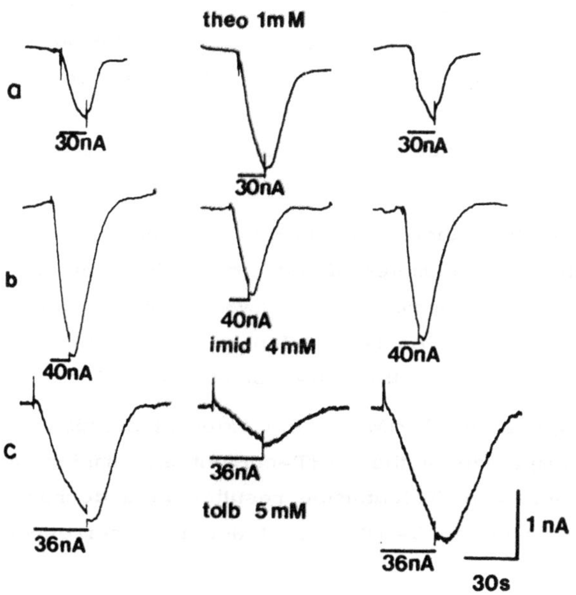


Fig. 3. Effect of theophylline (a), imidazole (b) and tolbutamide (c) on the cAMP-current. In every row the first record was obtained before the introduction, the second - 20 min after introduction of substances into external solution and the third one - 20 min after the start of washing by normal solution.

for the processes responsible for the rise of the cAMP-current was about 23.5 kcal/mol in the temperature range from 10 to 20$^{\circ}$C. The results obtained allow us to suggest that development of the cAMP-current actually reflects the activation of the cell cyclase system.

For elucidation of ionic nature of the cAMP-current, we studied the effect of holding potential on this current. It was found that cAMP-current consists of two components - an early and late ones. The early component has a reversal potential +20 mV and the late component shows reversal potential in the range of about -65 mV. Experiments with varying external ionic composition led to conclude that the early component of the cAMP-current is due to an increase in membrane conductance for sodium and calcium ions, whereas the late component - for potassium ions. In this case calcium component is suppressed rather effectively by cadmium ions.

One of the transmitters able to activate adenylate cyclase and to increase the cAMP level in the neuron is serotonin. Considering that iontophoretic cAMP injection into molluscan neurons evokes electrical responses similar to those found to serotonin application (6), the aim of our further study was to find out whether electrical responses to serotonin are mediated through cAMP.

Serotonin was applied under pressure to the neuronal soma through a micropipette with a tip diameter of 3-5 $\mu$m. Under voltage clamp conditions it led to the development of an inward current (5-HT-current) on the neuronal membrane. The reversal potential obtained by extrapolation in different neurons was in the range of -25 to +25 mV.

Addition of theophylline (1 mM) to the external solution caused an increase in the amplitude of the 5-HT-current and imidazole produced its substantial suppression. Tolbutamide resulted in a decrease of the rate of rise and decay of the 5-HT-current and in a corresponding decrease of its amplitude.

The observed dependence of the 5-HT-current on the presence of phosphodiesterase inhibitors or activators in the medium indicates that at least partly this current is associated with the elevation of the intracellular cAMP concentration. The effect of tolbutamide, an inhibitor of protein kinase reaction, on the 5-HT-current enables us to suggest that its development is related to activation of cAMP-dependent protein kinase, the phosphorylating action of which is necessary for the appearance of the corresponding ionic conductance on some functionally important proteins. These results can be regarded as a convincing argument in favour of the participation of adenylate cyclase system of the neuron in realization of the serotonin effect.

It is now accepted that the system of intracellular regulation represents a chain consisting of three messengers - neurohormone or neurotransmitter - cyclic nucleotides - calcium ions (7). It was Rasmussen who indicated for the first time in 1970 an important role of interaction of calcium ions and cAMP in the mechanism of hormone action.

To clear up the peculiarities of interaction of cAMP and calcium ions, we studied the effects of an increase of the intracellular calcium concentration on transmembrane current induced by cAMP injection into the neuron (cAMP-current).

Out of four microelectrodes inserted into the neuron, two were used for microiontophoretic injection of cAMP and/or calcium ions into the cell. At first several control cAMP injections were made and the cAMP-current was recorded. The subsequent iontophoretic injection of $Ca^{2+}$ ions elicited an outward transmembrane current whose amplitude varied in different neurons and depended on the size of the injecting current (Ca-dependent potassium current). When the outward current reached its stationary value, cAMP was injected again into the neuron and the cAMP -current was measured. Fig. 4 demonstrates the result of one of the experiments. As is seen, the amplitude of the inward cAMP-current on the background of $Ca^{2+}$ injection followed by the development of the outward current was increased by about 3 times. Moreover, the amplitude of the cAMP-current remained increased after the cessation of $Ca^{2+}$ injection and restoration of the steady-state level of the membrane current to the initial value. Subsequently, though there is a tendency to decrease, the amplitude of the cAMP-current was higher than the control level prior to the $Ca^{2+}$ injection into the neuron even after 1.5-2 h.

After repeated injections of $Ca^{2+}$ ions into the neuron or their prolonged injections a considerable deceleration of the rate of decay of the cAMP-current amplitude was found besides its increase.

It is known that the neuronal membrane has a well developed system of calcium potential-activated channels. Therefore, the effect of enrichment of the cytoplasm with $Ca^{2+}$ ions on the cAMP-current was studied during spike generation. In this case an essential increase in the cAMP-

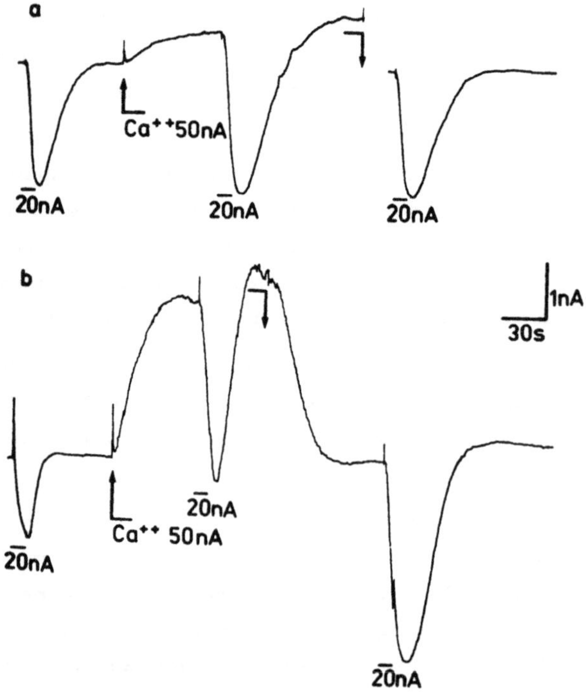


Fig. 4. Effect of intracellular iontophoretic injection of $Ca^{2+}$ ions on cAMP-current. Arrows denote the onset and the end of Ca ion injection. Ca injection current 50 nA.

current amplitude was observed about 10 s after cessation of stimulation. Every subsequent stimulation produced a progressive increase both in the amplitude and decay of the cAMP-current which, as a rule, did not restore their control levels during 2-3 h after the end of stimulation.

Similar results have been obtained with the use of other ways of increasing the intracellular concentration of $Ca^{2+}$ ions (external application of dinitrophenole, an uncoupler of oxidative phosphorylation in mitochondria, which produces liberation of calcium from them; external application of caffeine producing release of free calcium from intracellular sources).

The data obtained indicate the possibility of considerable potentiation of the cAMP-response upon elevation of the internal calcium concentration. They could be regarded as an indication of possibility of the increase of the effectiveness of those biologically active substances (transmitters, hormones, prostaglandins), which exert their effects through the cyclase system of the cell upon increasing the internal $Ca^{2+}$ level induced by either spike generation or calcium release from the intracellular sources.

One important property of potentiation of the cAMP-response upon elevation of the intracellular calcium concentration should be kept in mind. It is known that free calcium concentration in the neuron returns to its initial level in several seconds after the end of injection of these ions (8). At the same time, potentiated cAMP-responses remain for many minutes and hours after enrichment of the cytoplasm with $Ca^{2+}$ ions. Therefore, one may suggest that the leading role in the potentiation of cAMP-response is played not by the free calcium itself but by some other cytoplasmic processes initiated by the increase in the intracellular calcium level which change for a long time the state of the neuron. This process may be interpreted as a 'memory' of the neuron due to which the latter , as a result of spike generation, changes its ability to respond to biologically active substances exerting their action through the cyclase system.

One of the explanations of the potentiation of cAMP-responses upon increasing the intracellular calcium may be the presence of two phosphorylation centers in the channel-forming proteins responsible for the development of the cAMP-current - cAMP-dependent and $Ca^{2+}$-calmodulin-dependent. Phosphorylation of the first center upon increasing the intracellular $Ca^{2+}$ concentration may render the ionic channel into a 'preactive', non-conducting state, while the subsequent phosphorylation of the second center upon increasing cAMP concentration makes it conducting.

From the results presented a hypothesis can be put forward as regards the intracellular mechanism as one of the forms of memory, where the main element of associative connection might be ionic channels with two phosphorylation centers - cAMP-dependent and $Ca^{2+}$-calmodulin-dependent.

References

1. Greengard, P. 1978. Cyclic Nucleotides, Phosphorylated Proteins, and Neuronal Function. Raven Press, New York. p. 124.

2. Liberman, E.A., S.V. Minina, K.V. Golubtsov. 1975. Biophysics (Moscow) 20, 451-457.

3. Aldenhoff, J.B., G. Hofmeier , H.D. Lux, D. Swandulla. 1983. Brain Research 276, 289-296.

4. Hockberger, P., J.A. Connor. 1983. Science 219, 869-871.

5. Kanamori, T., T. Hayakawa, T. Nagatsu. 1976. Biochim. Biophys. Acta 429, 147-162.

6. Gerschenfeld, H.M., D. Paupardin-Tritsch. 1974. J. Physiol. 243, 427-456.

7. Cheung, W.Y. 1980. Science 207, 19-27.

8. Gorman, A.L.F., M.V. Thomas. 1978. J. Physiol. 275, 357-376.

# EXTERNAL CA IONS BLOCK NA CONDUCTING CA CHANNEL BY PROMOTING OPEN TO CLOSED TRANSITIONS

H.D. Lux
Abteilung Neurophysiologie, Max-Planck-Institut fuer Psychiatrie, D-8033 Martinsried

E. Carbone
Istituto di Cibernetica e Biofisica del C.N.R., I-16146 Genova

## Introduction

Ca transport through Ca channels is vital for a variety of cellular functions. For its duty, the channels must select Ca ions against usual majority ions such as $Na^+$. Indeed, Ca channels allow the influx of $Na^+$ and other alkaline ions (1-7) if the external level of free $Ca^{2+}$ is below micromolar values. The mechanism by which external $Ca^{2+}$ interferes with the flux of alkaline ions through Ca channels has now been directly studied on single channels of the low voltage-activated (LVA) $Ca^{2+}$ conductance (7-11) in vertebrate sensory neurons. Elevation of $Ca^{2+}_o$ causes prolonged closures and shortens open times for $Na^+$ currents through this channel. There is little effect on the single channel conductance, inconsistent with commonly held views. The open times for $Na^+$ decrease with increased $Ca^{2+}_o$ in a manner suggesting that one entering Ca ion blocks the channel for permeation of $Na^+$ ions. The probability that channels re-open for $Na^+$ is markedly reduced already at micromolar levels of $Ca^{2+}_o$ indicating an efficiently increased occupation of closed states.

We propose that $Ca^{2+}$-promoted changes in the state-occupancies of the Ca channel are responsible for the block of $Na^+$ currents and for the $Ca^{2+}$ specifity of this channel.

Receptors and Ion Channels

## Results

Unitary currents through Ca channels in excised membranes (outside-out patches) (12) of chick dorsal root ganglionic cells (DRG cells) were recorded under conditions where ordinary Na and K conductances were blocked by drugs (Tetrodotoxin, 3 µM) or absence of permeant ions. In this membrane preparation, the high threshold Ca current is known to run down within minutes (9-11, 13,14). Its block was supported in most experiments by applying Verapamil (100 µM) that preferentially blocks this Ca current (10,15,16). The fast inactivating Ca channel that is activated at lower voltages (LVA channel) (8) persists under these conditions and can be studied in isolation. Unitary $Ca^{2+}$ currents flowing through LVA channels are of small amplitude (about 0.4 pA) (7,8). Reduction of $Ca^{2+}_o$ in the presence of high $Na^+_o$ or $Li^+_o$ generated large and rapidly flickering inward currents through the channels (Fig.1). These currents were activated at more negative membrane potentials due to reduced external charge screening in low $Ca^{2+}_o$. If necessary, the shift was compensated for by changing the holding potential. Replacement of $Na^+$ (or $Li^+$) by choline removed the inward currents in low $Ca^{2+}_o$, as did the addition of the Ca channel blockers $Ni^{2+}$ (5 mM) and $Cd^{2+}$ (1 mM). Sample averages of the currents showed activation and inactivation time courses closely resembling those of the LVA Ca currents. These results indicate that these currents were carried by the alkaline ions flowing through LVA channels.

At $Ca^{2+}_o$ below 0.1 µM, the single channel $Na^+$ currents lasted on average 0.26 ± 0.06 ms, which is about a tenth of the mean open time of unitary $Ca^{2+}$ currents (7,8) through this channel. Openings were frequently followed by shortlasting closures of similar mean duration. These bursts of openings were separated by distinctly longer lasting closures (Fig.1). The average amplitude of the single channel events during depolarizations to -40 mV was 1.85 ± 0.35 pA, which was about 5 times larger than that recorded with isotonic $Ca^{2+}$ at corresponding potentials (7). Generally, these depolarizations produced the maximum current in sample averages or whole cells.

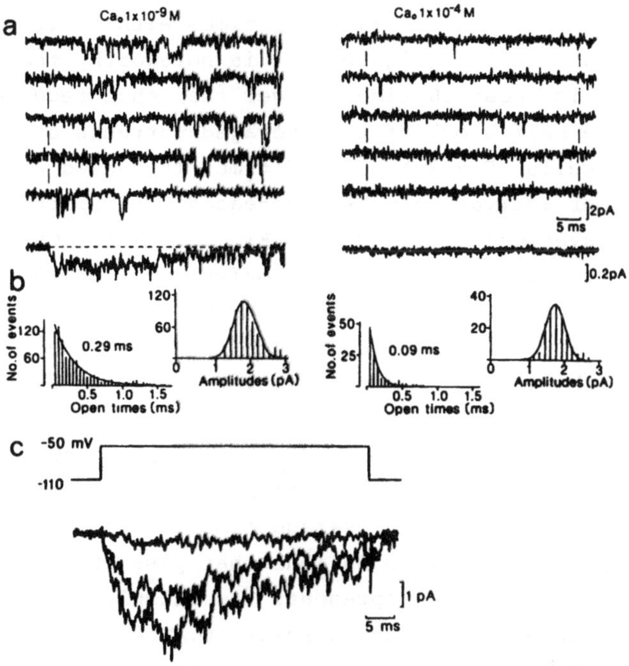


Fig.1: Block by external $Ca^{2+}$ of $Na^+$ currents through a LVA channel. a) Single channel $Na^+$ currents in an outside-out patch of chick DRG recorded during successive depolarizations to -40 mV in the presence of $1 \times 10^{-9}$ M $Ca^{2+}_o$ (left) and $1 \times 10^{-4}$ M (right). Bottom traces are sample averages of the currents (25 trials with no "blancs" in a), 73 trials with 17 "blancs" in b). Holding potential -110 mV in both cases. Bandwidth of current signals 3.6 kHz.

b) Same patch, amplitude and open time histograms of unitary $Na^+$ currents. Amplitude distributions fitted by Gaussian curves. Means were 1.81 pA ± 0.34 (S.D.) in a) and 1.73 pA ± 0.28 (S.D.) in b). Single exponentials were fitted to the open time distributions with time constants of 0.29 ms in a) and 0.09 ms in b).

c) Sample averages of single $Na^+$ currents of a patch at different external $Ca^{2+}$. The patch was exposed sequentially to solutions containing 140 mM NaCl and 10 mM $Ca^{2+}$ buffer; prepared with either EGTA ($10^{-9}$ M $Ca^{2+}$ lowest trace) or HEDTA ($1 \times 10^{-6}$, middle trace, and $1 \times 10^{-5}$ M $Ca^{2+}_o$, upper trace). Temperature 22°C.

Increasing $Ca^{2+}{}_{o}$ from nanomolar to 10 micromolar values strongly reduced the current amplitude of averaged samples (Fig.2a), while the amplitude of single channel currents was not significantly affected (see Figs 1 and 2b). The main effect on unitary currents was a decrease of mean open times with their values halved at 55 µM $Ca^{2+}{}_{o}$ (Fig 2b). It is noteworthy that this concentration is about 20 times larger than that required (2.3 µM) to produce half block of the averaged currents of samples and of whole cells (Fig.2a). Closed times increased and numbers of openings per activating pulse decreased in proportion to the reduction of averaged currents (see Fig.2c). With $Ca^{2+}{}_{o}$ $10^{-4}$ M, closures frequently over lasted the pulse duration (50 ms), and "blancs" were common (Fig.2). Thus, the primary reason for the reduction of macroscopic currents with increased $Ca^{2+}{}_{o}$ is a reduced availability of open time states of the channel for Na.

For given concentration ratios of Ca and Na ions, the average time of the transition from the open Na conductive to the closed state compares well with the average time at which an external Ca ion is expected to follow Na ions that pass the channel. The continuous line in Fig.2b represents the calculated mean open time of the channel under such assumption. The apparent $K_D$ of 55 x $10^{-6}$ M for the shutting of the Na-permeable channel suggests a rate constant for Ca entry of 2.4 x $10^{4}$ $s^{-1}$. This corresponds to a molar value of 4.6 x $10^{8}$ $M^{-1}s^{-1}$ which is near values expected for diffusion-controlled $Ca^{2+}$ entry (5).

Ba ions were found to act as Ca ions at similar concentrations, but Mg ions which do not carry currents through this channel were ineffective, even at millimolar concentrations. Membrane patches subjected to high internal free $Ca^{2+}$ (50 to 500 µM) behaved like patches dialysed with low free $Ca^{2+}$ ( $10^{-9}$ M) showing the same changes in the distributions of closed and open states. It thus appears that internal Ca ions are much less effective in blocking Na currents.

The action of external Ca ions on the lifetime of open states for Na is already limited by the diffusional access of Ca ions to their channel. It can be concluded that the blocking action

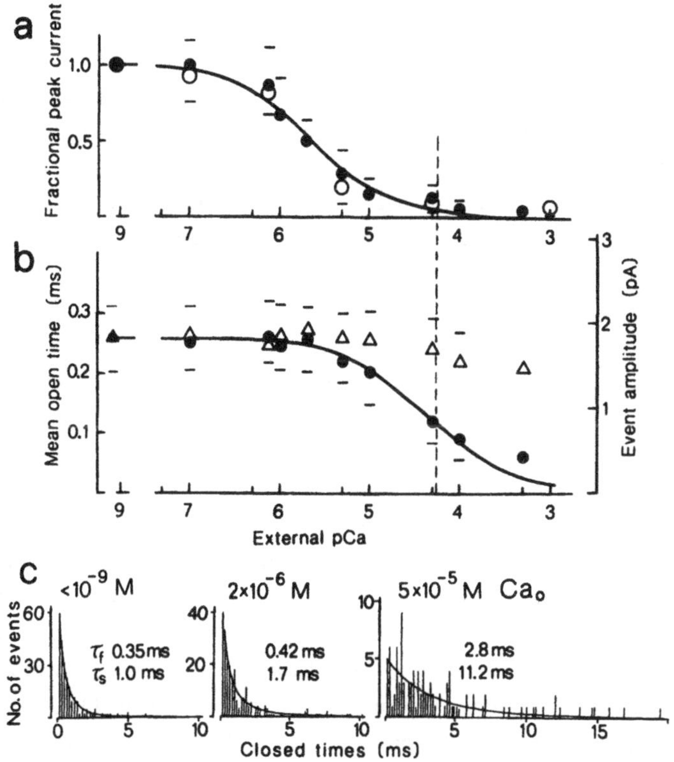


Fig.2: Parameters of $Na^+$ currents as a function of -log $Ca^{2+}_o$.
a) Averages of current samples ( ) of channel recordings. Open symbols display means of currents from whole DRG cells. Currents are given as fraction of values received at $Ca^{2+}_o$ $10^{-9}$ M. The continuous line is calculated for a one-to-one stoichiometry, with half block at $Ca^{2+}_o$ = 2.3 μM.
b) Amplitudes ( ) and mean open times ( ) with S.D. (bars) of 4 to 7 determinations each. Bandwidth limitations were responsible for the depression of recorded amplitudes of the relatively short events observed at $Ca^{2+}_o$ 5 x $10^{-5}$ M. Continuous line displays expected mean open times if equalled to
$0.26 \times (1 + 3 \times 10^3 \times Ca^{2+}_o / Na^+_o)^{-1}$ (ms), with 3 x $10^3$ the number of charges transferred during an average opening of 0.26 ms and 1.85 pA. Half value of mean open time is at 5.5 x $10^{-5}$ M $Ca^{2+}_o$ (dashed line).
c) Closed times received from single channel events of a patch at three $Ca^{2+}_o$. Double exponentials with minimum $\chi^2$ were fitted to the distributions with time constants indicated.

of $Ca^{2+}{}_o$ at micromolar levels on average or whole cell Na currents is mediated by Ca occupation of the channel at times when it is nonconductive for Na ions. This could be due to an external selectivity filter of high Ca specifity as previously proposed (3,17). Recent double binding site models (5,6) are able to account for the selectivity changes of Ca channels, but they are concerned with a decrease of the single channel conductance for $Na^+$ with increasing $Ca^{2+}{}_o$ that is responsible for the observed reduction of macroscopic Na currents. The block of the Na conductance is explained by high affinity binding of Ca ions to either one of two similar sites of the Ca channel while double occupation by Ca ions promotes $Ca^{2+}$ flow by electrostatic repulsion. In our case, increasing external or internal $Ca^{2+}$ had little effect on single LVA channel conductance. In particular, we failed to see a significant effect of high internal $Ca^{2+}$ on time distributions of events. It thus appears that internal Ca ions met a barrier rather than an internally accessible binding site as previously proposed. Our conclusion towards primary effects on state transitions favour a model (18) in which the probability of a given transition is a function of the binding of the permanent ion to a channel site (19,20). This view derives considerable support already by the result that open-closed fluctuation of the channel differs greatly when monovalent or bivalent ions are the current carriers.

References

1. Garnier, D., O. Rougier, Y.M. Gargouil, E. Coraboeuf. 1969. Pflügers Arch. 313, 321-342.

2. Edwards, C. 1981. Neuroscience 7, 1335-1366.

3. Kostyuk, P.G., S.L. Mironov, Ya.M. Shuba. 1983. J. Membrane Biol. 76, 83-93.

4. Almers, W., E.W. McCleskey, P.T. Palade. 1982. J. Physiol. 332, 52-53P.

5. Almers, W., E.W. McCleskey. 1984. J. Physiol. 353, 585-608.

6. Hess, P., R.W. Tsien. 1984. Nature 309, 453-456.

7. Carbone, E. & Lux, H.D. J. Physiol. (in press)

8. Carbone, E., H.D. Lux. 1984. Nature 310, 501-502.

9. Carbone, E., H.D. Lux. 1984. Biophys. J. 46, 413-418.

10. Fedulova, S.A., P.G. Kostyuk, N.S. Veselovsky. 1985. J. Physiol. 359, 431-446.

11. Nowycky, M.C., A.P. Fox, R.W. Tsien. 1985. Nature 316, 440-443.

12. Hamill, O.P., A Marty, E. Neher, B. Sakmann, E.F.I. Sigworth. 1981. Pflügers Arch. 39, 85-100.

13. Fenwick, E.M., A. Marty, E. Neher. 1982. J. Physiol. 331, 599-635.

14. Cavaliê, A., A. Ochi, D. Pelzer, W. Trautwein. 1984. Pflügers Arch. 398, 284-297.

15. Boll, W., H.D. Lux, H.D. 1985. Neurosci. Lett. 56, 335-339.

16. Bossu, I.L., A. Feltz, I.M. Thomann. 1985. Pflügers Arch. 403, 360-368.

17. Kostyuk, P.G., S.L. Mironov, P.A. Doroshenko. 1982. J. Membrane Biol. 70, 181-189.

18. Carbone, E., H.D. Lux, unpublished.

19. Läuger, P. 1985. Biophys. J. 47, 581-591.

20. Ciani, S. 1984. Biophys. J. 46, 249-252.

# EFFECTS OF CHANGING EXTERNAL CALCIUM CONCENTRATION ON CALCIUM CURRENT IN ISOLATED SMOOTH MUSCLE CELL

V.Ya.Ganitkevich, S.V. Smirnov, M.F. Shuba
Department of Nerve-Muscle Physiology, A.A.Bogomoletz Institute of Physiology of the Ukrainian Acad. Sci., Kiev, USSR

## Introduction

External calcium ions affect the excitability of smooth muscle cells. The most important properties of external Ca ions are their ability to carry inward current during excitation of cell membrane (1,2,3,4) and to influence a threshold of excitation (5). We have studied the basic effects of external calcium ions on calcium current ($I_{Ca}$) in isolated single smooth muscle cell.

## Methods

The technique of cell isolation was similar to described earlier (1). Patch-clamp technique in a whole-cell configuration was used for voltage clamp of cell membrane in Cs-TEA solution for internal perfusion of cell. External solution of the following composition was used (in mM): 110 NaCl, 20 CsCl, 2.5 $CaCl_2$, 10 HEPES, 6 glucose; pH was adjusted to 7.2 with TEA-OH. External solutions containing different concentrations of Ca or Ba ions were prepared by addition of the appropriate amount of $CaCl_2$ or $BaCl_2$ to Ca-free external solution. Experiments were performed at 22-24°C. Series resistance was compensated and it was less than 2 MOhm. External solutions were changed as in (6).

## Results

When external Ca ions concentration was increased from 2.5 mM, the following changes in $I_{Ca}$ could be observed: i) an increase

Receptors and Ion Channels

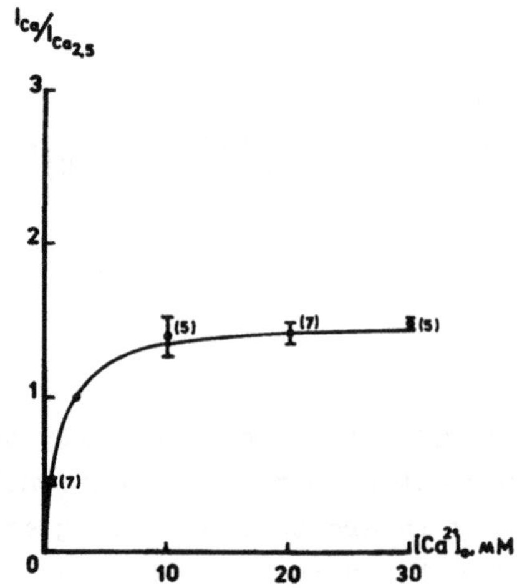


Figure 1. Concentration dependence of calcium current peak amplitude in respect to $I_{Ca}$ when external calcium ions concentration was 2.5 mM. Mean $\pm$ s.e. is indicated by points and vertical bars. The number of experiments is indicated near each point. Solid line represents the Langmuir curve with $K_d$= 1.17mM.

of maximal peak amplitude of $I_{Ca}$; ii) a shift of the I-V curve for $I_{Ca}$ to more positive potentials; iii) a considerable acceleration of $I_{Ca}$ inactivation. Opposite changes were seen when the external concentration of calcium ions was decreased. Concentration dependence of the peak amplitude of $I_{Ca}$ was studied in respect to a peak amplitude of $I_{Ca}$ when the external calcium was 2.5 mM. This approach was used because different maximal $I_{Ca}$ were observed in different cells. When the relative peak amplitude of $I_{Ca}$ was plotted against the external Ca ions concentration, it was found that rapid saturation of $I_{Ca}$ amplitude occured with increasing external Ca concentration (Fig.1). This dependence fits well the Langmuir curve with the apparent binding constant of 1.17 mM. Its mean that in physiological external $Ca^{++}$ions concentration (2.5 mM) calcium channels in smooth muscle cells were nearly saturated, so $I_{Ca}$ amplitude can be rised only by 50% with increasing the external calcium. Saturation seems to be a common property of the calcium channels (for review see 7,8). However, the larger apparent $K_d$ has been usually reported.

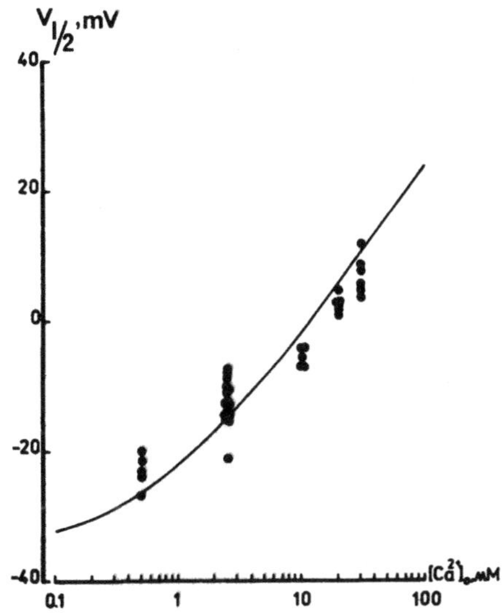


Figure 2. Dependence of $V_{1/2}$ of $I_{Ca}$ on calcium ions concentration in external solution. Solid line is the theoretical curve. Each point represents measurement from one cell.

Change in the potential, at which maximal peak amplitude of $I_{Ca}$ was observed upon varying the external Ca concentration, was due to a well-known stabilizing effect of $Ca^{++}$ ions on the cell membrane. The reason for this is the change of the membrane surface potential (9). To measure the changes in surface potential, we used the potential of $V_{1/2}$, at which $I_{Ca}$ had a peak amplitude equal to a half of maximal. When the external $Ca^{++}$ concentration was increased, $V_{1/2}$ was progressively more positive comparing to $V_{1/2}$ in the low external $Ca^{++}$(Fig. 2). When external Ca ions (2.5 mM) were replaced by equimolar amount of Ba ions, the current-voltage relation for the inward current was shifted by about 7 mV to more negative potentials. This indicates that $Ca^{++}$ ions exerted a stronger effect on the surface charges than $Ba^{++}$ ions. Assuming that $Ba^{++}$ ions do not bind to surface charges and exert their influence due to screening effect (10,11,12), we calculated the surface charges density ($\sigma$) in the vicinity of calcium channels using Gouy-Chapman theory.

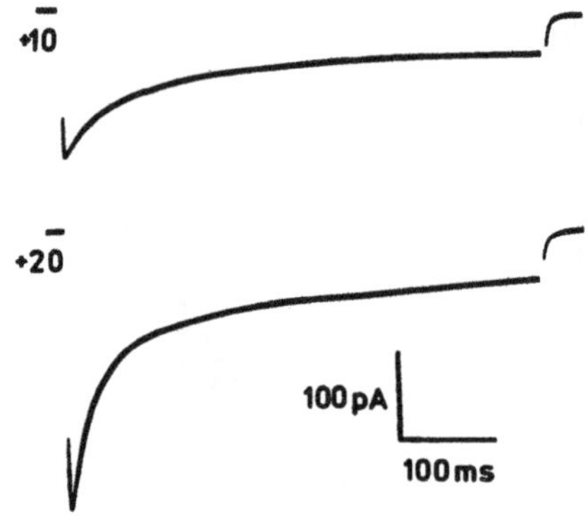


Figure 3. $I_{Ca}$ at the peak of I-V curves with 2.5 mM (upper trace) and 20 mM ( lower trace ) of external calcium. Membrane potential (in millivolts) is indicated by numbers near each current trace.

A reasonable fit of experimental $V_{1/2}$ values to theoretical curve at different external Ba concentrations was obtained assuming $\sigma$ is equal to 0.012 e/$Å^2$. This allowed us to fit the changes in $V_{1/2}$ found at different external $Ca^{++}$ concentrations assuming that the constant ( $K_{Ca}$ ) for calcium binding to surface charged groups is equal to 0.035 $M^{-1}$. Theoretical curve is shown by solid line in Fig. 2.

As surface membrane potential was changed, the nearmembrane concentration of $Ca^{++}$ ions seemed to be also changed. So, it is necessary to take into account surface potential changes when studying the concentration dependence of $I_{Ca}$. According to the mentioned values of $\sigma$ and $K_{Ca}$, it was found that saturation of $I_{Ca}$ can be largely explained by saturation of nearmembrane concentration of calcium ions. So, it looks that binding of Ca ions in the external mouth of calcium channel occurred with a much lower affinity. Thus, it is now possible to give a quantitative description of external calcium ions effects on $I_{Ca}$ in smooth muscle cells.

The another effect we observed when the calcium ion concentration in the external solution was changed was the change in $I_{Ca}$ inactivation kinetics. Comparison of $I_{Ca}$ inactivation time course upon varying $Ca^{++}$ concentration was made with the correction of surface potential changes, assuming that Ca channel gating

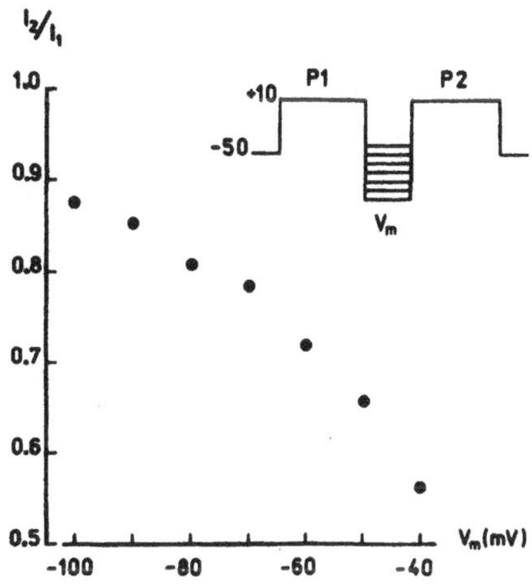


Figure 4. Potential-dependence of calcium current recovery from inactivation. The scheme of experiment is shown in the inset.

was not affected. It was found that a lowering of external $Ca^{++}$ concentration slowed down $I_{Ca}$ inactivation, while the elevation of external $Ca^{++}$ concentration accelerated it (Fig. 3). This finding supports our conclusion that $I_{Ca}$ inactivation in smooth muscle cells is associated with Ca entry (1). Detailed sequence of events resulting in inactivation of calcium current is unknown. Some our findings may indicate that $I_{Ca}$ inactivation is Ca-dependent to a large extent. For example, relation between fractional current inactivation and Ca entry was independent on the membrane potential. This relation can be fitted well by a binding-site model suggested for Ca-mediated inactivation (14, 15). However, we found that recovery of $I_{Ca}$ from inactivation was potential-dependent, and acceleration of $I_{Ca}$ recovery was observed upon hyperpolarization of the membrane (Fig. 4). So, the phenomenon of Ca-mediated inactivation in smooth muscle seems to be more complicated than a simple accumulation of internal calcium ions and needs further detailed investigation. Moreover, as was recently found in neurones (13), the possibility exists that this process may be mediated via dephosphorylation of calcium channels

References

1. Ganitkevich, V.Ya., S.V. Smirnov, M.F. Shuba. 1985. Doklady Acad. Sci. USSR 282, 717-720.

2. Mitra, R., M. Morad. 1985. Science 229, 269-272.

3. Klöckner, U., G. Isenberg. 1985. Pflüg. Arch. 405, 340-348.

4. Droogmans, G., G. Callewaert. 1986. Pflüg. Arch. 406, 259-265.

5. Bülbring, E., T. Tomita. 1969. Proc. Roy. Soc. B 172, 121-136.

6. Krishtal, O.A., V.I. Pidoplichko. 1980. Neuroscience 5, 2325-2327.

7. Hagiwara, S., L. Byerly. 1981. Ann. Rev. Neurosci. 4, 69-125.

8. Kostyuk, P.G. 1980. Neuroscience 5, 945-959.

9. Ohmori, H., M. Yoshii. 1977. J. Physiol. 267, 429-463.

10. Kostyuk, P.G., P.A. Doroshenko, V.N. Ponomarev. 1980. Doklady Acad. Sci. USSR 250, 464-467.

11. Wilson, D.L., K. Morimoto, Y. Tsuda, A.M.Brown. 1983. J. Membr. Biol. 72, 117-130.

12. Byerly, L., P.B. Chase, J.R. Stimers. 1985. J. Gen. Physiol. 85, 491-518.

13. Eckert, R., J.E. Chad. 1984. Progr. Biophys. Mol. Biol. 44, 215-267.

14. Standen, N.B., P.R. Stanfield. 1982. Proc. Roy. Soc. B 217, 101-110.

15. Plant,T.D., N.B. Standen, Ward, T.A. 1983. J.Physiol. 335, 189-212.

# ACTIVATION BY HISTAMINE IONIC CHANNELS IN THE MEMBRANE OF HUMAN ENDOTHELIAL CELLS.

P. Bregestovski, A. Bakhramov
Cardiology Research Center, Moscow, USSR.

## Introduction

Monolayer of endothelial cells forms the lining of the vessels and plays a number of important physiological functions, such as providing substances exchange between blood and tissue, metabolic activity, synthesis of mediators, humoral regulation of smooth muscle cells exitability, etc.
The membrane of endothelial cells contains receptors for such hormones and transmitters as serotonin, catecholamines, adenosine, acetylholine, histamine (1). Relationships between receptor activation and changes of membrane permeability in these cells are poorly investigated. For instance, histamine was shown to effect endothelial cells membrane depolarisation (2) and its application results in increase in intracellular calcium concentration (3). However, relationship between calcium influx and changes of the membrane permeability is not clear.
The using of conventional voltage clamp techniques is rather complicated because endothelial cells are of comparatively small size and flattened shape. Penetration of a small cell with microelectrodes caused injure of the membrane, decrease in the resting potential, changes the intracellular solution content. Development of the patch-clamp techniques allows to overtake some of these difficulties (4). It is possible to study whole-cell currents of the small size cells, to analyze the nature of ionic currents, mechanisms of its activation, effects of blockators. Using this techniques the effect of histamine on the membrane of human endothelial cells has been studied. The results obtained indicate that application of histamine induces an influx of calcium ions which may activate, in turn, $Ca^{2+}$-dependent ionic channels.

Receptors and Ion Channels

## Materials and Methods

The experiments were performed on endothelial cells from human umbilical vein. Cells were isolated enzimatically and cultivated for 1 - 7 days on Petri dishes (5). The studies were curried out in cell-attached, whole-cell and inside-out configurations (4). The composition of the external solution (in mM): NaCl - 140; KCl - 2.8; $MgCl_2$ - 2; $CaCl_2$ - 1; HEPES (Na) - 10; pH-7.4. The composition of main "intracellular" solution (in mM): KCl - 140; $MgCl_2$ - 2; EGTA - 1.1; $CaCl_2$ - 0.55 (pCa-7); HEPES (K) - 10; pH-7.4. In some experiments concentration of the free calcium varied from 0.1 uM to 10 uM.

Currents were recorded using an EPC-7 amplifier (List-Electronic, FRG) on the type-recorder (Bruel & Kjer, Denmark), and analyzed with microcomputer. The experiments were performed at room temperature (20 - 23°C).

## Results and Discussion

Resting potential of investigated cells was, on average, -30 mV. Current-voltage (I-V) relationships were nearly linear over the range of membrane potentials $\pm$60 mV. At positive potentials in some cells only 1.5 - 2 fold increase in slope conductance was registered. For instance, in the cell representing at the Fig.1, the slope conductance (G) over the range -70 - -30 mV was about 1.7 nS and at the range 0 - +60 mV G=2.5 nS. This character of I-V curve indicates that the membrane of endothelial cells posesses a few, if any, voltage-gated ionic channels.

In about 10% of the studied cells the membrane conductance was reversibly elevated by 3-10 times after application of 10 uM histamine (Fig.1). The effect of the drug developed relatively slow: the rise time of the response was about 3-5 min. The washout was also slow: complete restoration of the conductance occured in 10-15 min after washing with normal solution. I-V curve for histamine-activated currents was nearly linear. Reversal potential ($E_r$) ranged between -20 ÷ 0 mV, showing that histamine activates cation- or cation- and anion-selective channels. To elucidate the mechanism responsible for the action of histamine we studied its effect

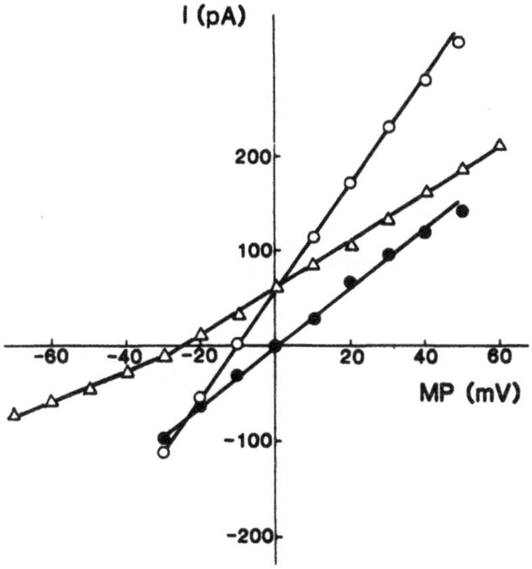


Fig.1. Histamine-induced currents in the whole-cell record mode. (Δ) I-V relationship in the absence of histamine; (O) I-V relationship in 10 min after addition of 10 uM histamine; (●) differential I-V relationship, characterizing the real effect of histamine.

on the level of single ionic channels.

In cell-attached configuration pipettes were filled with "intracellular" solution and histamine (usually 10 uM) was added to the bath solution. After establishment of cell-attached mode most of the patches were silent. After addition of histamine to external solution some of them (less than 10% of patches tested) showes activation of ionic channels. Two types of channels were recorded after the bath application of the drug (Fig.2). The reversal potential of each type of channels was respectively close to $E_K$ or $E_{Cl}$ as determined by experimental conditions. I-V curve was nearly linear, the slope conductance for both types was 20-30 pS. Average open time was 5-7 msec and did not depend markedly on the membrane potential.

Histamine was effective only in the presence of calcium in the bath solution (Fig.3.). In $Ca^{2+}$-free solution and in the absence of histamine the membrane was silent (Fig.3, upper trace). During 6 min application of $Ca^{2+}$-free solution with 10 uM of histamine channels also were not observed (middle trace). In several seconds after addition of $Ca^{2+}$ (final concentration 1 mM), ionic channels with elementary conductance of about 20 pS were activated (lower trace).

Thus, one can suggest that either calcium ions are required for histamine receptor activation or histamine causes entrance of cal-

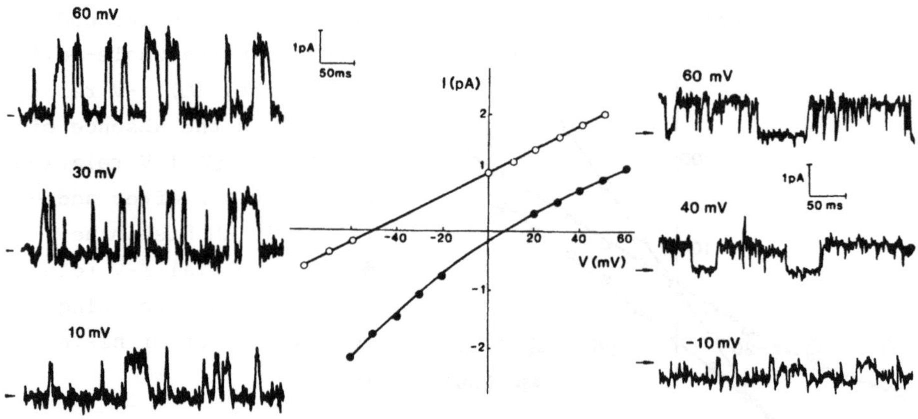


Fig.2. Histamine-induced single-channel current in cell-attached configuration. Left and right, single channel currents at different membrane potentials. Pipette potentials are indicated above the traces. Close state of channels is indicated with an arrow. Centre, single-channel I-V relationship. The slope conductance for outward currents is about 20 pS. (●) currents possesing presumably $K^+$-selectivity; (O) currents possesing presumably $Cl^-$-selectivity.

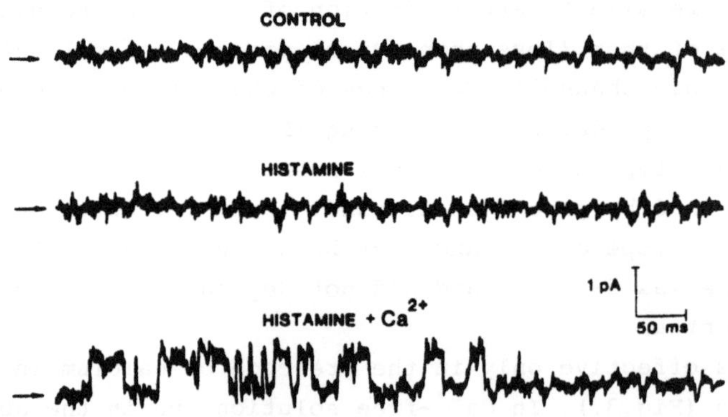


Fig.3. $Ca^{2+}$-dependence of histamine effect. The upper trace shows lack of the channel activity in external solution with 0.1 uM $Ca^{2+}$. The middle trace, 6 min after addition to this solution of 10 uM histamine. Note the absence of single channel currents. The bottom trace, the channel activity in 30 sec after addition to external solution of 1 mM $Ca^{2+}$. Cell-attached configuration.

cium ions into the cell which, in turn, may activate $Ca^{2+}$-dependent ionic channels. The latter suggestion is more likely and is in good agreement with earlier observation made on the guinea-pig aorta endothelium. It has been shown that calcium ions are required for the pronounced effect of histamine (2) and this drug increases several times calcium influx (3).

Our experiments with calcium ionophore A23187 provided support for this suggestion. Application of 1 uM A23187 resulted in the activation of single ionic channels with the amplitude and the kinetics similar to those described earlier for histamine.

Experiments with inside-out patches provided direct evidence for the existence of $Ca^{2+}$-activated ionic channels in the membrane of endothelial cells. At calcium concentration 0.1 uM from cytoplasmic side of the membrane ($[Ca^{2+}]_i$) the channels were unlike to be activated. At $[Ca^{2+}]_i$ more than 0.5 uM the channels were operate frequently. Fig.4 shows ionic currents at different membrane potentials and I-V characteristics of $Ca^{2+}$-activated ionic channels. Elementary conductance of channels in symmetrical potassium solution was about 20 pS.

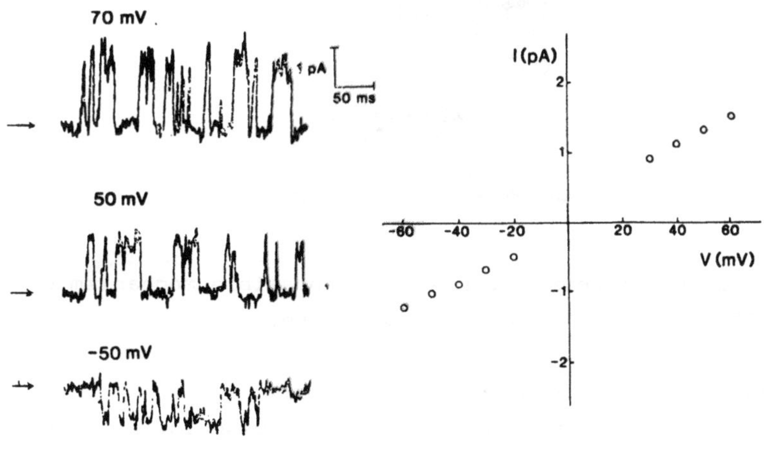


Fig.4. Inside-out recording of $Ca^{2+}$-activated ionic channels in human endothelium. Left, currents at different membrane potentials (70, 50 and -50 mV). Arrow indicates the close state of channel. Right, I-V relationship.

Two types of $Ca^{2+}$-activated ionic channels were registered. For one type $E_r$ and $\gamma$ depended on potassium concentration in the solution. Substitution of potassium ions for sodium in the cytoplasmic solution results in complete disappearance of outward currents and decrease of $\gamma$. For the other type of channels such a substitution produced no effect on its characteristics.

These data suggest the following scheme of histamine effect on the endothelial cell membrane (Fig.5). Interaction of the drug with receptor activate calcium flow into the cell (presumably through the receptor-operated ionic channels). Elevation of the cytoplasmic calcium level results in the activation of calcium-dependent potassium and presumably cloride channels, which increase the membrane conductance.

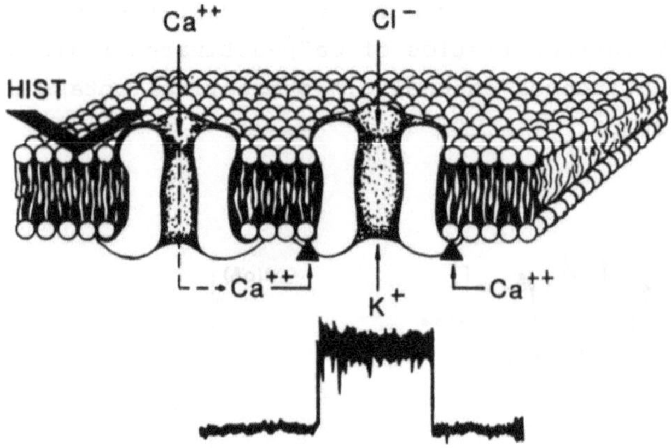


Fig.5. Schematical representation of a possible mechanism of histamine effect on endothelial cell membrane.

These results arise a number of questions:

- what is the mechanism responsible for calcium influx induction: is it due to receptor activation of calcium channels or is caused by some other factors;
- why the effect of histamine was observed only on 5-10% of the studied cells: due to heterogeneity of cell population in the vessel or alteration of the membrane properties during isolation and cultivation;

- what physiological role receptors for histamine and $Ca^{2+}$-activated ionic channels in the membrane of endothelial cells play in the vessel function?

These problems require further investigations.

The authors wish to acknowledge Drs. S. Danilov, A. Antonov and I. Moldabaeva for contributing culture of endothelial cells.

References

1. Freudenberg, N., Riese, K., Freudenberg, M. A. 1983. In: The Vascular Endothelial System. Gustav Fisher Verlag, Stuttgart, New-York, p. 21.

2. Northover, B. J. 1980. Adv. Microcirc. 9, 135.

3. D'Amore, P., Shepro, D. 1977. J. Cell. Physiol. 92, 177.

4. Hamill, O. P., Marty, A., Neher, E., Sakmann, B., Sigworth, F. 1981. Pflügers Arch. 391, 85.

5. Allikmets, E. Yu. and Danilov, S.M. 1986. Tissue Cell. 18, p.121.

# BLOCK OF SODIUM CHANNELS WITH CHEMICALLY MODIFIED GATING

W. Ulbricht
Physiologisches Institut, Universität Kiel, Kiel, FRG

## Introduction

It is generally accepted that blocking agents and gate modifiers act on different sites of the sodium channel. Hence one would not expect changes in block after chemical modification of gating. This, however, is not always the case as can be shown in experiments employing combinations of the blocking agents tetrodotoxin (TTX) and benzocaine (Benzo) with gate modifiers veratridine (Vera), *Anemonia sulcata* toxin II (ATX II) and chloramine-T (Cl-T).

## Methods

Voltage clamp experiments were done on myelinated nerve fibres of the frog, *Rana esculenta*, either in a standard chamber (1) or in a fast-exchange setup (2). Leakage and capacity currents were subtracted by an analogue device. Potentials are given as deviations, V, from the normal resting potential, depolarizations being positive. All solutions contained 10 mM TEA to suppress $K^+$ currents. Chloramine-T (0.6 mM) was applied for ca. 1 min while the membrane was continuously hyperpolarized by 20 mV (3).

## Results

### Rate of block of modified channels

When it became known that after treatment with Cl-T the nodal membrane continued to pass $Na^+$ current during a sustained depolarization (4), it was of interest, in continuation of earlier

Receptors and Ion Channels

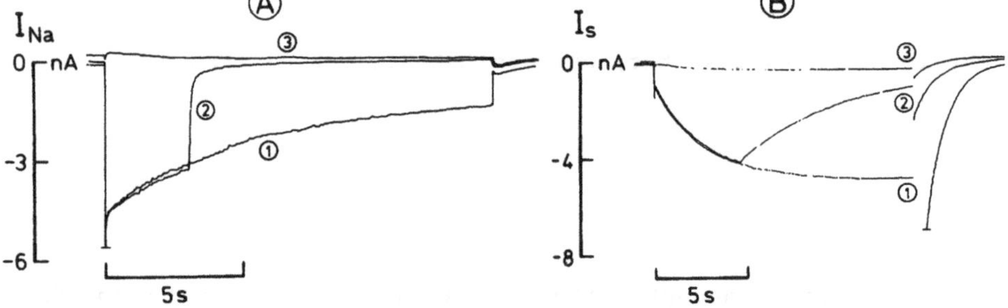


Fig. 1. Rate of action of 1 mM Benzo. A. On a node of Ranvier treated with Cl-T. The peak sodium current (-25.5 nA) is cut off and only the persistent component is shown. 20.1°C. From (2) B. In the presence of 60 µM Vera. The peak current is cut off and only the secondary slowly increasing current $I_s$ and the large tails are shown. A different fibre at 19.3°C. From (2)

experiments on the rate of local anaesthetic action (5), to determine the effect of a sudden application of Benzo to channels kept open by this treatment. The result is seen in Fig. 1A which presents current records obtained during 3 consecutive pulses of 14 s duration. At this slow time base the early peak $I_{Na}$ deteriorates to a vertical line most of which is cut off. Trace 1 shows the slowly declining "persistent" current in the control, trace 2 the fast decrease in current when 3 s after the start of the pulse 1 mM Benzo was applied; trace 3 was obtained ca. 30 s later (2). Analysis of trace 2 yields a half-time of current block of 0.06 s, in full agreement with the earlier experiments on repetitively pulsed membranes (5).

When we repeated this kind of experiment on sodium channels kept open by Vera we were surprised by the very slow time constant (5.6 s at 19°C) with which the Vera-induced slow current $I_s$ declined on suddenly applying 1 mM Benzo as illustrated by Fig. 1B. Here again the early peak current does not show; it is followed by a secondary slow current increase. On repolarization a large, slow current tail is observed which has been cut off in trace 1. Trace 2 shows the effect of a sudden application of 1 mM Benzo 5 s after the start of the impulse, trace 3 was obtained after equilibration in the Benzo solution where the steady inward current was only 9% of that in trace 1. Interestingly, application of only 25 µM Benzo little increased the time constant of the $I_s$ decline (to 5.9 s in the experiment of Fig. 1B) in contrast to what one would expect for reaction rate-limited, but also for access-limited time courses of block. Moreover, recovery from block by 1 mM Benzo on washing was approximately as fast as the onset. Finally, cooling which slows and reduces $I_s$ profoundly (6) also reduced the onset of Benzo block of $I_s$ with an unusually large $Q_{10}$ of 3.2. These and other results can be explained if one postulates that a channel kept open by Vera cannot be blocked by Benzo. What one observes in trace 2 of Fig. 1B is the rate with which veratrinized channels close spontaneously, since closed channels are blocked and cannot reopen. If one assumes that the conversion of (normal) open channels to "persistently" open channels more or less reflects binding of Vera to a specific site as has been proposed by others (7,8), it would then be mutually exclusive of Benzo binding to a blocking site, an interesting aspect worth pursuing.

It should be noted that Vera does not seem to interfere with all blocking agents. For instance, the rate of TTX action on current tails observed in Vera during trains (0.2 Hz) of 2-s pulses was not different from that determined in the absence of the alkaloid (9). Similar results were obtained when, in the presence of Vera, a concentrated TTX solution was suddenly applied during a 14-s impulse. $I_s$ promptly declined with a time constant as calculated from the rate constants of the TTX-channel reaction determined in the absence of alkaloid (2). Slight changes in the kinetics of TTX block, however, may have escaped our detection since no control measurements without Vera were made on the same preparation. This limitation is prompted by our unexpected observation that after Cl-T treatment the onset rate of TTX block is slowed (10). This is illustrated for the onset and offset of the action of 10 nM TTX in Fig. 2 where the open symbols refer to measurements before, filled symbols after Cl-T treatment. The time constants are given in the inset. The mean values from 6 fibres were 26.4 s before and 39.3 s after treatment; the respective mean offset time constants were 89.3 s and 82.1 s (18-20°C). The reason for the moderate change in

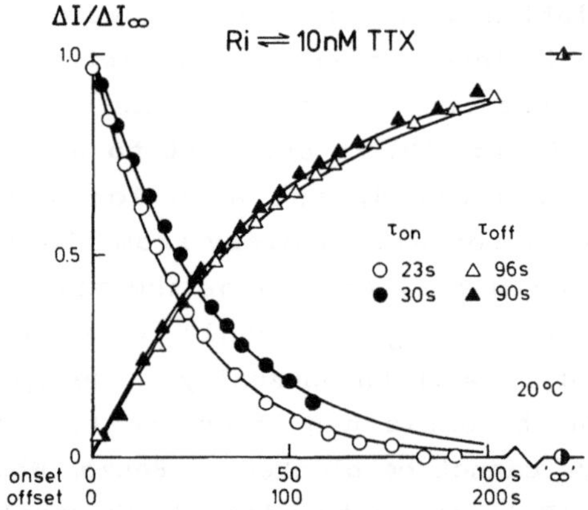


Fig. 2. Rate of onset (circles) and offset (triangles) of the action of 10 nM TTX before (open symbols) and after (filled symbols) Cl-T treatment. Ordinate, change, ΔI, of peak current, normalized to maximum change, $\Delta I_{\infty}$. Abscissa, time after solution change. Note different time scales for onset and offset. Exponential curves calculated with time constants given by inset. Unpublished experiment of J. Schmidtmayer and W. Ulbricht

kinetics is unclear, in particular whether it is a side-effect of Cl-T treatment or linked to the Cl-T-induced inhibition of Na channel inactivation.

Extent of block of modified channels

As mentioned, Cl-T treatment slows the inactivation and renders it incomplete as can be clearly seen in the records of Fig. 5. It was of interest to see whether peak and persistent current (at the end of a 15-ms pulse) were equally reduced by TTX. This was indeed found which argues against the possibility that the persistent current component flows through a different type of non-inactivating channels (unlikely also for other reasons; see ref. 3) which differ in their TTX sensitivity as has been proposed for the diphasic inactivation of untreated nodes (11).

The situation is quite different if the block is brought about by Benzo which reduces the persistent component more than the peak

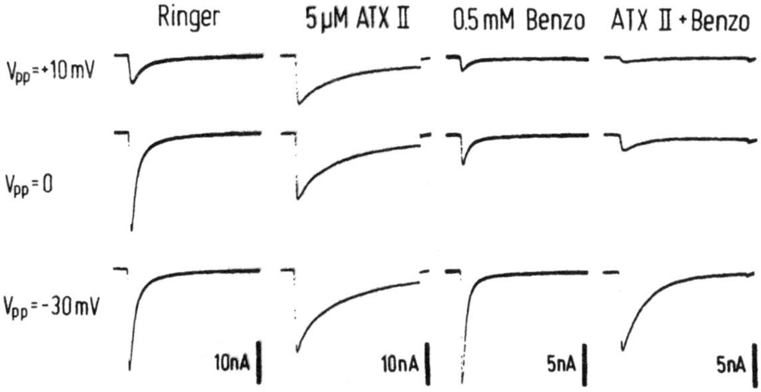


Fig. 3. Effect of 0.5 mM Benzo in the presence and absence of 5 µM ATX II. Original records of sodium current during 15-ms impulses, following 100-ms prepulses of $V_{pp}$ = -30, 0 and +10 mV. Unpublished experiment of J. Schmidtmayer and W. Ulbricht at 16°C

current. This is clearly seen in the bottom row of Fig. 3 which describes the combined effects of 5 µM ATX II and 0.5 mM Benzo. In this mixture there is hardly any persistent current to be seen whereas the peak current is reduced to ca. 50% (note the difference in current scale between ATX II and the mixture). The figure also gives a summary impression of the drug-induced changes of inactivation. The middle row was obtained without prepulse, the bottom row with a hyperpolarizing prepulse ($V_{pp}$ = -30 mV), the top row with a depolarizing presulse ($V_{pp}$ = +10 mV). The latter obviously has less reducing effect in ATX II than in the control whereas in Benzo there is a massive inactivation already at $V_{pp}$ = 0. This Benzo effect is also observed in the mixture (4th column).

The dependence on $V_{pp}$ of peak $I_{Na}$, normalized to its maximum value following a strong hyperpolarizing prepulse, is presented for the 4 solutions in Fig. 4. Circles refer to anaesthetic-free solutions, triangles to solutions containing 0.5 mM Benzo; open symbols denote results in the absence of toxin, filled symbols in the presence of 5 µM ATX II. Note that the curve through the filled circles does not reach zero because of the incomplete inactivation in ATX II (12). The main feature is the large shift of these curves by Benzo to more negative prepulse potentials. The shift at

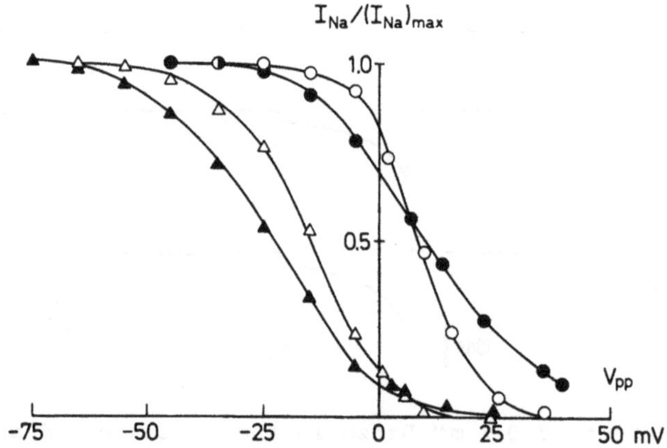


Fig. 4. Inactivation curves i.e. peak sodium current normalized to maximum value following strong hyperpolarizing prepulse vs. prepulse potential. ○ Ringer solution, △ 0.5 mM Benzo, ● 5 µM ATX II, ▲ 5 µM ATX II + 0.5 mM Benzo. From a different node than in Fig. 3; unpublished experiment of J. Schmidtmayer and W. Ulbricht at 17.3°C

the midpoint of the curves was -22.5 mV before and even -35.6 mV after introduction of ATX II. The mean values (±S.E.M.) from 4 preparations were -23.1 ± 1.9 mV and -30.2 ± 2.7 mV, respectively. $(I_{Na})_{max}$ was reduced to 0.55 ± 0.05 and to 0.58 ± 0.04 (16-17°C) in the presence of ATX II which, obviously, did not significantly influence peak current block.

Quite similar results were obtained in a study of Benzo action after Cl-T treatment (13). 0.25 and 1 mM Benzo led to a mean shift of the inactivation curve of -18.9 and -31.7 mV (6 fibres at 15-17°C) after treatment as compared to -15.6 and -22.7 mV before treatment (7 fibres). The mean reduction of $(I_{Na})_{max}$ was to 0.75 and 0.40 before and to 0.73 and 0.42 after treatment in these experiments. The persistent current seen after treatment was again more reduced than the peak $I_{Na}$ as illustrated by Fig. 5 which was obtained with a similar pulse protocol as in Fig. 3.

Our Benzo results before inhibition of inactivation can be interpreted in terms of the modulated-receptor hypothesis (14) which

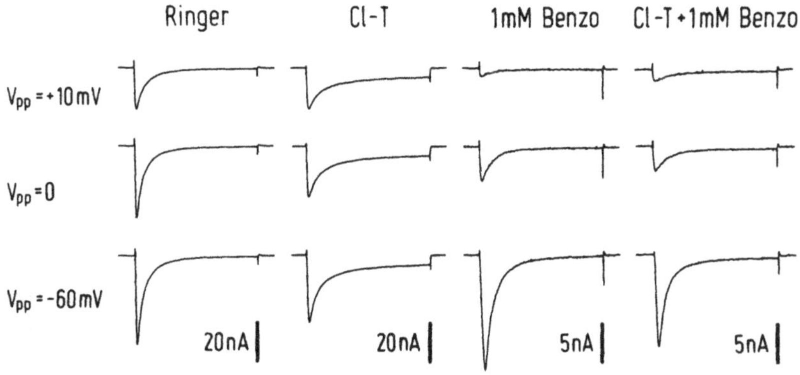


Fig. 5. Effect of 1 mM Benzo before and after treatment with 0.6 mM Cl-T. Records of sodium current during 15-ms depolarizing impulses of constant amplitude following 30-ms prepulses of -60, 0 and +10 mV in bottom, middle and upper row. Unpublished experiment of T. Meeder and W. Ulbricht at 16.2°C

assumes that affinity for the anaesthetic depends on the functional state of a channel. Reduction by Benzo of peak $I_{Na}$, following strong hyperpolarizing prepulses, then reflects block of resting channels with an equilibrium dissociation constant $K_R$. The fraction, p, of channels left unblocked is given by $p = 1/(c_R + 1)$ where $c_R = [\text{Benzo}]/K_R$. The shift, $\Delta V_h$, of the inactivation curve is due to the higher affinity for Benzo of inactivated channels. With $c_R$ known, one can calculate the corresponding equilibrium constant, $K_I = [\text{Benzo}]/c_I$, with the relation $\Delta V_h = k \ln[(c_R+1)/(c_I+1)]$ where k is the slope factor of the inactivation curve (15). Our results yield $K_R = 0.7$ mM and $K_I = 0.04$ mM. This calculation neglects the normally very transient open state. In the presence of ATX II or after Cl-T treatment, however, this state has to be considered; its affinity, expressed by $K_O$, can only be estimated at the time being. $K_R$ clearly is unchanged and if $K_I$ is unaffected, we obtain $K_R \gg K_O \geq K_I$. Unequivocal determination of $K_O$ and $K_I$ would require a full kinetic analysis of the interconversion of channel states in the presence of Benzo which has not yet been done. Nevertheless, there is reason to assume that $K_R$ and $K_I$ are independent of the distribution between states (drastically changed in favour of the open state by Cl-T) rendering these constants a valulable means to characterize chemically the two main closed states, resting and inactivated, of the sodium channel.

Acknowledgement

The experiments were supported in all stages by the Deutsche Forschungsgemeinschaft. Help by Ms Dieter throughout the experiments and with the figures and by Ms Ach for typing is gratefully acknowledged.

References

1. Nonner, W. 1969. Pflügers Arch. 309, 176.
2. Ulbricht, W., M. Stoye-Herzog. 1984. Pflügers Arch. 402, 439.
3. Schmidtmayer, J. 1985. Pflügers Arch. 404, 21.
4. Wang, G.K. 1984. J. Physiol. 346, 127.
5. Rimmel, C., A. Walle, H. Keßler, W. Ulbricht. 1978. Pflügers Arch. 376, 105.
6. Ulbricht, W. 1969. Pflügers Arch. 311, 73.
7. Sutro, J.B. 1986. J. Gen. Physiol. 87, 1.
8. Khodorov, B.I. 1985. Progr. Biophys. molec. Biol. 45, 57.
9. Ulbricht, W. 1977. In: Biochemistry of Sensory Functions (L. Jaenicke ed.). Springer-Verlag, p. 351.
10. Ulbricht, W., J. Schmidtmayer. 1986. Pflügers Arch. 406, R 28.
11. Benoit, E., A. Corbier, J.-M. Dubois. 1985. J. Physiol. 361, 339.
12. Ulbricht, W., J. Schmidtmayer. 1981. J. Physiol. (Paris) 77, 1103.
13. Meeder, T., W. Ulbricht. 1985. Pflügers Arch. 405, R 52.
14. Hille, B. 1977. J. Gen. Physiol. 69, 497.
15. Bean, B.P., C.J. Cohen, R.W. Tsien. 1983. J. Gen. Physiol. 81, 613.

# POTASSIUM CURRENTS IN THE ISOLATED SINGLE SMOOTH MUSCLE CELL MEMBRANE

V.A. Buryi, M.F. Shuba, A.V. Zholos
Department of Nerve-Muscle Physiology, A.A. Bogomoletz Institute of Physiology of the Ukrainian Acad. Sci., Kiev, USSR

## Introduction

Potassium outward current ( $I_K$ ) in smooth muscle cells is of special interest, since it controls the amplitude and duration of action potentials, as well as takes part in excitability regulation (1,2,3,4). This current is activated almost simultaneously with calcium inward current ( $I_{Ca}$ ) and consists of more than one component. In experiments performed on multicellular preparations the outward current was reported to consist of an initial inactivated component and subsequent noninactivated component. The inactivation of outward current was shown to be voltage-dependent (1,2). In addition, the inactivated $I_K$ exhibited some properties inherent for calcium-activated $K^+$ current ( $I_{K/Ca/}$ ) (2,5). Due to theoretical and experimental difficulties in measurements and separation of currents in multicellular smooth muscle preparations, the date obtained were limited and contradictory (6). In the present paper $I_K$ was investegated in single smooth muscle cell using whole cell patch clamp recording technique which allows a quantitative analysis of the results. $I_K$ was separated by elimination of $I_{Ca}$ with $Ca^{2+}$ channel blockers or using $Ca^{2+}$-free solution. But in this case $I_{K/Ca/}$ was also removed simultaneously with $I_{Ca}$ and recorded $I_K$ contained only a voltage-dependent component ( $I_{K/V/}$ ). Combining this approach with graphic subtraction of net $I_{Ca}$ recorded in the same cell we were able to separate $I_K$ on $I_{K/V/}$ and $I_{K/Ca/}$ components.

Receptors and Ion Channels

## Methods

Experiments were performed on single smooth muscle cells isolated from the guinea-pig taenia coli using collagenase. Details of cell isolation procedure have been described elsewhere (7). A suspension of isolated cells was transferred to an experimental chamber ( volume of 50 $\mu$l ) mounted on the stage of an inverted microscope. After adhesion of cells to the glass bottom of the chamber they were continuously superfused at 36°C with Hepes buffered Krebs solution containing (in mM): 120.4 NaCl; 5.9 KCl; 1.2 $MgCl_2$; 2.5 $CaCl_2$; 5 HEPES-NaOH (pH 7.3) and 11.5 glucose.
Ionic currents were recorded with the patch-clamp technique (8) in the whole cell configuration. Fire-polished patch pipette was filled with solution containing (in mM): 85 KCl; 30 $KH_2PO_4$; 5 $MgSO_4$; 5 $Na_2ATP$; 5 creatine; 20 taurine; 20 glucose; 3 EGTA and adjusted with KOH to pH 7.3. The patch electrodes had resistance of 1-1.5 MOhm. The clamp worked with a settling time of less than 1 ms. A correction for background current has been applied throughout.

## Results

Under voltage-clamp conditions, current traces recorded for different depolarizing steps were rather complex (Fig. 1). All clamp steps set between -30 mV and +35...+45 mV showed net inward current (Fig. 1B), which peaked within 1 - 5 ms and changed into an outward current. Both the amplitude and rate of rise of the outward current strongly increased with more positive clamp steps. Net outward current at -20...-10 mV appeared only after 100-150 ms, whereas at more positive clamp steps the inward current changed into an outward one in 5-10 ms and reached a peak after 10-20 ms. Afterwards the outward current inactivated to a steady state level. As a rule, the inactivation time course was complex but roughly it could be divided into fast and slow components with half times of decay of about several tens and several hundreds of milliseconds, respectively. The amplitude of both components as well as their rates of decay showed a very large variability in different cells. In addition, the fast component was found to decrease

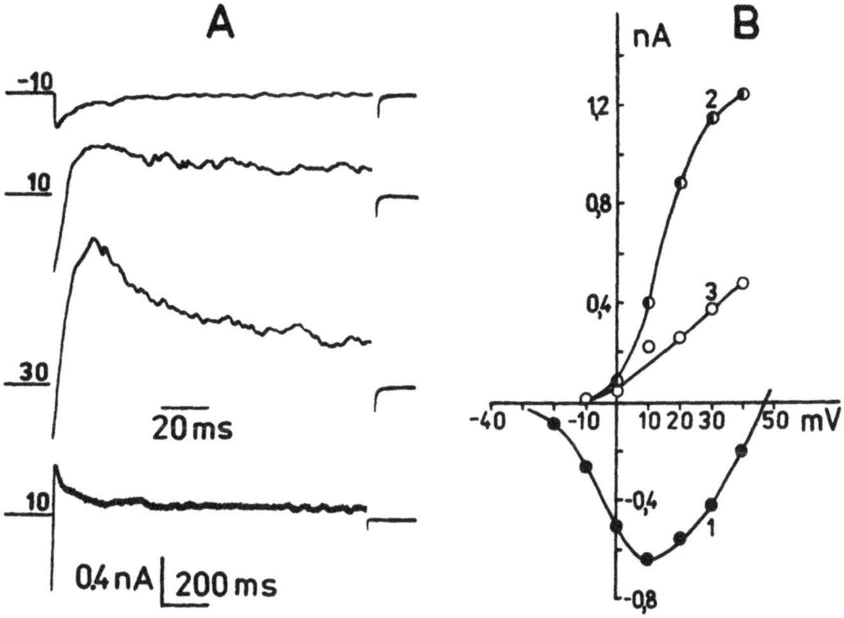


Figure 1. Voltage dependence of the total transmembrane current from single smooth muscle cell. A, a typical current traces elicited by depolarizing steps from -50 mV to the indicated level. B, current-voltage relationship for the peak of inward (1), outward (2) currents and the current at the end of depolarizing steps (3).

strongly with lowering temperature to 20°C. In some cells the current-voltage relation for peak outward current showed saturation which can be attributed to $I_{K/Ca/}$ (9). To demonstrate $K^+$ origin of the outward current, we determined its reversal potential in $K^+$ rich solution. It was found to be equal to $K^+$ equilibrium potential. Outward current was also sensitive to $TEA^+$. But even at high concentrations of $TEA^+$ the block of $I_K$ was incomplete. Fig. 2 presents the membrane current separated into two parts by substitution of external $Ca^{2+}$ with $Mg^{2+}$ ions which cannot permit through Ca-channels. The absence of noticeable increase in the outward current which could be expected from elimination of $I_{Ca}$ suggests simultaneous remowal of $K^+$ current activated by $I_{Ca}$. Hence, the difference between currents recorded in normal and $Ca^{2+}$-free solutions (shown by dashed line in Fig. 2B) represents

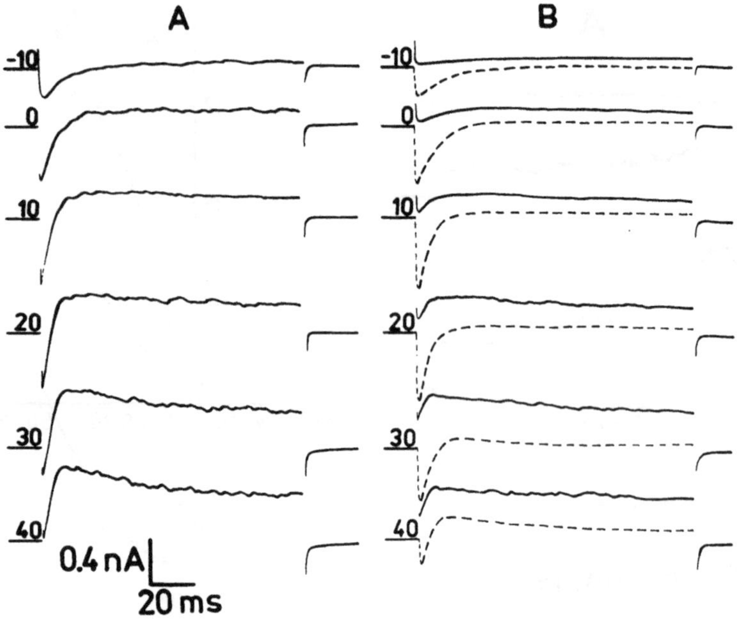


Figure 2. Separation of $I_{K/V/}$ from $I_{Ca}$ and $I_{K/Ca/}$.
A, membrane currents recorded in control solution. B, $K^+$ currents in the same cell recorded in Ca-free solution. Dashed lines are results of paired subtractions of records B from A. They represent sums of $I_{Ca}$ and $I_{K/Ca/}$.

a sum of $I_{Ca}$ and $I_{K/Ca/}$. Becouse both these currents are related in physiological conditions the analysis of their sum is very important for the understanding of the mechanism of electrical excitability. Since $I_{Ca}$ inactivates very slowly (10), the decay of $I_{Ca}+I_{K/Ca/}$ is determined almost completely by activation of $I_{K/Ca/}$ which demonstrates voltage-dependence (Fig. 2B) becoming faster with more positive clamping steps. At potentials between 0 mV and +10 mV the magnitude and time course of $I_{K/Ca/}$ in a short time ( 30-15 ms ) became comparable with those for $I_{Ca}$. At more negative potentials $I_{K/Ca/}$ was smaller, while at more positive values larger than $I_{Ca}$. Similar results were obtained when $I_{Ca}$ was blocked by Co ions (3 mM). Since it is imposible to record $I_{K/Ca/}$ alone, we tried to separate this current by graphic subtraction of $I_{Ca}$ from $I_{Ca}+I_{K/Ca/}$ obtained from the same cell.

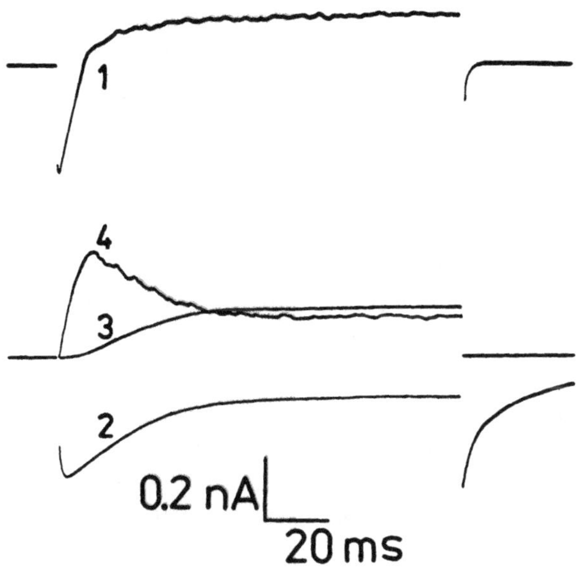


Figure 3. Components of membrane current from a single taenia coli smooth muscle cell. 1, total membrane current recorded in normal solution. 2, net $I_{Ca}$ recorded in K-rich solution.
3, $I_{K/V/}$ recorded in normal $Co^{2+}$-containing (3 mM) solution.
4, $I_{K/Ca/}$ as a result of subtraction of traces 2 and 3 from 1.
$V_h$=-50 mV; $V_m$= 0 mV.

The example of such an experiment is shown in Fig. 3. After recording a total membrane current (trace 1), the external solution was changed for high-$K^+$ solution, where Na ions were replaced by K ions to make their concentration equal to intracellular content. In this solution clamping step from -50 mV to 0 mV resulted in a net $I_{Ca}$ (trace 2). Then the cell was returned to normal solution with Co ions (3 mM) added after recovery of the current to an initial level. In this solution the voltage-dependent component of $I_K$ could be recorded (trace 3). Subsequent subtraction of traces 2 and 3 from 1 resulted in a net $I_{K/Ca/}$ (trace 4). This current reached a maximum in 10 ms and then decayed with time course and magnitude comparable with $I_{Ca}$. Due to such relationship between these currents, any change in $I_{Ca}$ under physiological conditions

would be compensated by corresponding change in $I_{K/Ca/}$. As a result, the total membrane current would be unchanged. Thus, $I_{K/Ca/}$ can be considered as a factor of effective negative feed-back which exerts a stabilizing effect on excitation process.
In contrast to $I_{K/Ca/}$, a voltage-dependent $K^+$ current remaining after elimination of $I_{Ca}$ showed large variations in different cells. Like a net outward current, it displayed rather complex time course of inactivation with fast and slow components declined to a steady state level (Fig. 2). We were unable to separate these components pharmacologically.
The steady state inactivation curve reveals that 60% of the current is available at the resting potential of -50 mV and that holding the potential at -80 mV brings the availability close to 100% (Fig. 4). The rate of removal of $I_{K/V/}$ inactivation significantly varies in different cells. The process fits to a single exponential with a time constant from several tens to several hundreds of milliseconds. The rate of activation of the current

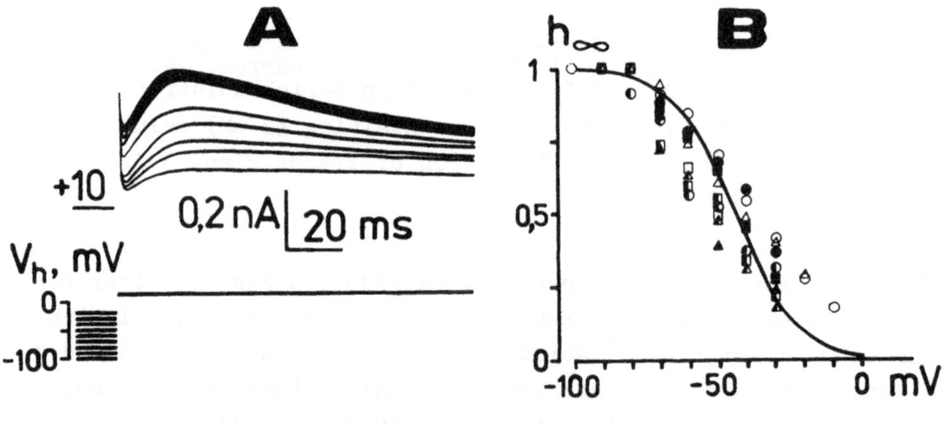


Figure 4. Steady state inactivation of voltage-dependent $K^+$current A, $I_{K/V/}$ recorded during voltage steps at different $V_h$ (as shown in bottom) to +10 mV. B, normalized currents plotted as a function of $V_h$. The curve was calculated by equation:

$$h_\infty = \frac{1}{1 + \exp(\frac{V+44}{10})}$$

is temperature-dependent and accelerates with increasing of clamp steps. Between 0 mV and +40 mV the activation process has a time constant of 5 - 14 ms at 36°C and 20 - 50 ms at 22°C.
We conclude that excitability in smooth muscle is regulated mainly by a voltage-dependent component of $I_K$ (11).

References


1. Shuba, M.F., V.A. Buryi. 1984. Fiziol. Zh. 30, N5, 545-557.
2. Vassort G. 1975. J. Physiol. 252, N3, 713-734.
3. Buryi, V.A. 1977. In: Physiology and Pharmacology of Smooth Muscle, Bulg. Acad. Sci., Sofia, 32-37.
4. Bury, V.A. 1979. In: Abstr. of papers of the 2nd inter. symp. "Physiology and pharmacology of smooth muscle", Varna, p.44.
5. Inomata, H., T. Mimata. 1983. In: Vascular Neuroeffector Mechanisms, 4 inter. Symp. (J.A. Bevan et al., eds.). Raven Press, New York. pp. 91-96.
6. Inomata, H., C.Y. Kao. 1976. J. Physiol. 255, N2, 347-378.
7. Buryi, V.A., A.V. Zholos, M.F. Shuba. 1986. Bull. Exp. Biol. Med. 3, pp. 270-273.
8. Hamill, O.P., A. Marty, E. Neher, B. Sakmann, F. Sigworth. 1981. Pflügers Arch. 391, pp. 85-100.
9. Meech, R.W., N.B. Standen. 1975. J. Physiol. 249, 211-239.
10. Ganitkevich, V.Ja., S.V. Smirnov, M.F. Shuba. 1985. Biol. Membrany. 2, N12, pp. 1225-1234.
11. Zholos, A.V., Buryi, V.A., M.F. Shuba. 1986. Biol. Membrany. 3, N8, pp. 807-814.

# PURIFICATION AND PROPERTIES OF THE TTX-SENSITIVE PROTEIN FROM BOVINE BRAIN SOLUBLE FRACTION

V.K.Lishko, V.A.Zhukareva

Department of neurochemistry, A.V.Palladin Institute of Biochemistry, Kiev, USSR

M.K.Malysheva

Department of Neurochemistry, A.A.Bogomoletz Institute of Physiology, Kiev, USSR

## Introduction

It was shown previously (I) that the cytoplasmic fraction of excitable tissues contains a specific hydrophilic protein with a channel forming activity. It was demonstrated that this protein induced in liposomes sodium selective pore activated by veratridine and inhibited by tetrodotoxin (TTX). It was appeared (2) that effect of TTX could be obtained even in absence of veratridine. Half-maximal effect was obtained approximately at 5-6 nM TTX. This value is very close to the effective TTX concentration in the experiments with the nerve cells. The most intriguing fact was the ability of the TTX-sensitive protein (TTX-P) to incorporate into liposomic membrane spontaneously without detergent or any other influences disturbing the phospholipid bilayer. It was shown that the penetration of TTX-P into phospholipid membrane is a vectorial process that results in determined orientation of TTX-sensitive pore.

In view of high specificity to TTX and Na-selectivity we had suggested that TTX-P was concerned to the voltage-dependent sodium channels beeing a precursor of its subunits or a product of its degradation. In this presentation we describe the purification of TTX-P from calf brain and some of its properties.

Results

To study the influence of TTX-P on the $^{22}Na$ permeability the liposomes prepared by ultrasonication of brain phospholipids suspension with cholesterol (20% w/w), have been used (2). Brain phospholipids were obtained as described in (2). $^{22}Na$ and TTX were included in the medium during sonication. $^{22}Na$ out-flux from the liposomes was studied using dialysis technique (I). TTX-P activity was estimated as a protein-phospholipid ratio that caused half-maximum increase in the sodium permeability of the liposomes. To induce the TTX-sensitive channel the liposomes were preincubated with TTX-P for 2 h at 4°C in buffer I containing 0,25 M sucrose, 40 mM imidazole-HCl, pH 7,4, I0 mM NaCl, 0,2 mM EDTA. For sodium dodecyl sulfate polyacrylamide gel electrophoresis the samples were boiled in 2% SDS plus 5% 2-mercaptoethanol. Electrophoresis was based on the method of Laemmly (3) using 3% stacking gel and 6-I0% running gel. For the analysis of native proteins a running gel with a linear 3-I2% acrylamide gradient was used.

The purification of TTX-P was carried out according to the following protocol.

Grey matter of calf brain (500 g) was homogenized in the 750 ml of the buffer I containing the protease inhibitors; 0,I mM phenylmethyl-sulphonyl fluoride, I μM pepstatin, I mM iodoacetamide, I mM O-phenanthroline. Homogenate was centrifuged for I hr at I50 000 x g.

To the supernatant I20 ml of the swollen DEAE-servacel 23SH, equilibrated in 40 mM imidazole buffer, pH 7,4 was added. After 30 min ion-exchanger was removed by centrifugation. As was published earlier (4) the TTX-P was eluted from DEAE-servacel between NaCl concentration from 0,I5-0,3 M, pH 7,4. To the protein fraction, desorbed from DEAE-servacel NaCl was added to final concentration of 0,4 M. This solution was passed through the WGA-Sepharose 4B column (I,0 x I5 cm), equilibrated by 0,4 M NaCl, 20 mM imidazole, pH 7,4. The flow rate was 90 ml/h. Almost all channel forming activity was bound and eluted by the same solution but containing 20 mM N-acetylglucosamine. The rate of elution was 30 ml/h. Fractions with maximal protein concentration were combined.

At this point of purification molecular weight of the proteins have been measured. Analysis of the native proteins by gradient gel electrophoresis shows three bands of 700 kDa, 350 kDa and 200 kDa. It was demonstrated that channel forming activity was connected with the two last bands. Previously these proteins have formed aggregates because after boiling in detergent in the presence of 5% mercaptoethanol one protein fraction with a molecular weight around 55000 could be seen only. The high molecular weight aggregates were isolated on Sepharose 4B column. 4 ml of the active fraction (protein concentration 7 mg/ml) collected after affinity chromatography were passed through Sepharose 4B column (I,7 x 50 cm) equilibrated by 0,25 M NaCl, 20 mM imidazole, pH 7,4.

The results of purification are summarised in Table I.

Table I. Purification of TTX-sensitive protein from grey matter of calf brain.

| Step | Protein | | TTX-sensitive activity |
|---|---|---|---|
| | mg | % | µg protein/mg lipid |
| Soluble cytoplasmic fraction | 6600 | I00 | 40 |
| DEAE-Servacel, 23 SH | 800 | I2 | 5 |
| WGA-Sepharose 4B | 7 | 0,I | 0,5 |
| Sepharose 4B | 5 | 0,07 | - |

Fig. I demonstrates a typical experiment showing functional activity of purified TTX-P. It was shown previously (2) that sodium flux throught proteoliposome membrane was affected only by intravesicular TTX. Fig. I shows the rate of $^{22}Na$ outflux from the liposomes modified with TTX-P (0,5 µg protein/ mg lipid) in the presence of TTX. These data indicate that TTX immobilized in the vesicles decreased Na outflux from proteoliposomes till the value of control liposomes.

Purified TTX-P was used to study the binding of $[^3H]$-TTX with the soluble and liposome integrated form of the protein. Toxin binding assay was carried out by rapid gel filtration procedure described by Levinson et al. (5). The protein or proteolipo-

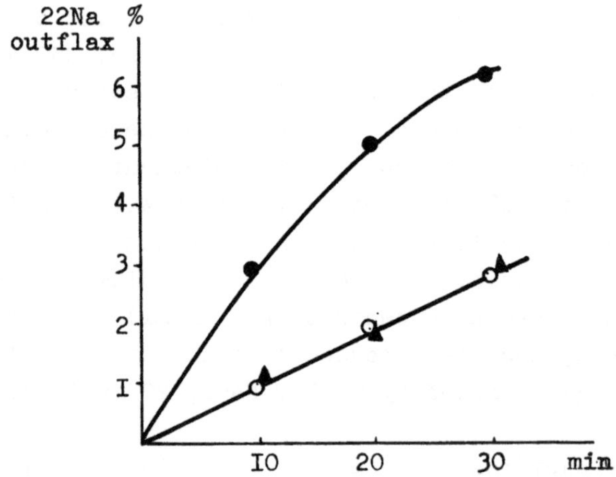


Fig I. Effect of TTX on $^{22}$Na outflux from the proteoliposomes.

-o- liposomes
-●- proteoliposomes
-▲- proteoliposomes containing IOO nM TTX

somes dissolved in I% Lubrol WX were incubated with I70 nM/L [$^3$H]-TTX (specific activity 8 Ci/mM) with or without 5 $\mu$M unlabeled toxin at 4$^\circ$C for 60 min. The aliquots (50 $\mu$l) were centrifuged for 30 s in plastic 0,5 ml columns containing 60 mg swollen Sephadex G-50. Nonspecific binding was determined in the presence of excess of unlabeled toxin and subtracted from total binding. Radioactivity of the samples was measured in Rack Beta liquid scintillation counter (LKB).

Fig. 2 shows that neither soluble TTX-P nor liposomes have bound [$^3$H]-TTX. TTX binding activity has been demonstrated in the Lubrol solution of the proteoliposomes modified by TTX-P. The value of TTX-binding was 200 pmol of TTX/mg protein. A further series of experiments aimed to compare antigenic determinants of TTX-P and nerve cell membranes were carried out using ELISA test and rabbit anti-TTX-P-antisera.

Fig.3 demonstrates the interaction of antibodies to TTX-P with brain synaptosomal membranes and neuroblastoma cells. The

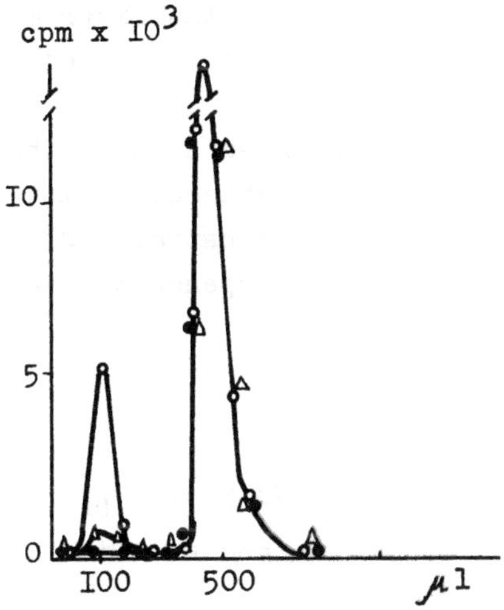


Fig. 2. Binding of [$^3$H]-TTX to the soluble TTX-P (-•-), liposomes (-Δ-) and proteoliposomes (-o-); peak I shows the radioactivity of lipid and protein fraction; peak 2 - free [$^3$H]-TTX.

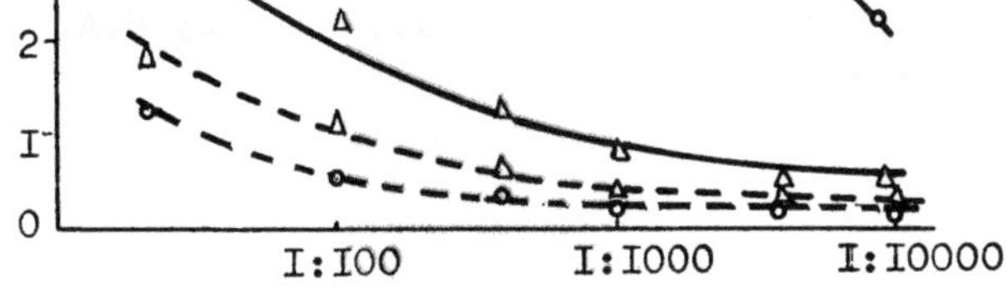


Fig. 3. Titration of antigens by anti-TTX-P-antisera.
Antigen used: -o-o- brain membranes
-Δ-Δ- liver membranes
Serum used: dotted line - intact rabbits, continuous line- TTX-P immunized rabbits

binding of antibodies was not observed with the liver membranes. These data suggest that TTX-P and nerve cell membranes have common antigen determinants.

In conclusion the data we have reported support the view that in nerve cell cytoplasma there is a channel forming TTX-sensitive protein. It can be isolated and demonstrates some properties that are inherent in sodium voltage-dependent channel.

Acknowledgement

We thank Dr. Grishin E.V. for providing $[^3H]$-TTX, Dr. Kolchinskaya L.I. for providing rabbit antiserum and Dr. Pinchuk J.V. for help in ELISA testing.

References

I. Malysheva M.K., Stefanov A.V., Chagovetz A.M., Lishko V.K. I982. Biochim. et Biophys.Acta. 688, 246.

2. Malysheva M.K., Lishko V.K., Zhukareva V.A., Lysenko V.V. I984. Neurophysiology. I6, 7I6.

3. Laemmly U.K. I970. Nature. 227, 688.

4. Lishko V.K., Malysheva M.K., Stefanov A.V., Chagovetz A.M. I982. In: Chemistry of Peptides and Proteins (W.Voelter et al., eds.). Berlin; New York: Walter de Gruyter & Co., 93.

5. Levinson S.R., Curatalo C.J., Reed J., Raftery M.A. I979. Anal.Biochem. I, 72.

# PROPERTIES OF RECEPTOR-OPERATED CALCIUM CHANNELS IN PLATELETS

P.V. Avdonin and V.A. Tkachuk
USSR Cardiology Research Center, Moscow 121552, USSR

## Introduction

The effects of multiple hormones and other biologically active substances on cells are mediated by a rise of cytoplasmic free calcium concentration ( $[Ca^{2+}]_i$) (1). The receptor-activated mobilization is mediated by a product of polyphosphoinositide metabolism, namely inositoltrisphosphate (2). However, the mechanism whereby the agonist binding to a receptor stimulates the transport of exogeneous calcium to the cytoplasm remains obscure. Moreover even the existence of a receptor-activated calcium current through the plasma membrane is disputed (1). In this study carried out on human platelets we have proved the existence of a receptor-operated calcium current through the plasma membrane and described its regulation by second messengers and pharmacological preparations.

## Methods

Human platelets separation, loading them with quin 2 and fluorescence measurements were performed as in (3). $^{45}Ca^{2+}$ uptake was determined according to (4). Platelet membrane isolation and measuring of GTPase activity were performed as in (5).

## Results

We have used two approaches to find out whether agonists can activate calcium current through the plasma membrane: namely, determined $^{45}Ca$ binding by cells and measured the concentration of $Ca^{2+}$ in the cytoplasm using quin 2. As is known, quin 2 is

Receptors and Ion Channels

accumulated in the cytoplasm creating a substantial additional buffer volume for $Ca^{2+}$. Therefore, if $^{45}Ca^{2+}$ actually penetrates in the cytoplasm, its incorporation by the quin 2-loaded cells must substantially exceed that of control cells. Indeed Fig.1 shows that PAF dramatically activates the incorporation of $^{45}Ca$ by platelets loaded with quin 2 whereas the same effect on control

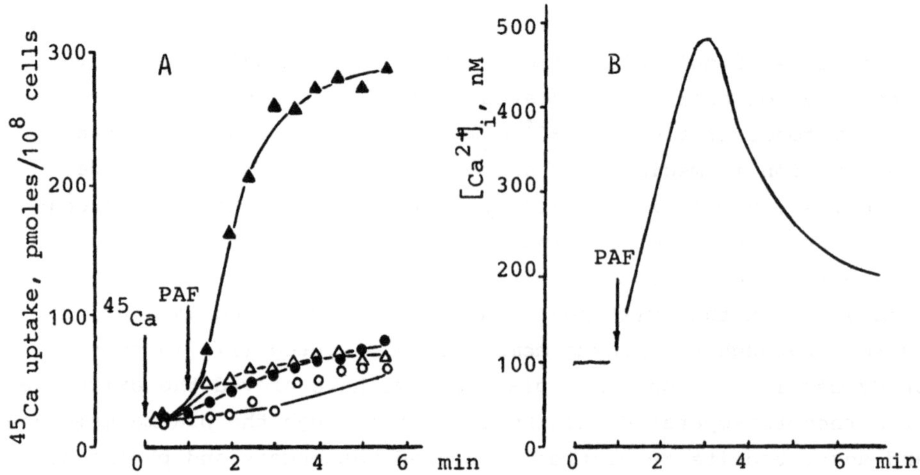


Fig.1. A. $^{45}Ca^{2+}$ uptake by control (o-o, △ - △) and quin 2-loaded (●-●, ▲ - ▲) platelets in the absence (o-o, ●-●) and presence (△ - △, ▲ - ▲) of $10^{-7}$ M PAF. B. PAF effect on $[Ca^{2+}]_i$ in quin 2-loaded platelets. $Ca^{2+}$ concentration in the medium was $10^{-4}$ M, intracellular quin 2 concentration was near 2 mM. $[Ca^{2+}]_i$ was calculated using the equation proposed in (6).

cells is much less marked. In the absence of agonists, however, quin 2 loading had no effects on $^{45}Ca$ binding by platelets. Simultaneously, the alterations in $[Ca^{2+}]$i occuring in response to PAF were registered by the quin 2 fluorescence on the identical experimental conditions (Fig.1B). The kinetics of $[Ca^{2+}]_i$ increase well correlates with the kinetics of $^{45}Ca$ incorporation. Thus, the obtained data demonstrate that PAF activates calcium current through the plasma membrane. The same effect is exerted by thrombin (4) and prostaglandin endoperoxide $H_2$ analogue U46619 (data not shown). What is the mechanism whereby the agonists stimulate $Ca^{2+}$ transport into platelets? The available evidence indicates that the receptor-mediated inflow of $Ca^{2+}$ is unrelated to activation of the potential-activated channels since depolarisation of platelet membrane by KCl doesn't increase $[Ca^{2+}]_i$ measured by quin 2, in the first place, and, secondly, the agonists do not have any substantial impact on the membrane potential (7,8). The sodium-calcium exchange can be also ruled out inasmuch neither a rise in the intracellular sodium concentration resulting from the inhibition of $Na^+,K^+$-ATPase by ouabain nor elevated sodium concentration in the surrounding medium affect $[Ca^{2+}]_i$ (7,8). Proceeding from these findings, one may conclude that in this case we are dealing with the third mechanism whereby $Ca^{2+}$ penetrates inside cells which is conventially termed receptor-operated calcium channels (ROCs) (9). Naturally, this term is rather tentative since we know nothing about the way of receptor coupling with putative channels and the structure of these channels.

However, there is additional evidence indicating that such channels actually exist. It was found that PAF and other agonists also stimulate the transport of other cations ($Mn^{2+}$ and $Ba^{2+}$) into platelets (4,10) (Fig.2). $Mn^{2+}$ possessing a higher affinity to quin 2 than $Ca^{2+}$supersedes and reduces the fluorescence, whereas $Ba^{2+}$ similarly to $Ca^{2+}$ increases the fluorescence of quin 2 (Fig.2). As is shown below, one and the same factors block the agonist-induced transport of all cations into platelets which proves that $Ca^{2+}$, $Ba^{2+}$ and $Mn^{2+}$ flow into platelets goes by the same pathway.

Regulation of receptor-operated channels by secondary messengers.

Fig.1 shows that the period of agonist-induced $Ca^{2+}$ transport into platelets is rather brief. This finding cannot be explained by the establishment of an equilibrium since the transmembrane gradient of $Ca^{2+}$ remains sufficiently high while the membrane potential is unaltered (7,8). Consequently there must be a mechanism for closing the ROCs. We assumed that the channel inactivation occurs via negative feedback mechanism. Second messengers appearing in the cytoplasm during the activation of receptors may serve as a signal. Along with $[Ca^{2+}]_i$ increase, platelet activators induce polyphosphoinositide hydrolysis leading to diacylglycerol formation. Protein kinase C (PK-C) serves as a target for it as well as for $Ca^{2+}$ (11,12). To determine the effect of PK-C on the ROCs we used a diacylglycerol analogue 4β-phorbol-12β-myristate-13α-acetate (PMA). As it was shown earlier, PMA taken in the concentrations

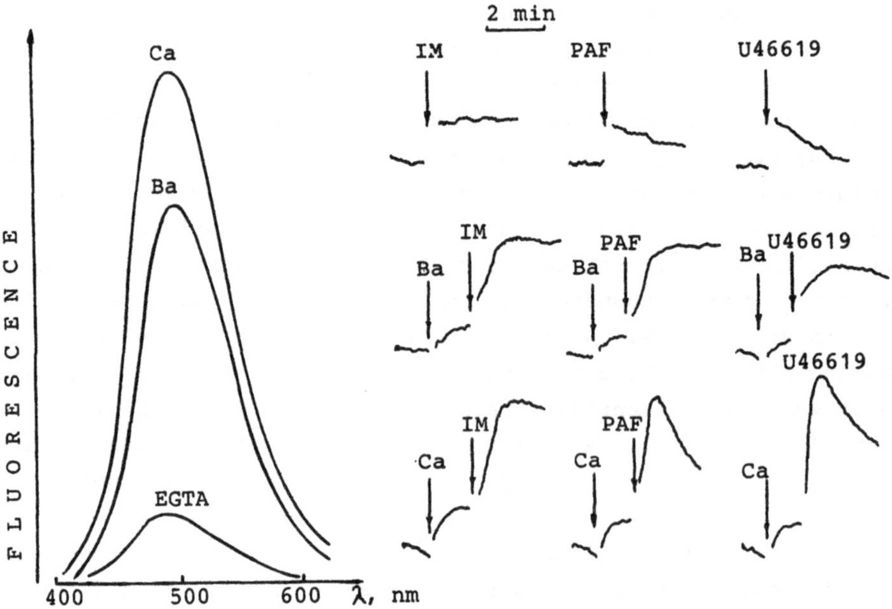


Fig.2. Effects of $Ca^{2+}$ and $Ba^{2+}$ on the fluorescence of quin 2. The fluorescence of a bivalent cation-free quin 2 was determined in the presence of 0.1 mM EGTA. The concentrations of quin 2, $CaCl_2$ and $BaCl_2$ were $10^{-4}$, $2x10^{-4}$ and $2x10^{-4}$M, respectively. Excitation wavelength was 340 nm. At the right fluorescence changes of quin 2-loaded platelets are shown in the medium with 5 mM $BaCl_2$, 1 mM $CaCl_2$ or without these bivalent cations in response to $5x10^{-7}$M ionomicin (IM), $10^{-7}$M PAF and $10^{-7}$M U46619.

stimulating endogeneous PK-C ($10^{-10}$-$10^{-8}$g/ml) inhibits the agonist-induced $[Ca^{2+}]_i$ increase (3). The effect of phorbol ester is explained by inactivation of the ROCs since it completely blocks the agonist-induced incorporation of $^{45}Ca$ (3) and current of $Ba^{2+}$ and $Mn^{2+}$ into platelets (Fig.3).

In what way does PK-C inactivate ROCs? As is known its substrate in plasma membrane is represented by a protein with molecular weight of about 40 kD (13). This protein has not been identified. However, it is assumed that it is actually an α-subunit of the GTP-binding protein transmitting signals from receptors through the plasma membrane (14). There are several types of membrane GTP-binding proteins with different α-subunits (15). All these subunits are characterized by the presence of a receptor-mediated high-affinity GTPase activity. PAF and other platelet activators also increase the activity of membrane GTPase (5,16,17). Therefore, if the $\alpha$-subunit coupled with the agonist receptors serves as a substrate for PK-C, one would expect to find a PMA effect on its GTPase activity. Indeed, the PAF-sensitive GTPase was inactivated in platelet membranes isolated after preincubation of platelets with PMA (Table 1). Contrarywise, the GTPase sensitive to $PGE_1$

Table 1. The Influence of PMA on Agonist-activated High-affinity GTP-ase of Human Platelet Plasma Membranes.
* $p < 0.01$

| | GTPase, pmol Pi/min/mg protein | |
|---|---|---|
| | Control | Preincubation with $10^{-6}$M PMA |
| without additions | 24.1±0.5 (3) | 23.9±0.4 (3) |
| $10^{-7}$M PAF | 30.9±0.6* (3) | 24.5±0.7 (3) |
| $10^{-5}$M $PGE_1$ | 29.4±0.6* (3) | 29.2±1.2* (3) |

belonging to the $\alpha$-subunit of another type remains unchanged. The obtained data corroborate the hypothesis that PK-C phosphorylates an $\alpha$-subunit of the GTP-binding protein. Further studies are required to determine the exact type of this subunit ($\alpha_i$ or $\alpha_o$). However, the available evidence indicates that it participates in the process of receptor coupling with calcium channels.
cAMP is another intracellular factor inhibiting an increase in $[Ca^{2+}]_i$ in response to aggregation inducers (4,8,18). According to some hypothesis this effect results from a calcium pump activation (18) though our data indicate that the cAMP effect is primarily related to blocking of the ROCs (Fig.3).
Effects of verapamil, nicardipine and calcium antagonists on the receptor-operated channels for bivalent cations. Since the ROCs perform an essential function playing important role in hormonal effects, we decided to find out whether these channels can be regulated by number of pharmacological preparations: potential-activated calcium channel blockers verapamil and nicardipine, calcium antagonists (chlorpromazine, (+)- and (-)-butaclamol (19)

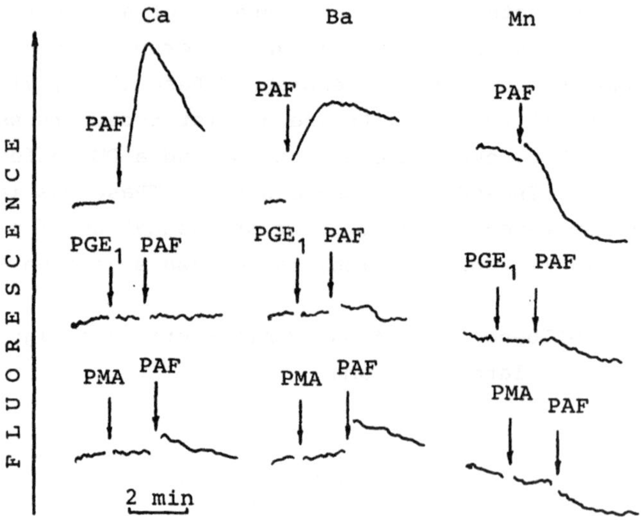


Fig.3. Blocking of $10^{-7}$M PAF-induced rise in $[Ca^{2+}]_i$ as well as $Ba^{2+}$ and $Mn^{2+}$ entry by $10^{-5}$M $PGE_1$ and $10^{-7}$M PMA.

and benzodiazepine receptor blockers: clonazepam, flunitrozepam and Ro5-4864, possessing anticalmodulin activity (20) ). Verapamil and nicardipine inhibit the PAF-induced $[Ca^{2+}]_i$ increase with $ED_{50}$ 3 and 1 µM respectively (Fig.4). Their action is directed at the ROCs since the same concentrations of these compounds block the inflow of $Ba^{2+}$ (Fig.5) though nicardipine also inhibits mobilization of the intracellular $Ca^{2+}$. It turned out that calmodulin blockers also inhibit the agonist-induced $[Ca^{2+}]_i$ increase in response to PAF (Table 2). The effect of verapamil, nicardipine and calcium antagonists are not specific with respect to PAF. They can be also seen in the presence of other inducers (data not shown). Since the main contribution into the $[Ca^{2+}]_i$ rise stimulated by this inducer is attributed to the exogeneous $Ca^{2+}$, one may conclude that calcium antagonists inhibit the activity of ROCs. Their action cannot be explained by phosphodiesterase inhibition since the cAMP level remained unchanged (data not shown). It is possible that the ROCs contain a protein resembling calmodulin and affording a target for these compounds. The obtained data made it

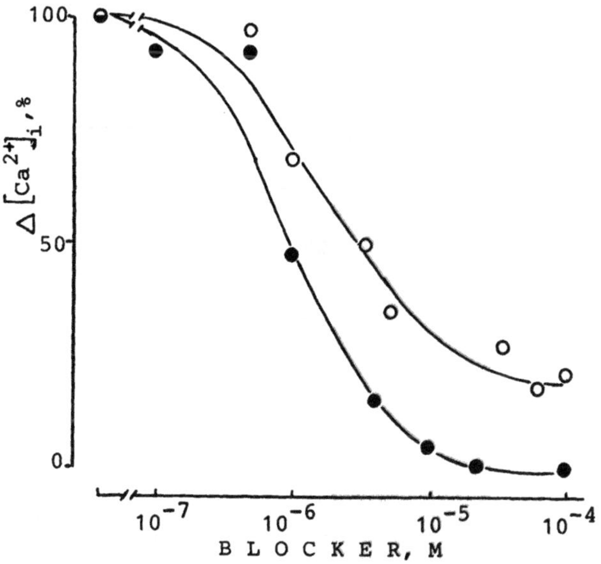


Fig.4. Blocking by verapamil (o-o) and nicardipine (●-●) of $3 \times 10^{-9}$M PAF-induced increase in $[Ca^{2+}]_i$. 100% corresponds to 330 nM.

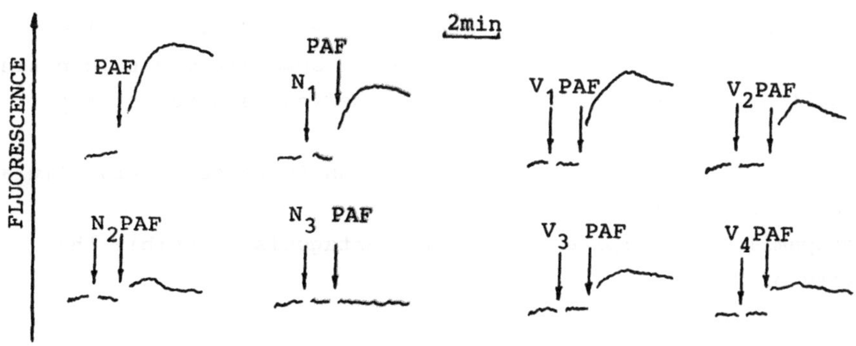


Fig.5. Blocking of $10^{-8}$M PAF-induced $Ba^{2+}$ entry by nicardipine ($N_1$ - $10^{-6}$M; $N_2$ - $2.5 \times 10^{-5}$M; $N_3$ - $5 \times 10^{-5}$M) and verapamil ($V_1$ - $10^{-6}$M; $V_2$ - $5 \times 10^{-6}$M; $V_3$ - $10^{-5}$M; $V_4$ - $10^{-4}$M).

Table 2. Blocking by Calcium Antagonists of PAF-induced Increase in $[Ca^{2+}]_i$.

| | $\Delta [Ca^{2+}]_i$, nM |
|---|---|
| $10^{-8}$M PAF | 680 |
| +$10^{-4}$M chlorpromazine | 165 |
| +$2.5x10^{5}$M Ro5-4864 | 360 |
| +$10^{-4}$M Ro5-4864 | 35 |
| +$10^{-4}$M clonazepam | 210 |
| +$10^{-4}$M flunitrozepam | 320 |
| +$10^{-5}$M (-)-butaclamol | 232 |
| +$10^{-4}$M (-)-butaclamol | 20 |
| +$10^{-4}$M (+)-butaclamol | 42 |

possible to arrive at the following conclusions.

1. PAF and other agonists activate the transport of $Ca^{2+}$, $Ba^{2+}$ and $Mn^{2+}$ ions into human platelets. It is assumed that these ions penetrate inside cells via specific ROCs. When platelets are saturated with quin 2, this pathway makes the major contribution to the $[Ca^{2+}]_i$ rise occuring in response to agonists.

2. Inactivation of the ROCs is performed by PK-C via negative feedback mechanism. A GTP-binding protein apparently participating in coupling of receptors with channels serves as a target for PK-C.

3. The ROCs in platelets are blocked by an increased intracellular concentration of cAMP.

4. Verapamil, nicardipine and calcium antagonists inhibit the activity of ROCs.

References


1. Gill, D.L. 1985. In: Cyclic Nucleotide and Prot.Phosphorylation Res., Vol. 19 (D.M.F.Cooper and K.B.Seamon, eds.). Raven Press, New York, p.307-324.

2. Berridge, M.J. 1984. Biochem.J. 220, 345-360.

3. Avdonin, P.V. and Altukhova, I.P. 1985. Biochemistry (USSR) 50, 1049-1054.

4. Avdonin, P.V., Boogry, M.E., Cheglakov, I.B., Mazaev, A.V.

and Tkachuk, V.A. 1986. DAN SSSR 289, 220-224.

5. Avdonin, P.V., Svitina-Ulitina, I.V. and Kulikov, V.I. 1985. Biochem.Biophys.Res.Commun. 131, 307-313.

6. Tsien, R.J., Pozzan, T. and Rink, T.J. 1982. J.Cell.Biol. 94, 325-334.

7. Doyle, V.M. and Ruegg, U.T. 1985. Biochem.Biophys.Res.Commun. 127, 161-167.

8. Avdonin, P.V., Men'shikov, M.Yu., Orlov, S.N., Pokudin, N.I. and Tkachuk, V.A. 1985. Biochemistry (USSR) 50, 1055-1062.

9. Berridge, M.J. 1982. In: Handbook of Experimental Pharmacology, vol. 58, pt.II (J.W.Kebabian and J.A.Nathanson, eds.). Springer-Verlag, Berlin, Heidelberg, New York. pp.227-270.

10. Hallam, T.J. and Rink, T.J. 1985. FEBS Lett. 186, 176-179.

11. Kikkawa, U., Takai, Y., Tanaka, Y., Miyake, R. and Nishizuka. 1983. J.Biol.Chem. 258, 11442-11445.

12. Rink, T.J. and Hallam, T.J. 1984. Trends Biochem.Sci. 9, 215-219.

13. Takai, Y., Kaibuchi, K., Matsubara, T. and Nishizuka, J. 1981. Biochem.Biophys.Res.Commun. 101, 61-67.

14. Katada, T., Gilman, A.G., Watanabe, J., Bauer, S. and Jakobs, K.H. 1985. Eur.J.Biochem. 151, 431-437.

15. Gilman, A.G. 1984. Cell 36, 577-579.

16. Aktories, K. and Jakobs, K.H. 1981. FEBS Lett. 130, 235-238.

17. Avdonin, P.V., Svitina-Ulitina, I.V., Leytin, V.L. and Tkachuk, V.A. 1985. Thromb.Res. 40, 101-112.

18. Zavoico, G.B. and Feinstein, M.B. 1984. Biochem.Biophys.Res. Commun. 120, 579-585.

19. Triggle, D.J. 1982. In: Calcium Blockers (S.F.Flaim and R.Zelis, eds.). Urban and Schwarzenberg, Baltimore, Munich. pp.121-134.

20. Baldenkov, G.N., Men'shikov, M.Yu. and Tkachuk, V.A. Biochemistry (USSR) (in press).

# III SECOND MESSENGER SYSTEMS

# ISOLATION, PHYSICO-CHEMICAL PROPERTIES AND RECONSTITUTION OF THE COMPONENTS OF ADENYLATE CYCLASE SYSTEM

V.L. Voeikov, V.Z. Slepak, I.P. Udovichenko
Moscow State University, Faculty of Biology, Moscow

## Introduction

Adenylate cyclase system is a multicomponent membrane system which consists of specific receptors recognizing extracellular chemical signals, GTP-binding regulatory proteins, $G_s$ and $G_i$, and the catalytic component. Hormone-receptor complex interacts with the respective G-protein, one of which ($G_s$) stimulates, and another ($G_i$) mediates inhibition of adenylate cyclase (AC). Many details of the mechanism of transmembrane signal transmission have been recently clarified due to isolation, structural analysis and reconstitution of β-adrenergic receptors (β-AR), G-proteins and AC (e.g. 1-3).

However the general picture of chemical signal transmission is far from being clear. It is now evident that G-protein family includes other members besides $G_s$ and $G_i$ (4), and that they are able to modulate not only AC but other effector protein activity (5). It also turnes out that hormone receptors are multifunctional proteins: at least some of them posess enzyme activity (6). This report focuses on some novel properties of β-AR and a G-protein isolated from bovine cerebellum.

## Results and Discussion

We have isolated some representatives of G-protein family, namely, $G_s$, β-subunit of G-proteins, and a low $K_m$ GTPase with the molecule weight 39 kD (P39) from bovine cerebellum. A similar protein has been recently isolated from bovine brain and has been referred to as $G_o$ (7).

Receptors and Ion Channels

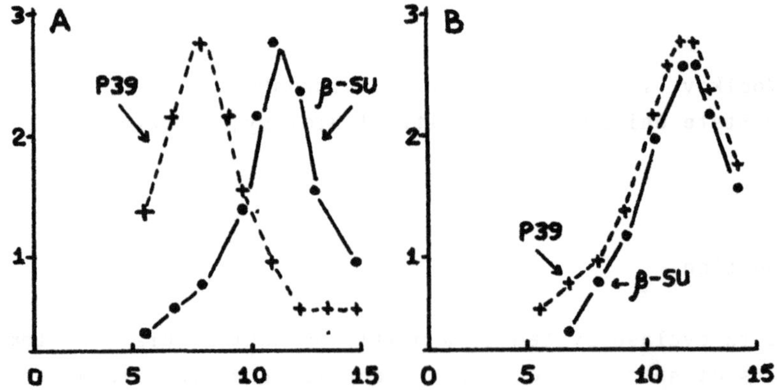


Fig. 1. Chromatography of the 1:1 mixture of pure P39 and β-subunit on heptylamine-Sepharose in the presence of GppNHp $10^{-4}$ (A) or in the absence of nucleotides (B). Abscissa-fraction number, ordinate-protein concentration, arbitrary units.

Our method of isolation of this protein differs from those generally used by others in some details, particularly in the test procedure. Fractions at different stages of purification were tested for GTPase rather then for GTP-binding activity. After the final stage of purification, chromatography on $G_7$-Sepharose, three main entities have been obtained: a low $K_m$ GTPase (P39), pure β-subunit of G-proteins and a fraction with $G_s$ activity. In order to test if P39 can interact with the β-subunit we studied the behaviour of their mixture on $G_7$-Sepharose (Fig. 1).

In the presence of guanyl-5'-yl-imidodiphosphate (GppNHp) the two proteins eluted from the gel independently, and in its absence they coeluted. Hence P39 like other subunits of G-proteins can bind β-subunit in the absence of a guanine nucleotide. Fig. 2 summarises the effects of β-subunit and $Mg^{2+}$ ions on GTPase activity of P39. While in the presence of β-subunit $Mg^{2+}$ did not affect GTPase activity of P39, in the absence of β-subunit $Mg^{2+}$ reduced $V_m$ and raised $K_m$ for GTP. β-Subunit lowed $K_m$ for GTP irrespective of $Mg^{2+}$. β-Subunit affects $G_o$ ability to bind guanine nucleotide in the opposite manner (7). Using rabbit polyclonal antibodies against P39 we studied its distribution in several biological tissues. P39 - Immunoreactive material was detected only in human and animal nervous

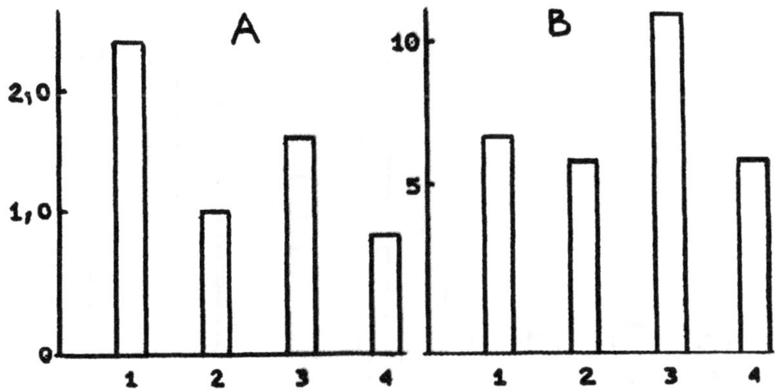


Fig. 2. Effect of $Mg^{2+}$, 5 mM (Bars 1 and 2) and β-subunit (Bars 2 and 4) on the GTPase activity of P39. A - effect on $K_m$ (value$\cdot 10^{-7}$ M), B - effect on $V_{max}$ (value$\cdot 10^{-8}$ mol/mg/hr).

tissues but not in several other tissues. The absence of P39 in rat reticulocyte membranes allowed to use these membranes for the study of P39 effects on β-AR dependent AC system. Fig. 3 demonstrates that P39 enhances AC stimulation by GTP. However absolute activity of AC stimulated by the β-agonist, isoproterenol (Iso), in the presence of GTP is attenuated by P39. Taking into consideration that P39 raises the basal activity of AC, fold stimulation of this enzyme by hormone is depressed from 11-12-fold to 4,5-fold. β-Subunit eliminated all P39 effects. It is interesting to note in this connection that AC in brain is characterized by high basal activity and low sensitivity to hormone stimulation. Thus addition of P39 to rat reticulocyte membranes makes their AC system more brain-like.

β-AR is another component of AC system which for a long time attracts attention of many investigators. We have developed a method for the preparative isolation of electrophoretically homogeneous β-AR from bovine cerebellum. β-AR was solubilized from cerebellum membranes with lauroyl sucrose (8) and purified using the novel affinity support, oxprenolol-Sepharose (9). The yield of the purified receptor was 18-23%. Its specific binding activity determined using β-antagonist, $|^3H|$ dihydroalprenolol ($|^3H|$ DHA), was 11,000 pmoles/mg protein. After SDS electophoresis only one protein band was revealed with the apparent molecular weight about 61 kD. The same band

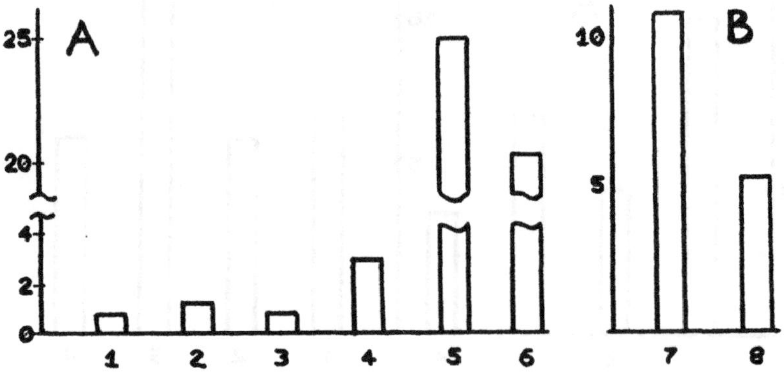


Fig. 3. Effect of P39 on GTP and Iso+GTP stimulation of AC in rat reticulocytes. A - AC activity, pmoles/mg/min; 1 - no additions; 3, 4, 6 - P39, 1 mg/ml; 2, 4 - GTP, $10^{-4}$ M; 5, 6 - Iso, $10^{-4}$ M + GTP, $10^{-4}$ M. B - Iso + GTP fold stimulation of AC; 7 - control; 8 - P39.

was identified after the photoaffinity labelling of the crude receptor preparation and by antibodies against the purified β-AR. Thus the method of purification allowed to obtain 10-15 nmoles of the electrophoretically pure β-AR beginning from 2-3 kg of the cerebellum grey matter. Purified β-AR and bovine brain were reconstituted into phospholipid vesicules and treated with GppNHp and the ligands of β-AR. Then the preparation of solubilized brain AC separated from endogeneous G-proteins was added into the reconstituted system and the enzyme activity was determined. After the treatment of proteoliposomes with Iso and GppNHp AC activity increased by 40-50%. β-Agonist, propranolol, abolished Iso effects. Hence the purified β-AR retains the ability for the functional interaction with $C_s$.

In the course of the development of the procedures for β-AR purification and reconstitution we noticed that some irreversible serine protease inhibitors decrease the radioligand binding to β-AR. This phenomenon was studied in more details. It turned out that $|^3H|$ DHA binding to β-AR was decreased after the membrane treatment with diisopropyl fluorophosphate (DFP) and phenylmethanesulphonyl fluoride (PMSF), which modify serine residues, and with Nα-p-tosyl-l-lysine chloromethyl ketone (TLCK), which modifies histidine residue in the active center of trypsin (Table 1). $|^3H|$ DHA binding to the recon-

Table 1. $|^3H|$-DHA Binding after the Treatment of the Preparation with an Inhibitor (% of the Respective Control)

| Preparation | Inhibitor | | | |
|---|---|---|---|---|
| | TLCK | TPCK | PMSF | DFP |
| Bovine cerebellum membranes | 73 | 100 | 79 | 92 |
| Reconstituted cerebellum receptor | 55 | 48 | 80 | 85 |
| Frog red cell membranes | 63 | 56 | N.D. | 100 |
| Intact frog red cells | 100 | 100 | 100 | 100 |

N.D. - not determined

stituted β-AR was inhibited by the same serine protease inhibitors to a greater extent and was severely depressed also by N-p-tosyl-l-phnylalanine chloromethyl ketone (TPCK), chymotrypsin inhibitor, which did not affect the membrane bound β-AR. Protease inhibitors did not affect β-AR binding properties in native erythrocytes. Thus the site of their action is likely to be faced into the cytoplasm.

As it is demonstrated in Table 2, protease inhibitors decrease β-AR affinity for both $|^3H|$ DHA and Iso not affecting $B_{max}$. It turns out that the affinity for the agonist is reduced much stronger than for the antagonist.

$|^3H|$ DFP labeled the purified β-AR reconstituted into phospholipid vesicules stochiometrically (about 1:1 mole/mole). Control experiments demonstrated that the labelling was specific. Prior incubation of the reconstituted β-AR with TLCK or Iso nearly completely abolished β-AR labelling with $|^3H|$ DFP (Fig. 4). Propranolol inhibited label incorporation to a lesser extent. The ability of serine protease inhibitors targeted at both serine and histidine residues of the active center to modify β-AR indicates that β-AR also poseses a specific site which is distinct from the binding site of the molecule.

Table. 2. Effect of TLCK on the Binding Parameters of β-AR

| Treatment | $|^3H|$ DHA | | Iso |
|---|---|---|---|
| | $K_d$ (M) | $B_{max}$ (pmol) | $K_d$ (M) |
| None | $2 \cdot 10^{-9}$ | 7.5 | $10^{-7}$ |
| TLCK, $10^{-4}$ M | $6 \cdot 10^{-9}$ | 7.3 | $10^{-6}$ |

This site may provide β-AR with some catalytic function, presumably a proteolytic one. In order to substantiate this supposition we compared the primary structure of bovine chymotrypsin and of the mammalian β-AR (2) Fig. 5 demonstrates that there are regions of significant homology between the two molecules in the viccinity of Asp-102 and His-57 constituting the active site of chymotrypsin, and the active Ser-195 of chymotrypsin even coinsides with

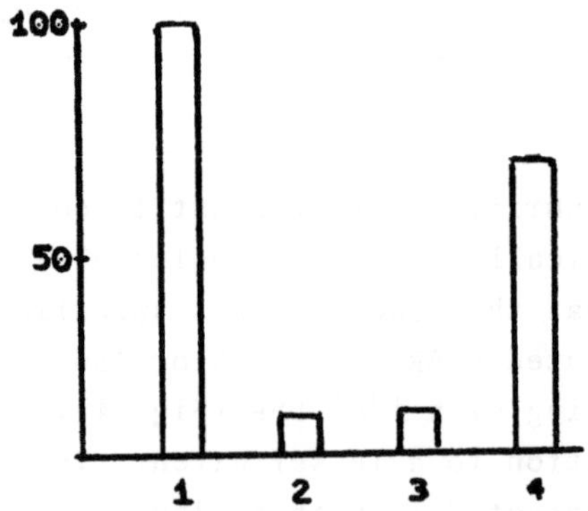


Fig. 4. $|^3H|$ DFP binding (B, % of the control) to reconstituted β-AR. 1 - control, 2 - PMSF, $10^{-4}$ M; 3 - Iso, $10^{-4}$ M, 4 - propranolol, $10^{-7}$ M.

| | | | | | | | | | | | | |
|---|---|---|---|---|---|---|---|---|---|---|---|---|
| β-AR | 399 | Val | Pro | Ser | Leu | Ser | Leu | Asp | Ser | Gln | Gly | |
| Chym | 188 | Val | Ser | Ser | Cys | Met | Gly | Asp | Ser | Gly | Gly | |
| | | | | | | | | | 195 | | | |
| β-AR | 140 | Lys | Tyr | Gln | Ser | Leu | Leu | Thr | Lys | Asn | Lys | Ala |
| Chym | 93 | Lys | Tyr | Asn | Ser | Leu | - | Thr | Ile | Asn | Asn | Asp |
| | | | | | | | | | | | | 102 |
| β-AR | 32 | Trp | Val | Val | Gly | Met | Ala | Ile | | | | |
| Chym | 51 | Trp | Val | Val | Thr | Ala | Ala | His | | | | |
| | | | | | | | | 57 | | | | |

Fig. 5. Regions of homology between β-AR (top line in each row) and bovine chymotrypsin A (bottom line). Coinsiding amino acid residues are underlined. Active site residues of chymotrypsin are numbered.

Ser-406 of the β-AR.

## Summary

Some representatives of the G-protein family and bovine cerebellum β-AR have been isolated and studied using reconstitution and other approaches. One of the isolated G-proteins (the molecule weight 39 kD) differs in several respects from those previously described. It interferes with the signal transmission in β-AR sensitive AC system. In the course of β-AR stidies data have been obtained which allow to suggest that β-AR may posess enzymatic, presumably proteolytic activity.

## References

1. Pfeuffer, E., R.-M. Dreher, H. Metzger, T. Pfeuffer. 1985. Proc. Nat. Acad. Sci. USA 82, 3086.

2. Dixon, R.A., B.K. Kobilka, D.-J. Strader, J.L. Benovic, H.G. Dohlman, T. Frielle, M.A. Bolanowski, C.D. Bennett, E. Rands, R.E. Deihl, R.A. Mumford, E.E. Slater, I.S. Sigal, M.G. Caron, R.J. Lefkowitz, C.D. Strader. 1986. Nature 321, 75.

3. Gilman, A.G. 1984. Cell 36, 577.

4. Neer, E.J., J.M. Lok, L.G. Wolf. 1984. J. Biol. Chem. 259, 14222.

5. Krause, K.H., W. Schlegel, C.B. Wollheim, T. Anderson, F.A. Waldvogel, P.D. Lew. 1985. J. Clin. Invest. 76, 1348.

6. Kasuga, M., F.A. Karlsson, C.R. Kahn. 1982. Science 215, 185.

7. Sternweis, P.C., J.D. Robinshaw. 1984. J. Biol. Chem. 259, 13806.

8. Hekman, M., D. Feder, A.K. Keenan, A. Gal, H.W. Klein, T. Pfeuffer, A. Levitzki, E.J.M. Helmreich. 1984. EMBO J. 3, 3339.

9. Voeikov, V.L., V.V. Gurevich, I.P. Udovichenko. 1984. Biol. Membrany 1, 65.

STRUCTURE OF CATALYTIC COMPONENT OF ADENYLATE CYCLASE SYSTEM REVEALED BY ELECTRON MICROSCOPY

V.V.Demin, A.V.Lunev, V.M.Lipkin, I.A.Kostonyan
Shemyakin Institute of Bioorganic Chemistry, USSR Academy of Sciences, Moskow 117871, USSR

## Introduction

Adenylate cyclase system of animals plays a key role in the mechanism of hormone regulation, it consists of at least three different components: hormone receptor, GTP-binding protein and adenylate cyclase or C-protein which converts ATP into cAMP. The catalytic component is still poorly studied. The C-protein is known to be an integral membrane protein, its single polypeptide chain has molecular mass ∿150 kDa (1). The present work is aimed at the electron microscopy study of the C-protein structure.

## Results

Adenylate cyclase was isolated from bovine brain cortex. The yield and enzyme activity of the protein at various stages of isolation are given in Table 1. To remove peripheral proteins, the membrane fraction obtained by the standard procedure (2) was treated with buffers containing 2 M NaCl and 1% digitonin. The membrane was solubilized with 10 mM zwitterion detergent CHAPS in 20 mM HEPES-Na buffer (pH 7.4). Additional purification was performed by DEAE-Sefacell chromatography. High hydrophobicity of adenylate cyclase allowed us to combine the ion-exchange and absorbtion chromatography: the protein was applied to the support and the column was washed with buffer containing 0.5 mM CHAPS + 3 M NaCl, then with the buffer containing 10 mM CHAPS. The enzyme was eluted with the buffer containing 10 mM CHAPS + 3 M NaCl. The final purification stage was HPLC on TSK-3,000. Electrophoresis in polyacrylamide gel in the presence of sodium dodecylsulfate showed that the preparation contained one polypeptide chain with molecular mass 150±10 kDa (Fig.1).

Receptors and Ion Channels

Table 1. Purification of Adenylate Cyclase From Bovine Brain Cortex

| Step | Specific* activity nM/mg·min | Total activity nM/min | Protein mg |
|---|---|---|---|
| Membranes | 0.1 | 1300 | 10000.0 |
| Membranes washed by 2M NaCl | 0.3 | 1300 | 4000.0 |
| Membranes washed by 1% digitonin | 0.7 | 1300 | 2000.0 |
| CHAPS extract | 0.7 | 1176 | 168.0 |
| DEAE-Sephacell chromatography | 330.0 | 578 | 1.8 |
| Precipitation by $(NH_4)_2SO_4$ | 80.0 | 102 | 1.3 |
| HPLC | 660.0 | 240 | 0.4 |

*Specific activity was measured in the presence of 100μM forskolinn(1).

The homogeneous C-protein effectively utilizes $Mn^{2+}$-ATP as a substrate (specific enzymatic activity ranges from 600 to 1,000 nM/mg·min).

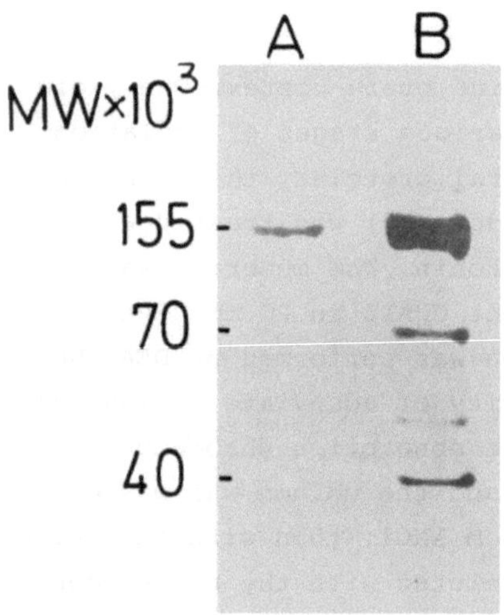


Fig.1. SDS-gel electrophoresis of bovine brain adenylate cyclase. A - adenylate cyclase; B - DNA dependet RNA-polymerase.

Specific enzymatic activity in case of $Mg^{2+}$-ATP is much lower (8-10 nM/mg·min), but it significantly increases (∿140 nM/mg·min) after reconstitution of the enzyme with purefifed GTP-binding protein in lipid membranes (1)(Table 2).

For electron microscopy analysis the isolated preparation of adenylate cyclase was reconstituted into plane membrane fragments by dialysis of 40 μl of the mixture of the solubilized protein (0.5 mg/ml) and azolectin (1-0.5 mg/ml) in the buffer containing 100 mM NaCl, 10 mM $MgCl_2$, 6 mM CHAPS against the detergent-free buffer.

Table 2. Response to Various Effectors of Purified Bovine Brain Adenylate Cyclase

| Effector* | Specific activity nM/mg.min | Stimulation % |
|---|---|---|
| $Mg^{2+}$ | 9 | - |
| $Mg^{2+}$ + NaF | 9 | - |
| $Mg^{2+}$ + NaF + GTP-binding protein | 140 | 1455 |
| $Mn^{2+}$ | 985 | - |
| $Mn^{2+}$ + NaF | 990 | 0.5 |
| $Mn^{2+}$ + calmodulin | 1325 | 34 |

*Effectors concentration: $Mg^{2+}$ - 15 mM, NaF - 10 mM, $Mn^{2+}$ - 10 mM, calmodulin - 4 μM. Reconstitution of GTP-binding protein performed as in (3).

Upon investigation of negatively stained membrane preparations the particles of 50-60 Å were found (Fig. 2 A,C,D). The structures of these particles were studied in detail by digital processing of their images including low-pass Fourier filtration (filtration radius 1/20 $Å^{-1}$) and cross-correlation analysis (4). Application of the cross-correlation function analysis allowed the identification of

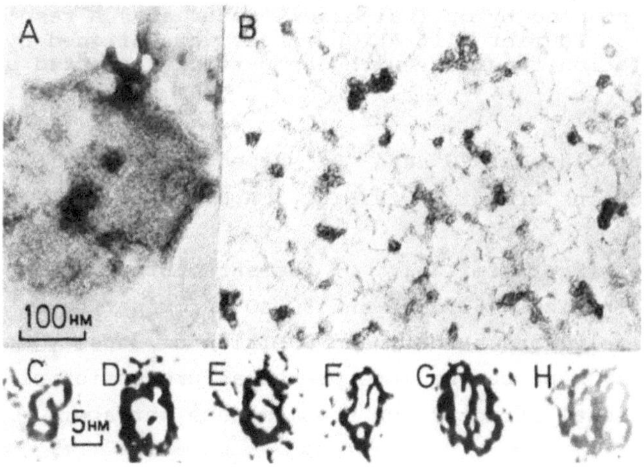


Fig. 2. Negatively stained adenylate cyclase: A,C,D - membrane reconstituted protein; B,E,F,G,H - solubilized protein.

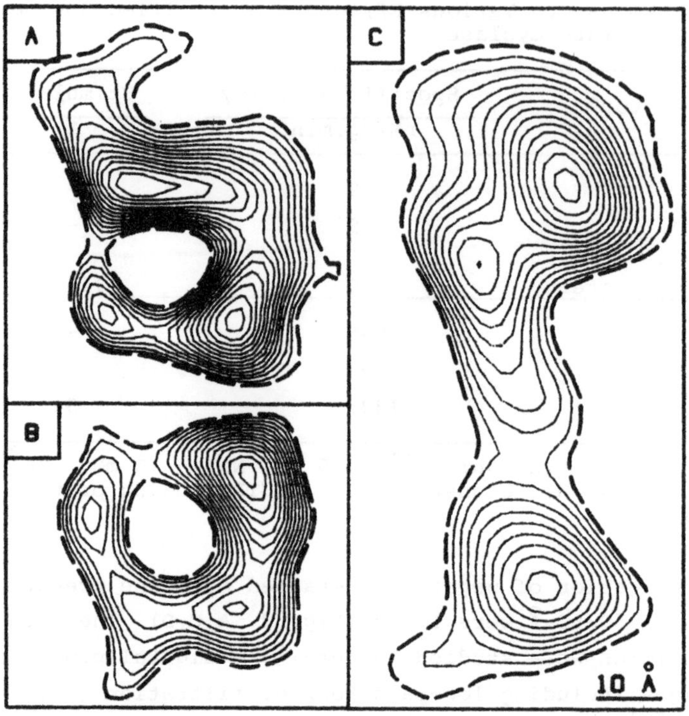


Fig. 3. Membrane (A,B) and side (C) projections of adenylate cyclase structure. Micrographs of small areas containing single particles were scanned by optical densitometer at 3 Å resolution. After low-pass Fourier filtration images were aligned by using the cross-correlation function, with one particle selected as a reference (3).

images of two classes: "C" and "L"-shaped particles (Fig. 2 C,D), their projections are given in Fig. 3 A,B.

Fig. 3 shows mirror similarity of the structures though they somewhat differ in sizes (60·50 Å and 50·40 Å for particles "C" and "L" respectively) and number, and position of density maxima. Obtained density maps can be interpreted as projection of protein three-dimensional structure on the membrane surface.

To identify other projections the negatively stained preparations of solubilized form of adenylate cyclase were investigated (Fig. 2 B, E, F, G, H). Several classes of repetitive structures were identified by means of digital processing of the images. Two of them - "C" and "L" - shaped particles - are identical to membrane projections. The others can be ascribed to tilted projections of the adenylate cyclase structure (Fig. 2 E,F). That also follows from their similarity to the structures obtained at the study of the tilted series of the membrane reconstituted preparations of the C-protein. One of projection found at the analyses of the solubilized protein has a rod shape (Fig. 2 G,H). Density map of rod (resolution 30 Å) obtained after the digital processing and statistic averaging is represented in Fig. 3C. The rod height is 100 Å. The rod ends dimensions (width of the upper part - 60 Å, width of the lower part - 45 Å) accord with the dimensions of membrane projections of the molecule. So, the rods, which are characteristic only for solubilized preparations, could be a side projection of the protein molecule.

Thus the electron microscopy study of the solubilized and membrane forms of the enzyme revealed three main projections of spatial adenylate cyclase structure: two membrane and one side projection. Existence of two membrane projections allows us to propose transmembrane character of the protein, which is in a good agreement with data obtained by Pfeuffer et al. (1). More over projection structure of adenylate cyclase rather similar to that of two transmembrane proteins: acetylcholine receptor (5) and fast sodium channel (6). So, we can conclude that "C" - and "L" - shaped particles are projections of adenylate cyclase structure on extra- and intracellular membrane surfaces.

Using the projection sizes we calculated the volume occupied by one protein particle and the corresponding molecular weight (specific protein volume - 1.3 $Å^3$/Da) (7). The calculated value of the molecular mass (110-170 kDa) is in a good accordance with that of the protein moiety of adenylate cyclase (1). The height of the molecule derived from its side projection considerably exceeds the usual thickness of the lipid bilayer that indicates the relatively small size of the membrane fragment of the molecule. This correlates with data on partial volumes of detergents bound to the protein which show that the hydrophobic area is small as compared to the hydrophilic regions (8,9). There are not direct evidences for the exact position of the membrane portion of the molecule. But similarity of the projection structures of adenylate cyclase with sodium channel and acetylcholine receptor allows one to suggest that intramembrane part of adenylate cyclase molecule located in its middle and most narrow part and significant parts of the polypeptide chain exposed at the both membrane surfaces.

References


1. Pfeuffer, E., S.Molner, T.Pfeuffer. 1985. EMBO J., 4, 3675.
2. Yeager, R.E., W.Heideman, G.B.Rosenberg, D.R.Storm. 1985. Biochemistry, 24, 3776.
3. Pfeuffer, T., B.Gaugler, H.Metzger. 1983. FEBS Lett., 164, 154.
4. Frank, J., A.Verschoor, M.Boublik. 1981. Science, 214, 1353.
5. Brisson, A., P.N.T. Unwin. 1985. Nature, 315, 474.
6. Ovchinnikov, Yu.A., V.V.Demin, E.V.Gfishin, S.N.Spadar. 1985. Biol. Membranes, 2, 957.
7. Henderson, R., P.N.T.Unwin. 1975. Nature, 257, 28.
8. Wahrmann, S.P., F.Gros, J.P.Pian, G.Schapira. 1980. Biochim. Biophys. Acta, 612, 421.
9. Neer, E.J. 1978. J.Biol. Chem., 253, 5808.

# PROTEIN KINASES AND THE DOPAMINERGIC SYSTEM

I. Pribilla, H. Krüger, U. Oberdieck and F. Hucho
Institut für Biochemie, Freie Universität Berlin, Thielallee 63, 1000 Berlin (West) 33.

*Summary*

*Incubation of bovine striatal membranes with a partially purified protein kinase C (PK-C) or cAMP-dependent kinase had no effect on agonist binding to the $D_2$-dopamine receptor. Most of the effects observed could be attributed to an enzyme-catalyzed modification of the ligand N-propylnorapomorphine. We purified a PK-C-inhibitor from bovine striatal soluble fraction and characterised it as a heat-resistent protein, with a native MW of ~ 40,000 Da. We propose that the inhibitor is a dimer, composed of two subunits with MW of 19,000 Da.*

## Introduction

There are two subtypes of dopamine receptors in the mammalian corpus striatum, $D_1$ and $D_2$, which differ in their pharmacological properties and their functions: while $D_1$-receptors stimulate adenylate cyclase via the ubiquitous cyclase stimulatory GTP-binding protein ($G_s$), the $D_2$-receptor couples to an inhibitory GTP-binding protein ($G_i$ or $G_o$), thereby lowering cyclase activity (1,2). When an agonist binds to one of these receptors, the corresponding G-protein dissociates from the receptor and starts to interact with the cyclase. The remaining "G-protein-free" receptor loses its high affinity for agonists if there isn't any other nonactivated G-protein coupling to it. The cyclase-regulating signal is terminated after a while by an intrinsic GTPase activity of the G-protein, leading to the resting GDP-form, which reassociates with the receptor.

Receptors and Ion Channels

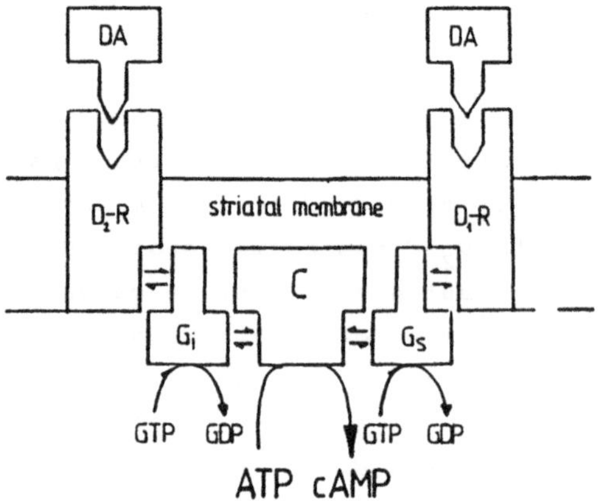


*Fig. 1: Components of the dopamine-responsive adenylate cyclase system. DA = dopamine; $D_1$, $D_2$ = dopamine receptor subtypes; G = guanine nucleotide regulatory component; C = catalytic unit; s = stimulatory; i = inhibitory.*

Several authors have reported that dopaminergic agonists inhibit inositoltrisphosphate production and prolactin release in the pituitary via $D_2$-receptors (3,4). This effect is cyclase independent, as one can interrupt the $G_i$/cyclase pathway by ADP-ribosylation of G with the *bordetella pertussis* toxin and still achieve inhibition of inositoltrisphosphate production (4). So besides the regulation of cyclase activity, $D_2$-receptors seem to be coupled differently to the activity of phospholipase C.
There are interactions and feedback regulations within the different second messenger systems. In platelet membranes, for example, the inhibitory G-protein ($G_i$) is a substrate of protein kinase C (PK-C) (5). The phosphorylated $G_i$ is no longer capable of inhibiting adenylate cyclase (6). Furthermore, protein kinase C is able to lower $\alpha_1$-adrenergic agonist binding by phosphorylation of the receptor.

Our aim was to investigate whether there is a phosphorylation effect on the agonist binding kinetics of the $D_2$-receptor in striatal membranes catalyzed by protein kinase C or cAMP-dependent kinase. While we failed to show any kinase effects, we did find a protein acting as a potent inhibitor of protein kinase C.

Methods

Agonist binding assay: The assay mixture contained 1 mg/ml membrane protein, 0.09 - 0.9 nM $^3H$-N-propylnorapomorphine, 10 μM pargyline, 0.1 % ascorbate and 100 nM ketanserin in 10 mM Mops buffer (pH 7.4), containing 120 mM NaCl, 5 mM KCl, 2 mM $CaCl_2$, 1 mM $MgCl_2$ (total assay volume 500 μl). Non sepcific binding was determined in the presence of 1 μM (+)butaclamol. The reaction was stopped after 30 minutes incubation at 30° C by filtration through a glass fiber filter (Whatman GF/C). The filter was washed with 5 volumes of cold assay buffer and bound radioactivity was determined by liquid scintillation counting.

Protein kinase C activity was determined according to (7).

For determining PK-C-inhibitor activity 10 μg protein of a sample were added to the PK-C assay mixture. The induced loss in PK-C activity was expressed as % inhibition achieved.

Purification of PK-C and PK-C-inhibitor: a) DEAE ion exchange chromatography on Whatman DE 52 resin, equilibrated with 20 mM TEA, 2 mM DTE, 5 mM EGTA and 2 mM EDTA.
b) Gel permeation of Pharmacia FPLC Superose 12 HR 10/30, equilibrated with 2o mM Hepes, 150 mM NaCl, 1 mM EDTA. Flowrate 0.5 ml/min; fraction size 1 ml.
c) Ion exchange chromatography on Pharmacia FPLC Mono Q HR 5/5 column, equilibrated with 20 mM Hepes, 1 mM EDTA; flowrate and fraction size as above.

Results

1) $^{3}$H-N-propylnorapomorphine binding of striatal membranes after preincubation with different kinases.

Striatal membranes were incubated for 10 minutes at 30$^{O}$ C with a fraction enriched in protein kinase C prepared from striatal soluble fraction or a probe enriched in cAMP-dependent protein kinase from the same tissue. The binding was assayed with the dopaminergic agonist $^{3}$H-N-propylnorapomorphine.

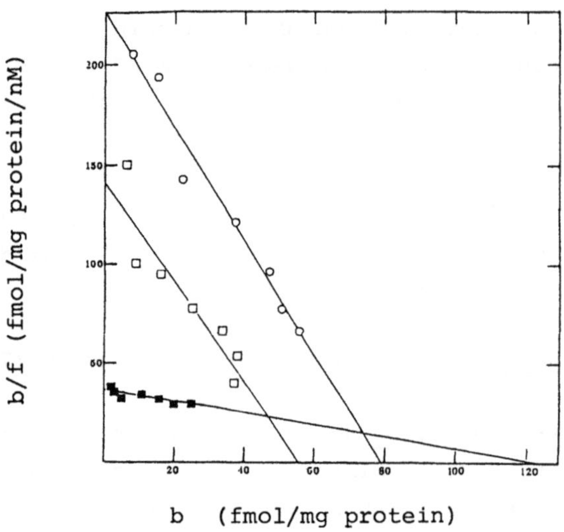


*Fig. 2: Scatchard analysis of $^{3}$H-NPA binding to bovine striatal membranes. Membranes were preincubated with:*

O-O-O *buffer*

□-□-□ *20 units of partially purified cAMPdPK/mg membrane*

■-■-■ *20 units of partially purified PK-C/mg membrane*

Incubation of membranes with the fraction enriched in protein kinase C results in a striking decrease in binding, while the cAMP-dependent kinase has no effect on the affinity and only slightly reduces the number of binding sites.

The effect of the protein kinase C enriched fraction turned out to be due to a ligand modifying activity of the kinase preparation. As there was no effect of PK-C-activating phorbolesters on the binding we concluded that there is no PK-C effect on the binding of the $D_2$-receptor. The observed effects (fig. 2) are due to an unidentified enzyme which alters the ligand, as was shown by thin layer chromatography.

2) Purification of a protein kinase C inhibitor from bovine striatum

The soluble fraction of bovine striatum was applied to a DEAE ion exchange chromatography. The column was eluted with a linear NaCl gradient (0-300 mM) and washed with 500 mM NaCl. The fractions of the high salt wash were pooled, boiled for 30 minutes and centrifuged. After dialysis of the supernatant the remaining heat-resistant proteins were separated on an FPLC-Superose 12 column. The inhibitory activity elutes as a single peak corresponding to a pool of proteins with molecular weights (MW) of about 40,000 Da.

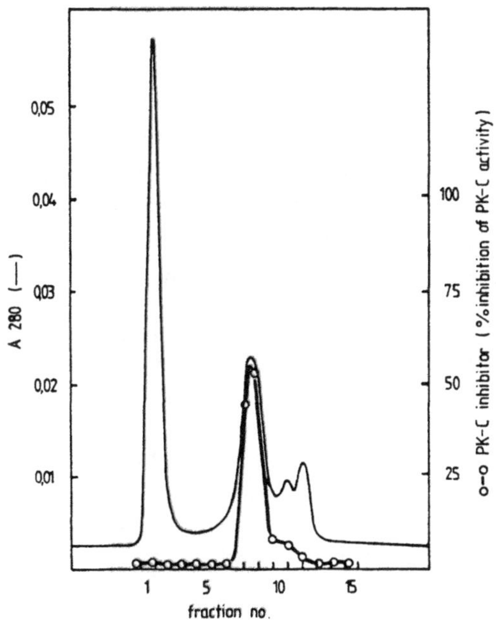


*Fig. 3: Gel permeation of heat-treated inhibitor fraction on FPLC-Superose column.*

The inhibitor fractions were pooled and concentrated on Amicon PM 10 membranes. The concentrate was applied to an FPLC ion exchange column (Mono Q) and eluted with an NaCl gradient (0-800 mM; two slopes). The inhibitory activity again elutes in a single peak (fig. 4), that corresponds to a single protein with an apparent molecular weight of 19,000 Da as judged by SDS-PAGE (fig. 5).

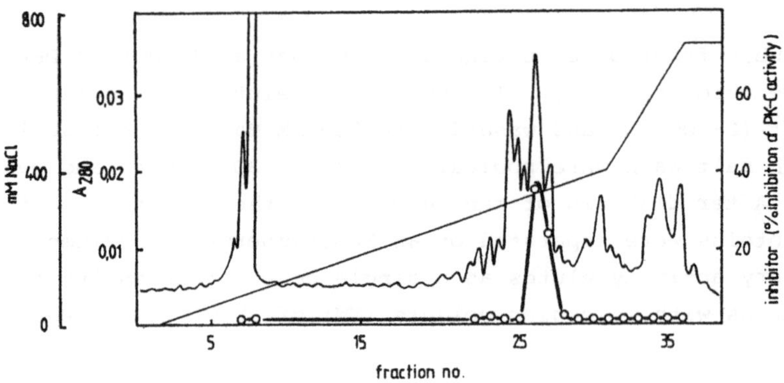


*Fig. 4: Ion exchange chromatography of PK-C inhibitor fractions on FPLC-Mono Q column.*

Fig. 5 shows a 15 % SDS-PAGE of protein fractions from some steps of the inhibitor purification. The supernatant of the boiled high salt wash of the DEAE column is already strikingly enriched in the 19 kDa band that turned out to be the inhibitor. The five-fold purification achieved by the two following steps (gel permeation, ion exchange chromatography) results in the pure inhibitor protein.

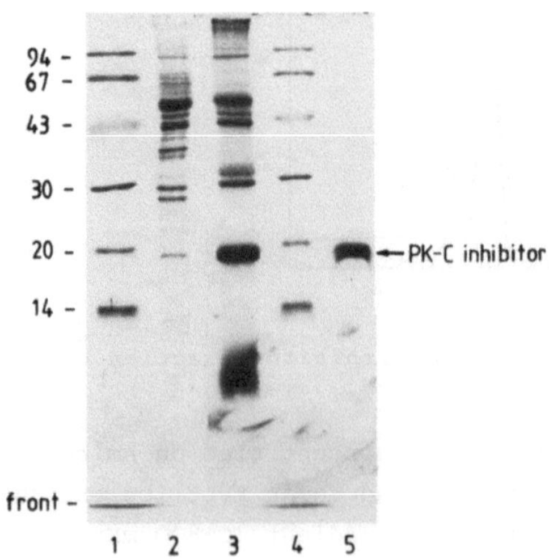


*Fig. 5:*
*Coomassie Blue Stain of 15% SDS-PAGE*

*lane 1 - marker proteins*
*lane 2 - crude soluble fraction*
*lane 3 - supernatant of boiled high salt wash from DE 52 column*
*lane 4 - marker proteins*
*lane 5 - pure PK-C inhibitor as pooled from Mono Q fractions*

3) Determination of the molecular weight of the PK-C inhibitor under nondenaturating conditions.

As there was a significant difference between the molecular weights determined from SDS-PAGE and gel permeation we rechromatographed the purified inhibitor on the Superose column after precise column calibration. The inhibitor elutes as a single peak of an apparent MW of 40,000 Da, accompanied by two minor impurities with MW 8000 and 3000 Da, respectively (fig. 6). As 40,000 Da is about twice the size that the inhibitor shows on SDS-PAGE, we propose that the PK-C inhibitor is at least a dimer, composed of two subunits with identical molecular weights.

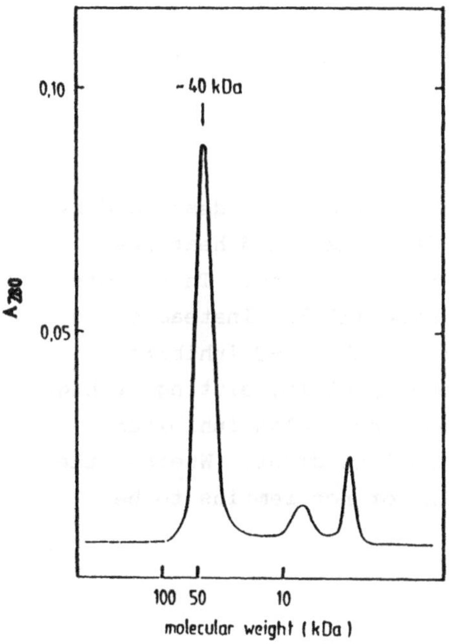


*Fig. 6: GEL PERMEATION OF THE PURIFIED PROTEIN KINASE C INHIBITOR ON A FPLC-SUPEROSE COLUMN.*
*Calibration: bovine serum albumin (67 kDa), ovalbumin (45 kDa), carboanhydrase (30 kDa), chymotrypsinogen (25,7 kDa), cytochrome C dimer (23.4 kDa), myoglobin (17,8 kDa).*

4) Concentration dependence of inhibition

The inhibition achieved by the PK-C inhibitor is a saturable function of the inhibitor concentration used (fig. 7). 40 - 50% of the PK-C molecules are not accessible to the inhibitor. Whether this might reflect isoenzymes of the PK-C or posttranslational modifications remains to be shown.

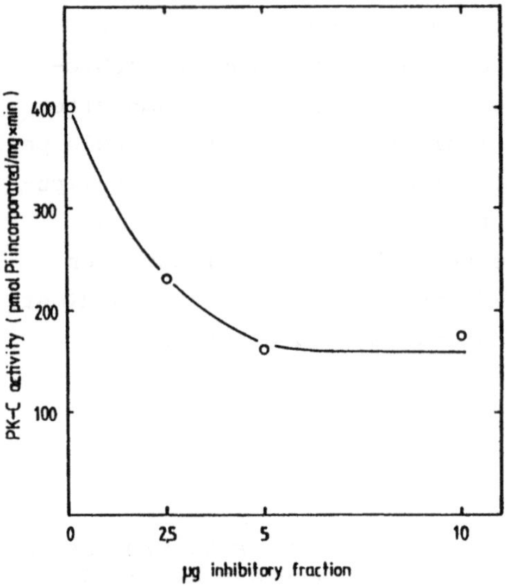


*Fig. 7: ASSAY OF PROTEIN KINASE C ACTIVITY IN THE PRESENCE OF INCREASING AMOUNTS OF HEAT-TREATED INHIBITOR.*

There has been another protein kinase C inhibitor described by Walsh and collaborators (8), that is a small and heat-resistant protein, showing a weak calcium binding activity. This protein differs from our PK-C inhibitor in size (17 kDa instead of 19 kDa) and ion exchange behaviour. While the PK-C inhibitor described here is a negatively charged protein, eluting at high salt concentrations from DEAE column, the "Walsh inhibitor" elutes in the very beginning of the NaCl gradient. Whether the two inhibitors are different proteins or not remains to be explored.

Acknowledgements

Financial support by the Deutsche Forschungsgemeinschaft and the Fonds der Chemischen Industrie is gratefully acknowledged.
H. Krüger is recipient of a Schering fellowship.

REFERENCES

1. Kebabian, J.W., et al. 1979. Nature 277, 93-96.

2. Weiss, S., et al. 1985. Mol. Pharm. 27, 595-599.

3. Strange, P.G., et al. 1985. Neurosci. Lett. 60, 267-272.

4. Kordon, C., et al. 1986. Biol. Chem. Hoppe-Seyler 367, 99.

5. Jacobs, K.H., et al. 1985. Eur. J. Biochem. 151, 425-230.

6. Katada, T., et al. 1985. Eur. J. Biochem. 151, 431-437.

7. Kikkawa, U., et al. 1983. Meth. Enzym. 99, 288 298.

8. McDonald, J.R., and Walsh, M.P. 1985. Biochem. J. 232, 559-567.

# INTERACTIONS BETWEEN PROTEINS INVOLVED IN THE ACTIVATION AND SUBSEQUENT DEACTIVATION OF PHOSPHODIESTERASE IN VISUAL ROD CELLS

H. Kühn

Institut für Neurobiologie, Kernforschungsanlage Jülich GmbH,
5170 Jülich, FRG

## Introduction

Cyclic GMP (cGMP) plays a key role in visual transduction in rod (1-3) as well as in cone (4, 5) cells of the vertebrate retina. So-called "light-sensitive" cation channels in the plasma membrane of the rod or cone outer segment are kept open in the dark (resting state) by binding cGMP (1-5), leading to partial depolarization of the cells. Absorption of light by rhodopsin, which is located in intracellular piles of disk membranes in the rod outer segment (ROS), leads to the activation of a cGMP-phosphodiesterase (PDE) (for recent reviews see refs. 6-8). This probably leads to a decrease in free cGMP concentration (9, but see also 10), and to closure of the cGMP-dependent channels (1-5, 11) and to hyperpolarization of the cell.

This short review restricts itself to describing only reactions in which photoactivated rhodopsin ($R^*$) directly participates. It will be shown that specific interactions of $R^*$ with three different proteins first lead to the amplified activation of PDE and subsequently to inactivation of the system. Many laboratories have contributed to our present knowledge; due to the limited space, only a few references can be given.

Receptors and Ion Channels

## Results and Discussion

### Light-dependent binding of three ROS proteins

Light absorption by rhodopsin causes cis-trans isomerization of its chromophore, 11-cis retinal. This leads to conformational changes not only in the chromophore-binding hydrophobic center of rhodopsin, but also at its cytoplasmic surface (reviewed in ref. 6). Such conformational changes are recognized by three ROS proteins (see Table 1). In the dark, these three proteins are either soluble (ii, iii), or peripherally membrane-associated (i). After illumination, they bind to $R^*$ and therefore resist extraction by aqueous buffers, in a reversible fashion (6, 12-14).

Table 1

Proteins that interact with photoactivated rhodopsin

| Name (synonyms) | (i) Transducin (GTP-binding protein, G-Protein, GTPase) | (ii) Rhodopsin-kinase (opsin-kinase) | (iii) 48 kD-protein (arrestin, S-antigen) |
|---|---|---|---|
| Native $M_r$ | 85 000 | 69 000 | 48 000 |
| Polypeptide $M_r$ | 41 000 (α)<br>37 000 (β)<br>8 000 (γ) | 68 000 | 48 000 |
| Number of copies per 1000 rhodopsins | ca. 100 | 1-10 | 100-1000 (25) |
| Solubility in darkness (physiological ionic strength) | membrane-associated | mostly soluble | soluble |
| Effects of nucleotides | GTP dissociates $T_\alpha$-GTP from $T_{\beta\gamma}$ and $R^*$ | ATP enhances dissociation (14) | ATP and GTP strongly enhance light-induced binding (14,24) |
| Function | activation of PDE | deactivation of $R^*$ | deactivation of phosph. $R^*$ |

(i) A guanine nucleotide binding protein (G-protein, "trans-ducin"), which has many structural and functional similarities with hormone receptor G-proteins, binds to $R^*$ in a 1 : 1 complex (13, 15); this enables exchange of GTP for previously bound GDP on the $\alpha$-subunit ($T_\alpha$) of transducin (16, 17). After nucleotide exchange, the protein complex dissociates into $R^*$, $T_{\beta\gamma}$, and $T_\alpha$-GTP (18) which then activates cGMP-phosphodiesterase (17). One $R^*$ can serially interact with several hundred molecules of transducin and catalyze their GDP/GTP exchange, thereby providing the first step of amplification of the photon signal (16, 17).

(ii) A protein kinase ("rhodopsin kinase"), which is independent of cyclic nucleotides or $Ca^{++}$, phosphorylates photobleached but not unbleached rhodopsin at multiple (maximally nine) serine and threonine sites (19). Seven potential phosphorylation sites are located near the carboxyl terminus of rhodopsin (20, 21), an additional site has recently been identified in the third cyto-plasmic loop, at Ser-240 (McDowell and Hargrave, personal communi-cation). Overall phosphorylation seems to be a slow reaction when an excess of rhodopsin has been photoisomerized (19), but it can be much faster - occurring in the range of seconds - if only a small proportion of rhodopsin has been photoisomerized, or if the ROS preparation is enriched with kinase (19, 26).

(iii) A soluble protein called "48 kD-protein" (12), or "S-anti-gen" (22), or "arrestin" (23), also binds to $R^*$, and particularly well to phosphorylated $R^*$ (24). This protein is very abundant in the rod cell; it has recently been reported that the molar ratio of 48 kD-protein to rhodopsin in the rod cell should be close to 1 : 1 (25). Upon light-adaptation of retinas, most of the 48 kD-protein is found to be shifted from the rod inner segment to its outer segment (25), consistent with its solubility in darkness and its binding to bleached and phosphorylated rhodopsin (24).

Competitions between the three proteins for binding to $R^*$

Competition between rhodopsin-kinase and transducin has been demonstrated to occur under special (unphysiological) conditions: in the absence of GTP, when the complex between $R^*$ and transducin is stable and long-lived, a strong inhibition of $R^*$ phosphorylation by the kinase can be observed at low bleaching levels (6). This inhibition does, however, not occur in the presence of GTP or GTP analogs (6). Under this (physiologically more normal) condition, the complex between $R^*$ and transducin is rather short-lived (15, 27); each cycle comprising transducin association to $R^*$, GTP binding to $T_\alpha$, and $T_\alpha$-GTP dissociation from $R^*$, takes only a few milliseconds (27), and it appears that $R^*$ is sufficiently "free" during these cycles to allow binding of kinase and incorporation of phosphates into $R^*$. This suggests that competition between transducin and kinase is physiologically unimportant (6).

In contrast, there is a significant competition between 48 kD-protein and transducin for binding to phosphorylated $R^*$ (24), and this competition is thought to be of physiological relevance (28).

Although light-induced binding of 48 kD-protein to unphosphorylated disk membranes has been observed earlier (12), this binding is rather weak and requi.res high bleaching levels, and temperatures above 20° C, to be observable (14). If rhodopsin is phosphorylated, 48 kD-protein binds much more strongly so that its binding can be observed also at lower bleaching levels and lower temperatures (24). The possibility cannot be excluded that unphosphorylated $R^*$ does not bind 48 kD-protein at all and that the previously observed binding in the absence of ATP (12, 14) was due to the presence of some residual phosphorylated rhodopsin which had not been completely dephosphorylated in vivo before preparation of the ROS. In any event, 48 kD-protein binds to phosphorylated $R^*$ much better than to unphosphorylated $R^*$. Not only phosphorylation, but also de novo photoisomerization of rhodopsin is required for this binding to occur (24).

In contrast to 48 kD-protein, transducin binds somewhat less strongly to phosphorylated than to unphosphorylated $R^*$ (ref. 24, and H. Kühn unpublished observations). However, it still binds, even when $R^*$ is highly phosphorylated (24), and thereby becomes activated in the presence of GTP to mediate the activation of PDE (28). Added 48 kD-protein then inhibits PDE activation (28), most probably by competing with transducin for interaction with the phosphorylated $R^*$. Inversely, an excess of transducin is also able to displace 48 kD-protein from its binding to phosphorylated $R^*$ (24). Hence, the binding of both 48 kD-protein and transducin to phosphorylated $R^*$ is easily reversible, and the binding equilibrium can be shifted in either direction depending on the molar ratio of 48 kD-protein vs. transducin present.

## Activation and deactivation of the cGMP enzyme cascade

To summarize the previous sections: Photoactivated rhodopsin ($R^*$) activates transducin by catalyzing the binding of GTP to transducin's $\alpha$-subunit ($T_\alpha$). Each cycle of transducin association with $R^*$, GTP binding to $T_\alpha$, and dissociation of $T_\alpha$-GTP from $R^*$ is so rapid that a single $R^*$ molecule can successively activate hundreds of $T_\alpha$ molecules. Active $T_\alpha$-GTP then activates the PDE by binding the inhibitory 13 kDal subunit of the PDE (29).

In order to reverse activation, it seems necessary that all the active precursors of PDE activation, namely $R^*$ and $T_\alpha$-GTP, be deactivated. (Another thinkable way of deactivation, namely a direct inhibition of the active PDE by some $R^*$-triggered mechanism, could not be convincingly demonstrated so far.)

The active transducin subunit, $T_\alpha$-GTP, inactivates itself by its intrinsic GTPase activity. The resulting $T_\alpha$-GDP then reassociates with $T_{\beta\gamma}$ and may be reactivated if active $R^*$ molecules are still present.

Several deactivation mechanisms of R* exist; they occur on different time scales. Metarhodopsin II (which is the active R*, see ref. 6 for a review) spontaneously but slowly decays, with a half-time in the range of a few minutes, into inactive photoproducts. A much faster deactivation is observed when ROS membranes are supplemented with ATP (30), and various lines of evidence have suggested that the effect of ATP is exerted by the phosphorylation of R* (30, 26, 28). Recent experiments, using a defined "reassociated system" consisting of previously highly phosphorylated and regenerated rhodopsin in washed disk membranes to which purified transducin and PDE were added in the absence of ATP, clearly demonstrated that the light-induced capacity of phosphorylated rhodopsin to activate the enzyme cascade is indeed significantly (3-5 times) lower than that of unphosphorylated rhodopsin (28). If purified 48 kD-protein was added, it potentiated the inhibitory effect of rhodopsin phosphorylation, leading to near-complete inactivation. In these experiments, the initial velocity of PDE was inhibited (up to 98 %) since rhodopsin was already phosphorylated prior to the light stimulus. If rhodopsin is previously unphosphorylated, the light-stimulated PDE activity in the presence of ATP is initially high (although not quite as high as in absence of ATP, see refs. 26, 28, 30) and becomes rapidly quenched with increasing phosphorylation of R*. ATP in the absence of rhodopsin-kinase has no effect (28), nor has 48 kD-protein in the absence of rhodopsin phosphorylation (28).

Thus, phosphorylation of R* by rhodopsin-kinase and ATP is a prerequisite for rapid deactivation of R*, and this deactivation is potentiated by the subsequent binding of 48 kD-protein.

Recent elegant electrophysiological experiments on "truncated" toad ROS have confirmed and complemented our biochemical view on the activation and deactivation of the light response of rod photoreceptors (2). They clearly show that GTP is required for the activation of the light response (activation of transducin), and ATP is required for its deactivation.

Acknowledgement

I thank my coworkers, U. Wilden and S.W. Hall, who have been actively involved in the work on rhodopsin phosphorylation and PDE deactivation; I thank E. Wüst and R. Esser for technical assistance, and A. Eckert for typing the manuscript. This work was in part supported by a grant SFB 160 from Deutsche Forschungsgemeinschaft.

References

1. Fesenko, E.E., S.S. Kolesnikov, A.L. Lyubarsky. 1985. Nature 313, 310-313.

2. Yau, K.W., K. Nakatani. 1985. Nature 317, 252-254.

3. Zimmermann, A.L., G. Yamanaka, F. Eckstein, D.A. Baylor, L. Stryer. 1985. Proc. Natl. Acad. Sci. USA 82, 8813-8817.

4. Haynes, L., K.W. Yau. 1985. Nature 317, 61-64.

5. Cobbs, W.H., A.E. Barkdoll, E. N. Pugh. 1985. Nature 317, 64-66.

6. Kühn, H. 1984. In: Progr. Retinal Research (N. Osborne and J. Chader,, eds.). Pergamon Press, Vol. 3, p. 123-156.

7. Fung, B.K.K. 1985. In: Molecular Mechanism of Transmembrane Signalling. (P. Cohen and M.D. Houslay, eds.). Elsevier North Holland, p. 183-214.

8. Stryer, L. 1986. Ann. Rev. Neurosci. 9, 87-119.

9. Cote, R.H., M.S. Biernbaum, G.D. Nicol, M.D. Bownds. 1984. J. Biol. Chem. 259, 9635-9641.

10. Kilbride, P., T.G. Ebrey. 1979. J. Gen. Physiol. 74, 415-426.

11. Koch, K.W., U.B. Kaupp. 1985. J. Biol. Chem. 260, 6788-6800.

12. Kühn, H. 1978. Biochemistry 17, 4389-4395.

13. Kühn, H. 1980a. Nature 283, 587-589.

14. Kühn, H. 1980b. Neurochem. Intern. 1, 269-285.

15. Kühn, H., N. Bennett, M. Michel-Villaz, M. Chabre. 1981. Proc. Natl. Acad. Sci. USA 18, 6873-6877.

16. Fung, B.K.K., L. Stryer. 1980. Proc. Natl. Acad. Sci. USA 77, 2500-2504.

17. Fung, B.K.K., J.B. Hurley, L. Stryer. 1981. Proc. Natl. Acad. Sci. USA 78, 152-156.

18. Kühn, H. 1981. In: Current Topics in Membranes and Transport. Vol. 15. (W.H. Miller, ed.). Academic Press, p. 171-201.

19. Wilden, U., H. Kühn. 1982. Biochem. 21, 3014-3022.

20. Hargrave, P.A., S.L. Fong, J.H. McDowell, M.T. Mas, D.R. Curtis, J.K. Wang, E. Juszcazak, D.P. Smith. 1980. Neurochem. Intern. 1, 231-244.

21. Ovchinnikov, Y.A. 1982. FEBS Lett. 148, 179-191.

22. Pfister, C., M. Chabre, J. Plouet, V.V. Tuyen, Y. DeKozak, J.P. Faure, H. Kühn. 1985. Science 228, 891-893.

23. Zuckerman, R., B. Buzdygon, N. Philp, P. Liebman, A. Sitaramayya. 1985. Biophys. J. 47, 37a.

24. Kühn, H., S.W. Hall, U. Wilden. 1984. FEBS Lett. 176, 473-478.

25. Broekhuyse, R.M., E.F.J. Tolhuizen, A.P.M. Janssen, H.J. Winkens. 1985. Current Eye Res. 4, 613-618.

26. Sitaramayya, A., P.A. Liebman. 1983. J. Biol. Chem. 258, 12106-12109.

27. Vuong, T.M., M. Chabre, L. Stryer. 1984. Nature 311, 659-661.

28. Wilden, U., S.W. Hall, H. Kühn. 1986. Proc. Natl. Acad. Sci. 83, 1174-1178.

29. Hurley, J.B., L. Stryer. 1982. J. Biol. Chem. 257, 11094-11099.

30. Liebman, P.A., E.N. Pugh. 1980. Nature 287, 734-736.

PHOSPHORYLATION OF THE NICOTINIC ACETYLCHOLINE RECEPTOR BY cAMP-DEPENDENT PROTEIN KINASE

M. Hillmann and F. Hucho

Institut für Biochemie, Freie Universität Berlin, Thielallee 63, 1000 Berlin (West ) 33.

## Introduction

External physiological stimuli control intracellular events in mammalian tissue. One major mechanism by which this is achieved is phosphorylation and dephosphorylation.

Protein phosphorylation is an important mechanism for regulating the gating properties of many species of ionic channels. At present, the nicotinic acetylcholine receptor (nAChR) is the best characterized ion channel. It can be phosphorylated by three different types of protein kinases: a cAMP-dependent (1), a $Ca^{2+}$/phospolipid-dependent (3), and a tyrosine-specific protein kinase (2).

Membranes from *Torpedo* electric tissue rich in AChR also contain a $Ca^{2+}$/calmodulin dependent protein kinase (4), but the receptor appears to not be a substrate of this enzyme.

Protein kinase activities of membranes rich in nAChR *Table 1:*

| Protein kinase activities | Phosphorylation sites*) | Amino acid residue | | Ref. |
|---|---|---|---|---|
| Membrane-bound cAMP-dependent protein kinase | γ-polypeptide chain | serine | 361 | 1 |
| | δ-polypeptide chain | serine | 354 . | |
| Tyrosine-specific protein kinase | β-polypeptide chain | tyrosine | 355 | 2 |
| | γ-polypeptide chain | tyrosine | 354 | |
| | δ-polypeptide chain | tyrosine | 372 | |
| $Ca^{2+}$/phospholipid-dependent protein kinase | α-polypeptide chain | serine | 333 | 3 |
| | δ-polypeptide chain | serine | 377 | |

*) predicted by Huganir et al. (2)

Receptors and Ion Channels

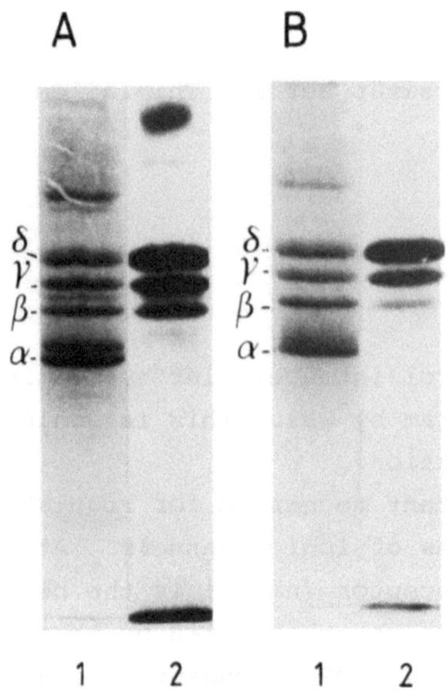


*Fig. 1: shows phosphorylation of membranes rich in AChR by endogenous protein kinases.*

*A Phosphorylation of AChR-rich membranes*

*B like A, but with purification by affinity chromatography*

*1 Coomassie blue protein stain*

*2 autoradiogram*

*The phosphorylation and purification of 2o - 30 µg AChR rich membranes was performed as described in (1) with the following modifications: solubilization of membranes by 1 % Triton X-100 (final concentration), phosphorylation in the presence of 1 mM Ouabain, 2 µM ATP (0.5 µCi/µl), incubation time: 30 min. SDS Gel electrophoresis: 10 % gel, Laemmli (5).*

Purification by affinity chromatography of the phosphorylated membranes shows that the γ- and δ-polypeptide chains are the predominant substrates. The δ- and γ-polypeptide chains are specifically phosphorylated by the cAMPdPK. We did not find any protein kinase C activity. Here we describe the purification of the cAMPdPK.

## Results and Discussion

<u>1. cAMP-dependence:</u> The enzyme exists in an inactive tetrameric $R_2C_2$-form and is activated after dissociation in the presence of cAMP (6,7). Fig. 2 shows the phosphorylation of an exogenous substrate (Kemptide) by solubilized membranes rich in AChR in dependence of cAMP.

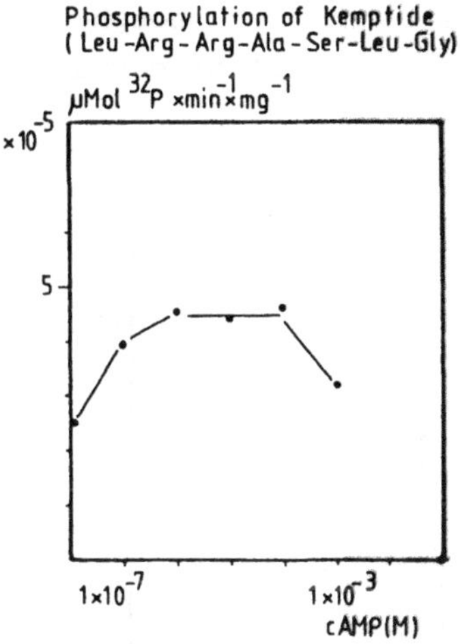


*Fig. 2: Effect of cAMP on Kemptide-phosphorylation*

Enzyme activity of AChR-rich membranes (preparation as described in (8)) was estimated by the method of Roskoski jr. (9).
Kemptide (100 μM) and AChR-rich membranes (20 μg), (2 mg/ml) were incubated with described reaction mixture (50 μl). After incubation (30 mins., 30° C) 40 μl aliquots were spotted onto phosphocellulose filter (P81, Whatman), the incorporation of radioactive phosphate was determined by measuring Cerencov radiation.

The protein kinase activity is moderately stimulated by cAMP. Maximum activation was achieved with a cAMP-concentration of 0.1-1 μM (80 %). The phosphorylation of Kemptide can be inhibited to 90 % by the specific protein kinase inhibitor; this proves that the Kemptide phosphorylation is mediated to an extent of 90 % by a cAMP-dependent protein kinase activity. The regulatory subunit of the enzyme is partially removed during purification or it is cleaved proteolytically; this accounts for the high basal kinase activity (in the absence of cAMP).

2. Purification: We have shown that the cAMPdPK is an integral membrane protein which is closely associated with the nAChR in the membrane. The membranes were extracted with Triton X-100 (final concentration 1 %). During solubilization the enzyme activity towards exogenous substrates increases, probably due to dissociation from the receptor and to an increase of accessibility of the catalytic site for exogenous substrates.
After solubilization the protein kinase is purified by chromatography on a Cibacron Blue Sepharose CL-6B column, and it is eluted with 0.25 M KCl. Therefore it can be classified as type II cAMPdPK (fig. 3). The protein-rich fractions could not be stimulated,

neither by cAMP nor by other effectors as $Ca^{2+}$ or phospholipids. The fractions only contain the catalytic subunit of cAMPdPK.

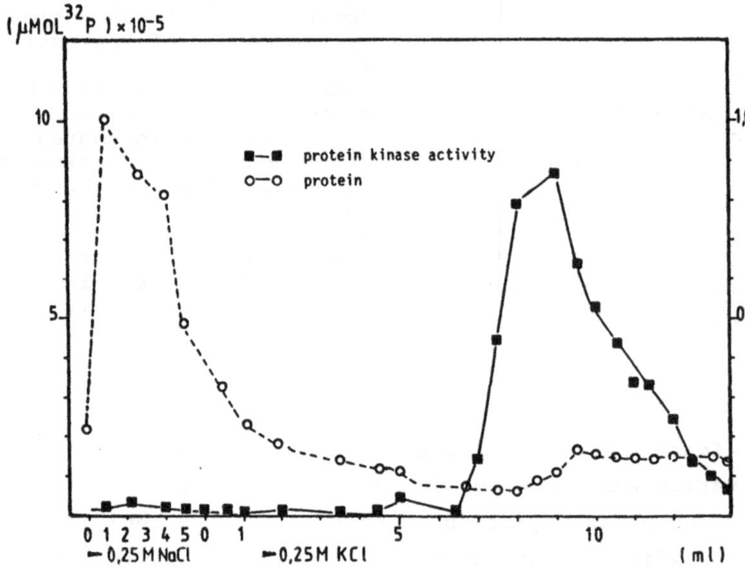


*Fig. 3: Cibacron Blue Sepharose CL-6B column elution profile*
*o---o protein (determined by the method of Peterson (19)*
*■—■ protein kinase activity*

*Conditions and procedures: The solubilized membranes (14 mg of protein in 7 ml) have been incubated with 0.1 mM cAMP (10 mins., 0 - 5° C for this and subsequent procedures unless otherwise specified) and applied to a Cibacron Blue Sepharose CL-6B column (0.9 x 11.5 cm), equilibrated with a buffer [(4 mM Mops (pH 6.8), 0,5 mM dithiothreitol, 5 mM $MgCl_2$, and 5 % glycerol (v/v)], to which 0.1 mM cAMP was added (10).*

Buffer A (3 x 1 ml) + 0.25 M NaCl was used to wash the AChR-protein from the column; buffer A (15 ml), containing 0.25 M KCl, was used to elute the catalytic subunit fraction. Protein kinase activity was measured as described in fig. 2. The respective fractions were combined and concentrated by using Amicon's microconcentrator. Fractions were stored at -20° C with 40 % glycerol.

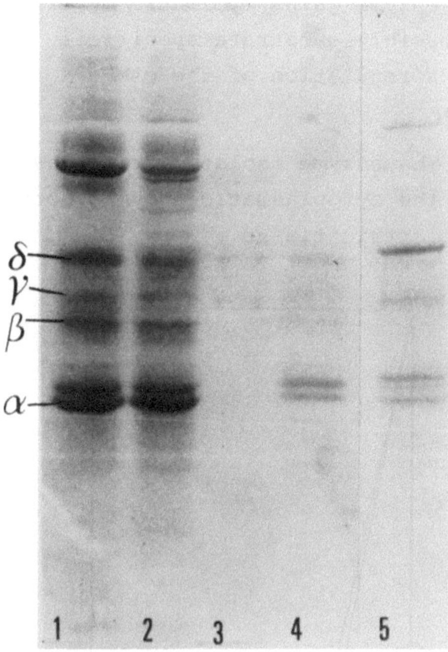


*Fig. 4:* *SDS-Polyacrylamid electrophoresis of samples from the purification steps, lo % Laemmli gel*

| | |
|---|---|
| *lane 1* | *AChR-rich membranes* |
| *lane 2* | *solubilized membranes* |
| *lane 3* | *protein not bound to the Sepharose column* |
| *lane 4* | *protein eluted by treatment with NaCl* |
| *lane 5* | *protein kinase-rich fraction* |

Treatment with 0.25 M NaCl removes the main part of the AChR from the column, but traces of AChR are still present in each fraction of the purification (fig. 4), this proves again the close association between AChR and protein kinase.

The catalytic subunit has been purified about 60-fold (compared with intact membranes) to a specific activity of $3.5 \cdot 10^{-3}$ units $mg^{-1}$ (1 unit = $1 \times 10^{-6}$ mol $^{32}P$-phosphate incorporation $\cdot$ $min^{-1}$, $30^{o}$ C). In exceptional cases a purification up to 370-fold was achieved. A calculation of the amount of AChR and protein kinase shows a 1 : 10 ratio (or 1 : 4). This stoichiometry indicates that the protein kinase is possibly involved in regulating receptor functions like desensitization.

The catalytic subunit has an estimated molecular-weight of 45,000. This estimation was performed by blotting the catalytic subunit with $^{125}I$-regulatory subunit (isolated from bovine brain).

<u>3. Substrate specificity</u>: As mentioned above, the protein kinase activity towards exogenous substrates increases during solubilization of the membranes rich in AChR. After purification - i.e., removing the natural environment - the specificity of the enzyme

decreases. This indicates that the enzyme gains specificity by its location in the membrane and that possibly substrate specificity is lost during enzyme purification; a regulation of the cAMPdPK by nAChR appears to be possible (11).

4. Comparison with other cAMPdPKs: The enzyme isolated from AChR-rich membranes has been compared to the cytoplasmatic enzymes both from bovine heart and from Torpedo electric tissue.

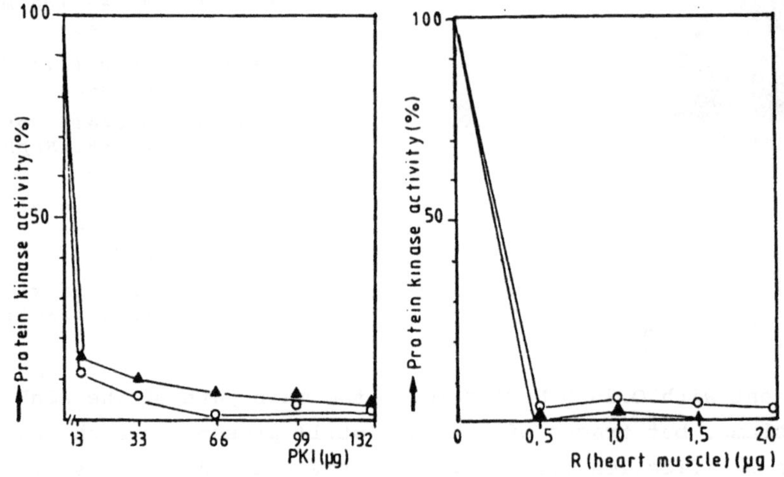


*Fig. 5: Inhibition of cAMPdPK by protein kinase inhibitor (bovine muscle, A) or regulatory subunit (B)*

*o—o cytoplasmatic enzyme*
*▲—▲ enzyme from AChR-rich membranes*

*Protein kinase activity was determined as described in fig. 2.*

The inhibition of our purified enzyme by the specific inhibitor protein (12) (up to 96%) is comparable with the inhibition of commercially available enzyme from bovine heart. Incubation of the enzyme with regulatory subunit of cytoplasmatic cAMPdPK of type I or II inhibits it completely.
The electric tissue of *Torpedo* is also a source of cytoplasmatic cAMPdPK. This enzyme and the purified catalytic subunit were used for immunological characterization with antiserum against the catalytic subunit of cytoplasmatic cAMPdPK from bovine heart (13).

This antiserum, however, reacted neither with catalytic subunit of cytoplasmatic cAMPdPK nor with membrane-bound cAMPdPK, nor does it react with AChR-rich membranes from *Torpedo*.

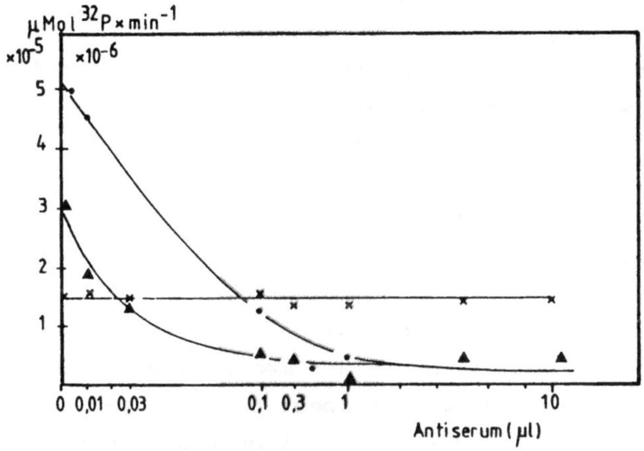


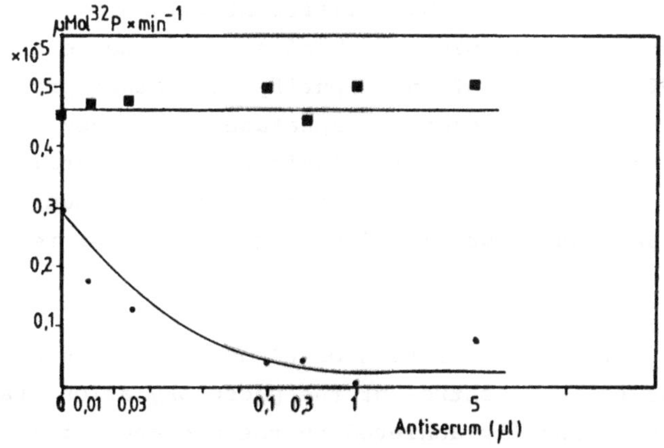


*Fig. 6: Immunotitration of cAMPdPK from Torpedo with antiserum*

▲——▲ / ●——● *control (cytoplasmatic C, bovine heart)*

■——■ *C of AChR-rich membranes (Torpedo)*

×——× *cytoplasmatic C (Torpedo)*

*Procedure and conditions: After incubation of antiserum- and enzyme-dilutions in a buffer A (10 mM K/PO$_4$, pH 7.4; 0,14 M NaCl, and 0.02 % NaN$_3$). Final volume: 50 µl (15 h, 4° C), 50 µl Protein A-Sepharose (0.107 g + 1.87 ml buffer A) were added and shaken*

*(1 h, 4° C). After centrifugation (8000 x g, 2 min.) the protein kinase activity of the supernatant was measured as described in fig. 2.*

Both cAMP-dependent protein kinases from *Torpedo* electric tissue react with regulatory subunits of membrane-bound or cytoplasmatic protein kinases and with the specific inhibitor of cAMPdPK. They are comparable with other cAMP-dependent protein kinases, but they differ with regard to their antigenic properties, i.e., they are not identical with other cAMP-dependent protein kinases. (It is also possible, though not very probable, that the antigenic epitope of the catalytic subunits of the *Torpedo* enzymes are covered by lipids or proteins).

It is not unusual that immunologically different forms of protein kinases exist. The cytoplasmatic and membrane-bound forms of cGMPdPK are also different with respect to their immunological properties. The regulatory subunits of membrane-bound cAMPdPK of type II (brain tissue) often have different immunulogical properties, similar to, for example, R-subunits of bovine heart, (14). R-II- subunits of the brain often co-purify with other proteins like MAP 2 or Calcineurin (a protein phosphatase), and they have more functions than just regulating ( = inhibiting) the catalytic subunit (15, 16). It is possible that the catalytic subunit of cAMPdPK of *Torpedo* has a special function in receptor regulation, too.

5. Regulation: If phosphorylation of nAChR plays a functional role, there has to be a control of the phosphorylation states of the AChR. This is usually achieved by the presence of a protein phosphatase, which is dephosphorylating the phosphoprotein. However, in our preparations we did not find any phosphatase activity.

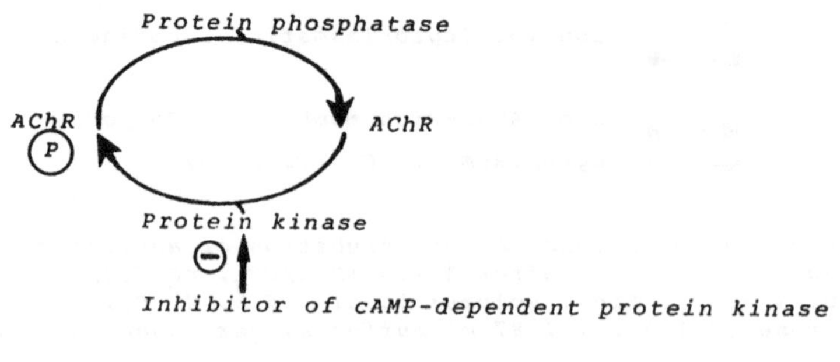

But we were able to isolate the specific cAMPdPK-inhibitor from the electric tissue of *Torpedo*. At present we have no idea as to how regulation of phosphorylation states by PkI could work. Greengard and Albuquerque (17, 18) reported a stimulation of AChR-desensitization by cAMP-dependent phosphorylation with an involvement of the adenylate-cyclase activating drug forskolin. With AChR-rich membranes or with the purified enzyme we could not find any effect of forskolin on the receptor phosphorylation.

Summary

We have shown that the cAMPdPK of *Torpedo* membranes rich in AChR is an integral membrane protein which is very closely associated with the nAChR in the membrane. There is evidence that the AChR regulates the activity of this enzyme. The purified catalytic subunits from *Torpedo* electric tissue show the same characteristics with regard to their reaction with protein kinase inhibitor and regulatory subunits as compared with other protein kinases, but they are not identical in respect to their immunological properties.

Acknowledgements

Financial support by the Deutsche Forschungsgemeinschaft (SBF 312) and the Fonds der Chemischen Industrie is gratefully acknowledged.

References

1. Greengard, P., and Huganir, R.L. 1983. Proc. Natl. Acad. Sci. USA 80, 1130-1134.

2. Huganir, R.L., et al. 1984. Proc. Natl. Acad. Sci. USA 81, 6968-6972.

3. Huganir, R.L., et al. 1983. Soc. Neurosci. Abstr. 9, 578.

4. Palfrey, H.C., et al. 1983. J. Biol. Chem. 258, 9496-9505.

5. Laemmli, U.K. 1970. Nature 15, 680-685.

6. Titani, K., et al. 1981. In: "Protein Phosphorylation" (O.M. Rosen, E.G. Krebs, Cold Spring Harbour Symp. 8, 19-29.

7. Beavo, J.A. et al. 1975. Adv. Cyclic Nucleotide Res. 5, 241-251.

8. Schiebler, W. and Hucho, F. 1978. Eur. J. Biochem. 85, 55-63.

9. Roskoski, R., Jr. 1983. Meth. Enzym. 99, 3-6.

10. Witt, J.J., Roskoski, R.,Jr. 1978. Biochemistry 14, 4503-4507.

11. Gordon, A.S. 1977. Proc. Natl. Acad. Sci. USA 74, 263-267.

12. Scott, J.C., et al. 1985. Proc. Natl. Acad. Sci. USA 82, 4379-4383.

13. Schwoch, G., et al. 1980. Biochem. J. 192, 223-230.

14. Weldon, S.L., et al. 1985. J. Biol. Chem. 260, 6440-6448.

15. Leiser, M., et al. 1986. J. Biol. Chem. 261, 1904-1908.

16. Kiss, Z., et al. 1986. Biochem. J. 234, 163-168.

17. Albuquerque, E.X., et al. 1986. FEBS Lett. 199, 113-120.

18. Huganir, R.L., et al. 1986. Nature 321, 774-776.

19. Peterson, G.L. 1977. Anal. Biochem. 83, 346-356.

# IV Pumps

# PHOTOELECTRICAL ACTIVITY OF BACTERIORHODOPSIN IN PLANAR LIPID BILAYER

V.S. Markin, V.M. Mirsky, Yu.A. Chismadzhev
Frumkin Institute of Electrochemistry USSR Academy of Sciences, Moscow, USSR

## Introduction

The understanding of functioning mechanism of BR - the molecular photochemical transformer - is impossible without quantitative study of its photoelectric characteristics. The most promising approach to this problem is assumed to be the reconstitution of BR into a planar bilayer lipid membrane (BLM) and the investigation of this system by means of a whole set of efficient experimental techniques devised for BLM. Some methods for the formation of photoactive BLM with BR were reported in (1-3), but the further investigations (4-7) have proved that the photoresponses observed are due to BR separated from the BLM by a layer of water ("third water").

In 1981 Bamberg et al. proposed a method of BR transfer into an organic solvent and formed BLM from this suspension (8). We proved that while forming BLM from such suspension by the monolayer method the transmembrane incorporation of BR into BLM occurs indeed and without the "third water" structure formation (9). The aim of this work was the study of BR suspension in an organic solvent formed according to (8) and the investigation of photoelectric characteristics of BR in BLM formed from the suspension.

## Experimental

The chemicals used included soybean phosphatidilcholine (azolec-

Receptors and Ion Channels

tine) by "Associated Concentrates", buffer MES by "Serva", dicyclohexilcarbodiimide by "Sigma", nigericin by "Calbiochem behring", KCl (special pure), decane (chemically pure) and other chemical (pure) by Reachim. 4,5,6,7-tetrachloro-2'-trifluormethylbenzimidazole (TTFB) was a gift from B.A.Tashmuhamedov. Purple membranes from Halobacterium halobium was a gift from L.N. Chekulaeva. Usually we used strain P-353 (Pushchino), some experiments were did on BR of strain $R_1M_1$, but the results were similar. We used method (8) with minor modifications (10) for the formation BR suspension in azolectine in decane solution (BRS). The original relationship of concentrates was 1 mg of BR, 33 mg of azolectine, 1 ml of decane. BLM was formed on the 0.3 mm diameter hole in a teflon film 5μ thick separating the two aqueous cell section. 2 μl BRS or azolectine solution in decane (33 mg/ml) per $sm^2$ were spread on the aqueous electrolyte surface (100 mM KCL, 10 mM MES, pH 6.3) and the electrolyte levels were raised higher than the hole in the film. The other experimental details were reported in (10-12). All the experiments were carried out at room temperature.

## Results

Investigation of BR suspension in azolectine in decane solution. The adsorption spectra of the same amount of BR as a purple membrane suspension (spectrum 1), BRS (spectrum 2) and the sample obtained similarly as BRS but without cooling while sonicating are shown on Fig.1. The first spectrum was recorded relatively to water, the second and third relatively to azolectine in decane solution. The band 360 nm in the latter spectrum corresponds to the free retinal. BRS spectrum contains the native BR adsorption band (560 nm) and the one corresponding to free retinal. The conclusion may be drawn comparing the spectra that while transferring bacteriorhodopsin into the organic phase only a slight denaturation of BR (apparently, dissociation into bacterioopsin and retinal) occurs. The absense of BR adsorption maxi-

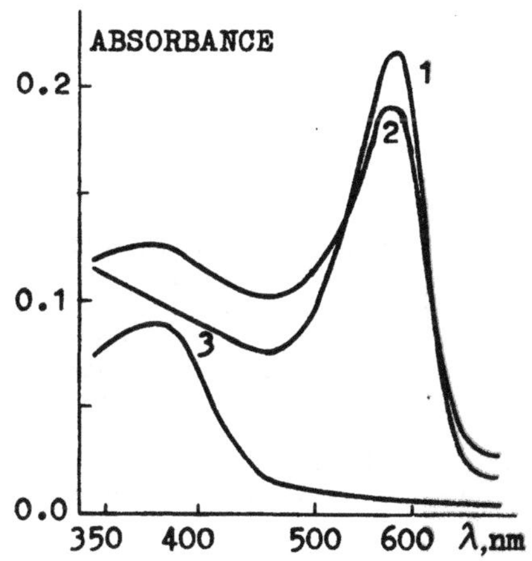


Fig.1.Absorbance spectrum of bacteriorhodopsin: 1- purple membranes in water, 2- bacteriorhodopsin in azolectine solution in decane, 3 - as (2), with bacteriorhodopsin denaturating by sonication without cooling.

mum shift in BRS suggests that the polarity of the chromophore surrounding has not changed. Assuming the extinction coefficient being the same one can estimate the yield of BR with native spectrum in the transfer into decane solution of azolectine as 70--90% (the same yield was obtained in the quantitative determination of the protein with Lowry method). If hexane was used instead of decane the almost complete denaturation of BR occured according to (8). The CD -spectrum of BRS (curve 1, fig.2) corresponds qualitatively to the CD-spectrum of purple membranes in water (curve 2) shaped typically for exciton interaction (13). This proves agregated (nonmonomolecular) state of BR in BRS. This conclusion was confirmed by BRS investigation with the dynamic light scattering method - the particle diffusion coeffi-

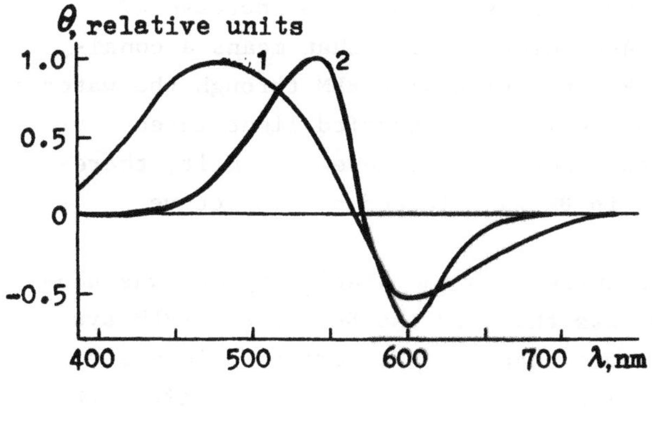


Fig.2. CD-spectra of bacteriorhodopsin in azolectine solution in decane (1) and of purple membranes in water electrolyte (2).

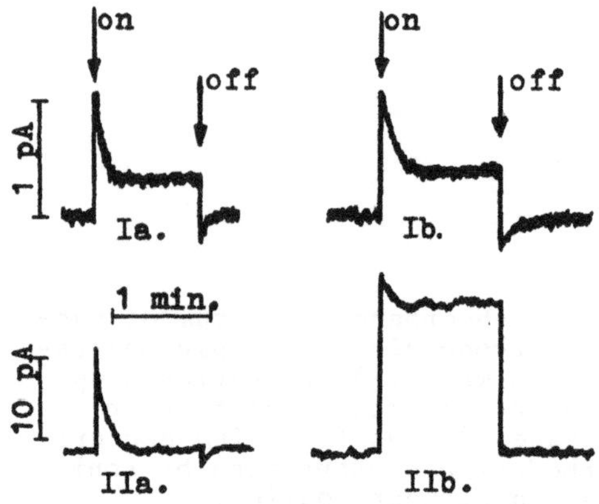


Fig.3. Photocurrent of BLM formed from suspension of bacteriorhodopsin in azolectine solution in decane. I - BLM according to Montal -Mueller, II - BLM according to Mueller-Rudin technique. a) without protonophore, b) with protonophore

cient in suspension was about $2.10^{-13}$ $m^2/s$ which corresponds to the size of particles about 200-800 nm.

Bacteriorhodopsin reconstitution in BLM. BLM of BRS and lipid monolayers generated the stationary photocurrent of about 0.3 pA (Fig.3-la). The photocurrent polarity always corresponded to the proton transfer to the part of cell without BR. Addition of protonophore TTFB did not change the stationary photocurrent though the BLM conductivity increased more than 2 orders of magnitude (Fig.3-lb). According to (14) it means that all the stationary photocurrent is due to BR in BLM only. This excludes the possibility of existence of sandwich-like structure with the "third water" in the system. For example fig.3-II shows the results of a similar experiment on BLM formed of BRS by Mueller - Rudin technique. It is shown that in this case the addition of the same quantity of protonophore leads to multiple increase of stationary photocurrent. According to (14) that means a considerable contribution of BR contacting with BLM through the water to the stationary photocurrent. In the studied light intensity range (up to 40 $mW/sm^2$) the photocurrent depended on it, therefore the proton transfer in BR was limited by the active centre functioning.

The ratio of initial photocurrent to the stationary one was about 4. It is considerably less than for the BR liposome-BLM system (6,10), but a little more than in (8), performed in a similar system. The addition of nigericin (2 μM) did not effect the initial photocurrent therefore the photocurrent peaks cannot be due to the rise of proton gradient in unstirred layers. It was assumed in (8), that the photocurrent peaks are due to capacity photoresponse of BR adsorbed at a teflon partition. Thus the discrepancies in the initial to stationary photocurrents ratio in our work and in (8) may be ascribed to athinner partition used in our work.

Forming BLM so that both monolayers were prepared of BRS, the photocurrent was not observed, though by analog differentiation of a cyclic current voltage characteristic (CVC) averaged for several periods we managed to show the existence of photoconductivity in this system (13). Apparently the absense of photocurrent is due to the opposite pumping of protons by equal amounts of BR in such membrane oriented in opposite directions. So the investigated method proposed by Bamberg et al. (8) results in the transmembrane incorporation of BR into BLM without the formation of sandwich-like structures with the "third water".

Current voltage characteristic of the BLM with BR. Typical record of the cyclyc CVC of BLM with BR in the dark and in the light are shown on fig.4. The CVC in the light (upper loop) compared to the dark one (lower loop) is shifted upwards by the photocurrent value and its slope increases by the photoconductivity value. Fig.4b shows the difference of cyclic CVC obtained

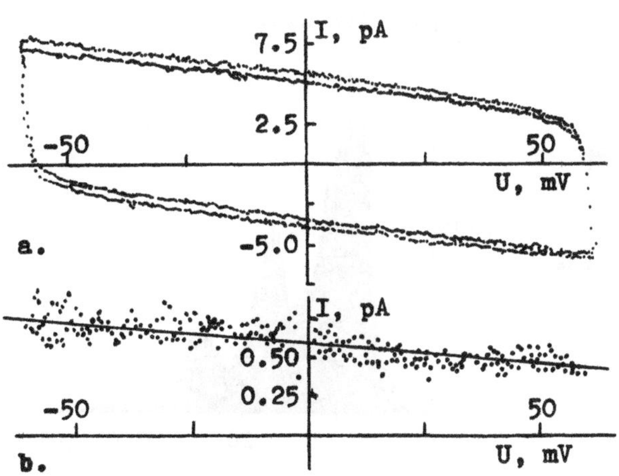


Fig.4. The cyclic current voltage characteristics of BLM with bacteriorhodopsin in light and in dark (a) and the difference of this characteristics

by digital subtraction and averaging as a dependence of BR photo current on the voltage applied. It is notable that in spite of a visible nonlinearity of cyclic CVC the photocurrent on voltage dependence is linear.

It was found that the photoconductivity strongly varies in a series of measurements at the same membrane and the data may be distributed into 3 groups with intervals of 15 pSm. A supposition arose that a mechanism exists in BLM with BR resulting in random discrete fluctuations of conductivity (we relatively name it "channel"), while the typical switching period exceeds the record time of a CVC. This supposition was proved by the experimental data. The membrane current record at a voltage clamp of 20 mV is shown on fig.5a. Typical switching time was several minutes (part of recording with more quick fluctuations is chosen for the figure ). The illumination did not affect the functioning of the "channel". Statistical analysis of current fluctuation in BLM with BR under voltage clamp was carried out to elucidate the discrete nature of these fluctuations. The distribution of BLM conductance obtained by computer processing of current during 22 minutes is shown on fig.5b. The big peak corresponds to the background conductance (all the "channels" are closed), the small peaks correspond to a membrane conductance with one or two open "channels".

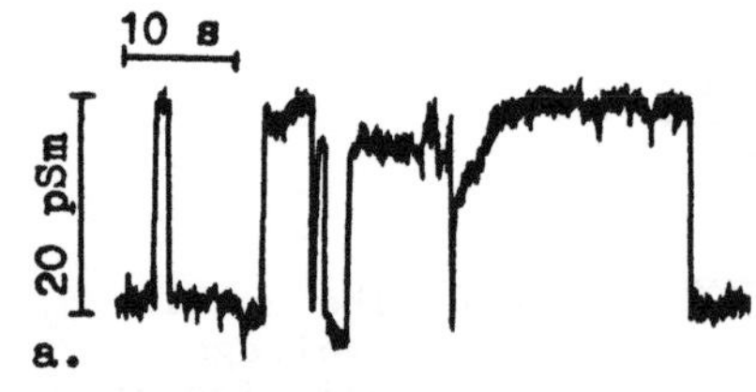


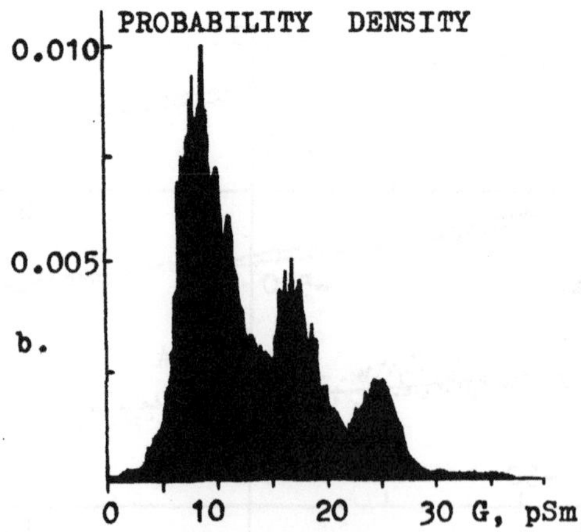


Fig.5. Fluctuations of the conductance of BLM with bacteriorhodopsin (a) and statistical distribution of this conductance (b)

To find out the properties of BR on the basis of BLM experiments one needs to know the degree of orientation of BR in BLM. It could be helped by use of suitable inhibitors of BR, but no such inhibitors are known at the moment. The experimental test of effect of dicyclohexylcarbodiimide (by adding up to 10 mM to the background solution) and of $La(NO_3)_3$ (by adding up to 16 mM into the same solution) proved that thes substances does not affect the photocurrent. But the linear extrapolation of CVC of BLM with BR to the zero current point gives higher voltage (220 mV) than for BR in liposomes-BLM systems. That suggests that the BR orientation in BLM is higher than in liposomes.
The linearity of the BR current voltage characterisic is an important result determining the choice of a possible energetic profile of the BR proton channel. The channel models with a several energetic barriers and the models with a number of equal barriers do not exhibit the necessary properties. We suggest that the most probable BR channel profile with linear current voltage dependence is the multibarrier channel with potential energy of protons linearly decreasing towards active centre. The detailed discussion of this model will be presented later.

Acknowledgements

The authors wish to express their gratitude to Dr. L.A. Podrez for performng the protein analysis, and Drs. V.S. Sokolov and V.I. Portnov for their helpful advice and fruitful discussions.

References

1. Zs. Dancshasy, B. Karvaly. 1976. FEBS Lett. 72, 136.

2. L.A. Drachev, A.D.Kaulen, S.A.Ostroumov, V.P.Skulachev. 1974. FEBS Lett., 39, 43.

3. L.A. Drachev, A.D. Kaulen, A.A. Kondrashin, E.A. Liberman, I.A. Nemechek, S.A.Ostroumov, A.Yu. Semenov, V.P.Skulachev, A.A. Yasaytis. 1974. Doklady Akadem. Nauk SSSR, 218, 481.

4. L.A. Drachev, V.N. Frolov, A.D. Kaulen, E.A. Liberman, S.A. Ostroumov, V.G. Ptakinova, A.Yu. Semenov, V.P. Skulachev. 1976. J.Biol.Chem. 251, 759.

5. A.D. Kaulen. 1978. Thesis of Dissertation. Moscow, Lomonosov University.

6. T.R. Herrman, G.W. Rayfield. 1978. Biophys. J., 21, 111.

7. E. Bamberg, H.-J. Apell, N.A. Dencher, W. Sperling, H. Stieve, P. Lauger. 1979. Biophys.Struct.Mech., 5, 277.

8. E. Bamberg, N.A. Dencher, A. Fahr, M.P. Heyn. 1981. Proc. Natl.Acad.Sci.USA, 78, 7502.

9. V.M. Mirsky, V.S. Sokolov, V.S. Markin. 1984. Elektrokhimia, 20, 876.

10.V.M. Mirsky, V.S. Sokolov, V.S. Markin, L.N. Chekulaeva. 1984. Biol.Membrany, 1, 1143.

11.V.M. Mirsky, V.S. Sokolov, E.I. Melnik, T.V. Diukova. 1983. Bioelectrochem.Bioenerg., 11, 327.

12.V.S. Sokolov, V.M. Mirsky, V.S.Markin, V.E. Kasarinov. 1986. Electrokhimia, 22, 959.

13.M.P. Heyn, P.-J. Bauer, N.A. Dencher. 1975. Biophys.Res.Commun., 67, 897.

14.V.M. Mirsky, V.S.Sokolov. 1984. Biofizika, 29, 246-249.

# POSITION AND ORIENTATION OF THE RETINAL CHROMOPHORE IN THE TWO-DIMENSIONAL PROJECTED DENSITY OF THE PURPLE MEMBRANE

F. Seiff, J. Westerhausen, I. Wallat, and M.P. Heyn
Biophysics Group, Dept. of Physics, Freie Universität Berlin, FRG

## Introduction

Structural information on the position and orientation of retinal is of considerable importance for an understanding of the photochemistry and the pumping mechanism of bacteriorhodopsin at the molecular level. Due to its low electron density X-ray diffraction and electron diffraction methods have not been successful in localizing the chromophore within the structure of bacteriorhodopsin. Some progress was achieved with neutron diffraction using perdeuterated retinal containing 28 deuterons (1,2). In these experiments the chromophore was replaced by perdeuterated retinal and its position was determined from the difference in neutron diffraction intensities between samples with deuterated and undeuterated retinal. The result of these experiments were contradictory (1,2). One of the major problems in such experiments is sample preparation. In the first set of experiments bacteriorhodopsin was bleached but the resulting retinal oxime was not removed from the membrane (1). This could cause an exchange of label. In the second set of experiments the retinal synthesis was suppressed by nicotine and a mixture of oxidation products of perdeuterated ß-carotene, including perdeuterated retinal, was added to the bacterial culture (2). In this way also polyenes of the wrong chain length could be incorporated in bacteriorhodopsin. As a reference sample normal purple membranes were used. The amount of information obtainable with perdeuterated retinal is expected to be limited. Retinal has an elongated polyene structure (Fig. 1), which makes an angle of about 20° with the plane of the membrane (3). The projected difference density is therefore expected to have a length of about 14 Å. With perdeuterated retinal only the center of deuteration of this rod-like difference density can be deter-

Receptors and Ion Channels

mined. More detailed structural information about the location of various parts of retinal may be obtained with partially deuterated retinals, provided such weak labels can be detected. We have synthesized two partially deuterated retinals with 10 and 11 deuterons in the polyene chain and the cyclohexene ring respectively (Fig. 1a and 1b).

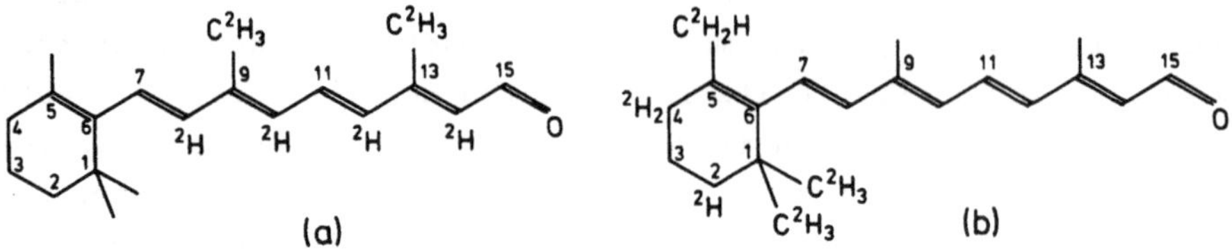


Fig.1. Chemical structures of the synthetic $[^2H_{10}]$ (a) and $[^2H_{11}]$ (b) retinals as determined by $^1$H-NMR and mass spectroscopy.

These retinals were added to the growth medium of strain JW5, a mutant of Halobacterium halobium which is deficient in the synthesis of retinal. In this way a well-defined labelled retinal was incorporated in bacteriorhodopsin without the necessity of chemical modification and the possible interference by retinal oxime. In order to check if the results of (1) were possibly due to the different sample preparation, samples were also prepared by bleaching purple membranes and regenerating the apomembranes with partially deuterated retinal. The retinal oxime was completely removed by repeated washing with bovine serum albumin. As a further improvement with respect to previous work all reference samples with undeuterated retinal were prepared in exactly the same way as the deuterated samples. Our results show that it is possible to localize weak labels containing only 10 or 11 deuterons and that the positions of different parts of the chromophore can be determined. A low-resolution map of the arrangement and orientation of the chromophore in the interior of bacteriorhodopsin is emerging.

## Materials and Methods

Synthesis and characterization of [$^2H_{10}$] retinal. [8,10,12,14,19,19,19,20,20,20-$^2H_{10}$] Retinal (Fig. 1a) was synthesized as described in detail (4). The 13-cis, 9-cis, and all-trans isomers of [$^2H_{10}$] retinal were separated by HPLC and characterized by mass spectroscopy, $^1$H-NMR, and UV spectroscopy. The mass spectrum showed one major peak (79%) at 294, and minor peaks at 293 (14%) and 295 (5%). The average number of deuterons incorporated was 9.94. The $^1$H-NMR spectrum of [$^2H_{10}$]-retinal showed three peaks for protons in the polyene chain that were assigned to the three protons at C-15, C-11, and C-7 and that occurred at the same chemical shift values as for fully protonated retinal. The UV spectrum in ethanol had its maximum at 380 nm and was identical to the spectrum for protonated retinal.

Synthesis and characterization of [$^2H_{11}$] retinal. [2,4,4,16,16,16,17,17,17,18,18-$^2H_{11}$] Retinal (Fig. 1b) was synthesized according to the reaction scheme of Fig. 2 starting from $d_6$-aceton. The reaction scheme is based on procedures developed by J. Lugtenburg and coworkers (5). $d_6$-aceton (1) was reacted with vinylmagnesiumbromide (2) in tetrahydrofuran and converted to dimethylvinylcar-

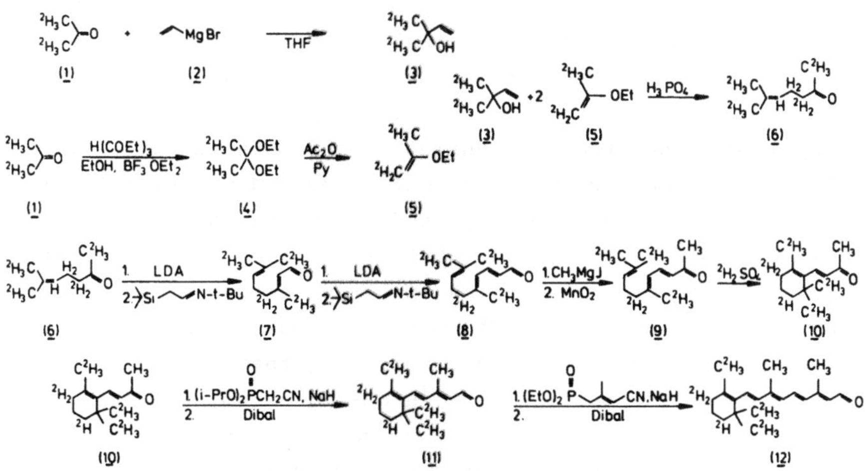


Fig.2. Pathway for the synthesis of [$^2H_{11}$] retinal (12) starting from $d_6$-aceton (1) and vinylmagnesiumbromide (2).

binole (3) with 32% yield (6). Diethoxypropane (4) was formed from $d_6$-aceton (1) and orthoformic acid ethylester in the presence of bortrifluoride (7) and converted to ethyl-1-methylethenylether (5) in the presence of acetic anhydride and pyridine (7). The Claisen reaction of 2 mols of (5) with one mol of (3) at 6 bar in an autoclave resulted with a yield of about 80% in deuterated 6-methyl-5-hepten-2-one (6) (8). Repeated Peterson olefination with LDA and the silyl compound (16) resulted in 3,7-dimethyl-2,6-octadienal (7) and finally in 5,9-dimethyl-2,4,8-decatrienal (8) with an overall-yield of about 59% (9,10). (8) was oxidized with methylmagnesium iodide and activated manganese dioxide to Ψ-ionone (9) (11), which was cyclized to deuterated ß-ionone (10) in the presence of deuterated sulfuric acid and nitromethane (12). ß-ionone (10) was converted to the deuterated $[^2H_{11}]$ retinal (12) in a four-step sequence involving the phosphonate compounds (13) and (15) and dibal (14)-reduction (5,13). All reactions involving metallo-organic compounds were performed under dry argon. Reactions with conjugated polyenes were performed in dim red light. The final product was purified by chromatography (5% ether/hexane, silica gel < 230 mesh) and characterized by UV-spectroscopy, $^1$H-NMR and mass-spectroscopy. The UV spectrum in ethanol had its maximum at 380 nm and had the same shape and extinction coefficient as that of undeuterated retinal. The $^1$H-NMR spectrum of the deuterated retinal (12) had the following features. The lack of a signal at $\delta$ = 1.03 ppm shows that the methyl groups of carbon 16 and 17 are fully deuterated. From the signal at $\delta$ = 1.44 ppm we conclude that the methyl group at C-5 contains one proton, which was introduced by an exchange reaction during the preparation of (6). Position 4 is furthermore completely deuterated and position 2 only to 50%. These results are to be expected on the basis of the scheme for the synthesis (Fig. 2) (7). Whether position 3 is deuterated cannot be decided from the $^1$H-NMR spectrum because of the overlap with the $H_2O$-peak at this $\delta$. The mass spectrum of the deuterated retinal had its main peak at 295 indicating that 11 deuterons were incorporated. On the basis of the $^1$H-NMR spectrum, the mass spectrum and the reaction scheme, we conclude that the endproduct of the synthesis corresponds to the structure represented in Fig. 1b.

Regeneration of Apomembrane. This procedure involving exhaustive washing with bovine serum albumin has been recently described (14).

Regeneration of Retinal⁻ Mutants. The mutant strain JW5, which is deficient in the synthesis of retinal, was grown under standard conditions. On days 4,5, and 6 of growth, all-trans-[$^2H_{10}$] retinal or fully protonated retinal was added to the growth medium. The absorption spectrum of the resulting purple membranes has the same ratio of absorbance at 280 and 570 nm (1.6) as native purple membrane and shows no sign of additional absorbance at ≈ 420 nm from a cytochrome b-type protein. To test whether all the available sites in the lattice were occupied by retinal, additional retinal was added to the isolated membrane patches. No further increase in absorbance at 570 nm was observed. Of the retinal added to the growth medium, 25% was incorporated in purple membranes. The mean patch diameter, as determined from the flash-induced transient dichroism, was ≈ 1 μm. The X-ray diffraction pattern of these samples was, accordingly, sharper and better resolved than for wild-type purple membranes.

Neutron Diffraction Experiments. Oriented purple membrane samples were prepared for neutron diffraction by applying a concentrated suspension on a thin quartz slide (0.3 mm) and by allowing it to dry slowly (24 hr) at 50% relative humidity. The resulting films covered an area of 8 x 20 mm and contained 9 mg of bacteriorhodopsin. Each slide was coated with purple membrane in this way on both sides. Ten slides formed a stack of total thickness 6 mm, containing 180 mg of bacteriorhodopsin. This stack was mounted in an aluminium sample holder. The neutron diffraction data were collected on the D16 diffractometer of the High Flux Reactor (Institut Laue-Langevin, Grenoble). A detailed description of this instrument has recently appeared (15). Briefly, a neutron beam of wavelength 4.52 Å is selected by a graphite monochromator. The sample stack is mounted on the θ-axis of the diffractometer with the normal to the quartz planes initially (θ = 0) parallel to the incident beam. Data were collected in a (θ, 2θ) scan in which the detector was moved in small angular steps synchronously with the sample, in such a way that the angular position of the detector

(2θ) is always twice that of the sample (θ). The angular resolution of the detector was 0.145°. Since the purple membranes are stacked parallel to the quartz slides but are randomly oriented around the axis perpendicular to the slide, the (θ, 2θ) scan provides a powder pattern of the in-plane diffraction from the two-dimensional bacteriorhodopsin lattice. The diffracted intensities were detected by a two-dimensional position-sensitive detector. The quality of the parallel orientation of purple membranes on the slides was determined by measuring the mosaic spread of the first-order lamellar diffraction. For the chain-deuterated samples the full width at half height of the mosaic spread was 12° for the retinal$^-$ mutant and 16° for the regenerated apomembranes. For the samples deuterated in the cyclohexene ring the mosaic spread was only 7°. The data for the chain-deuterated samples were collected at 50% relative humidity. The samples deuterated in the cyclohexene ring were dried at 80% relative humidity. Before the beginning of the diffraction experiments these samples were equilibrated in 100% relative humidity for at least 24 hr. During the diffraction experiments, these dark-adapted samples were enclosed in a cylindrical aluminium can at a relative humidity of 100%.

## Results and Discussion

The neutron diffraction data are presented elsewhere (14,16). The observed intensities could be indexed on a two-dimensional hexagonal lattice with unit cell dimension of 63 Å. The reflections are characterized by the two indices (h,k). The highest well resolved reflection observed was (7,1). Beyond (5,2) no differences in intensities between deuterated and undeuterated samples were observed. The resolution corresponding to (5,2) is 8.7 Å. Label positions can be determined, however, to an accuracy of about 1 Å (17). The intensities were converted into structure factors in the usual way. For nonequivalent reflections, which overlap in the powder pattern, the intensity was split into the squared structure factors according to their ratios in the electron diffraction pattern (18). The phase information was taken over from the EM work (18). The two approximations have recently been studied in detail and been shown to be acceptable for a weak label such as deuterated retinal (17). Fig. 3 shows the structure of bacteriorhodopsin based on the neutron diffraction intensities using these approximations. It is clear that the projected structure determined from the neutron diffraction data is the same in all its main features as the well known structure from electron diffraction (18,19). From the differences in intensities between deuterated and undeuterated samples, Fourier difference maps were calculated (14,16). For the chain-labelled retinal the Fourier difference maps for the $retinal^-$ mutant and the regenerated apomembrane samples had their maxima at very nearly the same position (14). The oval set of lines in Fig. 3, near helix 6, indicates the peak position for the center of deuteration of the chain (14). The circular set of lines, to the left of the oval set, shows the corresponding maximum for the retinal sample deuterated in the cyclohexyl ring. Both Fourier difference maps have secondary maxima. On the basis of a refinement procedure and model calculations, it could be shown that these secondary maxima do not correspond to true label density, but are due to intrinsic errors in the Fourier difference method as well as to cut-off and phase errors (16). The main purpose of the model calculations was to determine if the difference density had the correct amplitude expected for a label of 10 or 11 deuterons. This was indeed the case.

In terms of the previous experiments with perdeuterated retinal the results presented in Fig. 3 are clear cut. According to this figure the chromophore has its cyclohexene ring near helix 4 and points with its polyene chain to the right in the direction of helices 1 and 2. The center of deuteration of perdeuterated retinal lies between C-7 and C-8. The maximum in the difference density for the previous work with perdeuterated retinal thus has to lie between the two positions for the ring and the chain shown in Fig. 3. This is indeed the case for the results of Jubb et al. (2). King et al. (1) had this maximum difference density close to helix 2, however. Their result has to be incorrect. This error is most likely due to the low signal to noise ratio of their data. The quality of our data obtained at the high-flux reactor of the ILL is an order of magnitude better than that obtained at Brookhaven (1). Our results with regenerated apomembranes shows, however, that the method employed by King et al. can be sucessful provided the retinal oxime is removed.

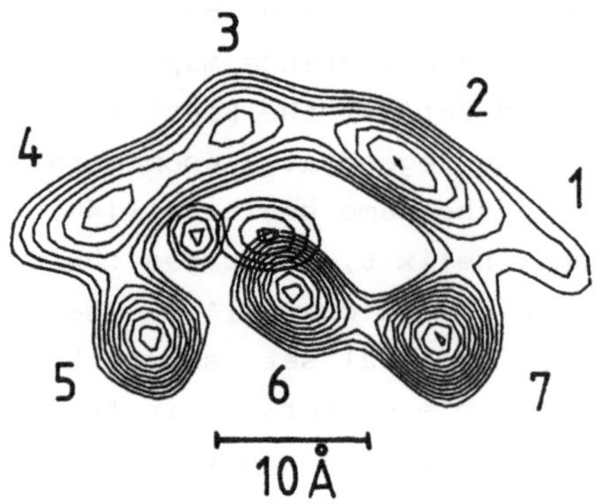


Fig.3. Summary of the neutron diffraction results for JW5 mutants regenerated with chain-deuterated (14) and ring-deuterated retinal. Superimposed on the structure of bacteriorhodopsin, as determined from the neutron diffraction intensities, are shown the 85%, 90%, 95%, and 99% contour lines for the positive difference density from these experiments. The oval set of lines near helix 6 corresponds to the center of deuteration of the polyene chain (C-11). The circular set of lines to the left corresponds to the center of deuteration of the cyclohexene ring.

Fig. 3 shows that the distance between the projected centers of deuteration of the chain (C-11) and of the ring (near the middle of the C-5-C-6 bond, inside the ring) is $\approx$ 4.9 Å. The expected distance is estimated to lie between 4.3 and 5.7 Å. This calculation takes into account that the 6-s bond has the planar trans conformation (20) and that the polyene chain makes an angle of $\approx$ 20° with the plane of the membrane (3). The uncertainty is mainly due to lack of information about the orientation of the plane containing the chain and the ring with respect to the plane of the membrane. The result of Fig. 3 about the projected distance between the two centers of deuteration is thus fully consistent with our present knowledge about the conformation and orientation of the chromophore. The direction from the cyclohexene ring to the Schiff base is from left to right in Fig. 3. It is tempting to draw a line through the two difference peaks and to extrapolate to the position of the Schiff's base taking into account the 20° orientation of the polyene chain. Such an extrapolation is subject to at least two uncertainties: the lack of geometrical information mentioned above and the effect of the 50% 13-cis retinal in our dark-adapted sample. The result of the extrapolation is that the Schiff's base nitrogen is located halfway between the axes of helices 2 and 6. The maximal distance of the lysine nitrogen from the helical axis, assuming the lysine is extended perpendicular to the axis, is ≈ 8 Å. Only the axes of helices 2 and 6 fall within a circle of radius 8 Å drawn around this point. Since retinal is attached to lysine-216 of helix G in the sequence, it follows that G is either 2 or 6. Since the axes of the other helices in Fig. 3 (3,1,7) fall clearly outside the circle, it is unlikely that this conclusion will be altered. The result that the chromophore is located in the interior of bacteriorhodopsin was also obtained using fluorescence energy transfer, a method of considerably lower spatial resolution (21,22).

References


1. King, G.I., P.C. Mowery, W. Stoeckenius, H.L. Crespi and B.P. Schoenborn. 1980. Proc. Natl. Sci. USA 77, 4726.

2. Jubb, J.S., D.L. Worcester, H.L. Crespi and G. Zaccai. 1984. EMBO J. 3, 1455.

3. Heyn, M.P., R.J. Cherry and U. Mueller. 1977. J. Mol. Biol. 117, 607.

4. Ermann, P. 1982. Dissertation, Universität Erlangen-Nuernberg, FRG.

5. Lugtenburg, J. 1985. Pure a. Appl. Chem. 57(5), 753.

6. Ramsden, H.E., J.R. Leebrick, S.D. Rosenberg, E.H. Miller, J.J. Walburn, A.E. Balint and R. Cserr. 1957. J. Org. Chem. 22, 1602.

7. Sancy, G. and R. Marbet. 1967. Helv. Chim. Acta 50, 1164.

8. Sancy, G. and R. Marbet. 1967. Helv. Chim. Acta 50, 2091.

9. Albavella, J.P. 1977. J. Org. Chem. 42, 2009.

10. Corey, L.J., D. Enders and M.G. Bock. 1976. Tetrahedron Letters 7.

11. Attenburrow, J., A.F.B. Cameron, J.H. Chapman, R.M. Evans, B.A. Hems, A.B.A. Jensen and T. Walker. 1952. J. Chem. Soc., 1104.

12. Beilsteins Handbuch d. org. Chemie (1967) Bd. 1, 2075.

13. Dugger, R.W. and C.H. Heathcock. 1980. Synth. Commun. 10(7), 509.

14. Seiff, F., I. Wallat, P. Ermann and M.P. Heyn. 1985. Proc. Natl. Acad. Sci. USA 82, 3227.

15. Institut Laue-Langevin. 1983. Neutron Beam Facilities at the HFR, available from the Scientific Secretary, Institut Laue-Langevin, 156X, 38042 Grenoble Cedex, France.

16. Seiff, F., J. Westerhausen, I. Wallat and M.P.Heyn. 1986. Proc. Natl. Acad. Sci. USA 83, in press.

17. Plöhn, H.-J. and G. Büldt. 1986. J. Appl. Cryst. 19, 255.

18. Unwin, P.N.T. and R. Henderson. 1975. J. Mol. Biol. 94, 425.

19. Hayward, S.B. and R.M. Stroud. 1981. J. Mol. Biol. 151, 491.

20. Harbison, G.S., S.O. Smith, J.A. Pardoen, J.M.L. Courtin, J. Lugtenburg, J. Herzfeld, R.A. Mathies and R.G. Griffin. 1985. Biochemistry 24, 6955.

21. Kouyama, T., Y. Kimura, K. Kinosita and A. Ikegami. 1982. J. Mol. Biol. 153, 337.

22. Rehorek, M., N.A. Dencher and M.P. Heyn. 1983. Biophys. J. 43, 39.

# THE LIGHT-ENERGIZED $H^+$-PUMP BACTERIORHODOPSIN: A MODEL SYSTEM FOR FUNCTIONAL TRANSMEMBRANE RECONSTITUTION OF ION CHANNELS, RECEPTORS, AND PUMPS

Norbert A. Dencher

Biophysics Group, Department of Physics, Freie Universität Berlin,
Arnimallee 14, D-1000 Berlin 33, FRG

## Introduction

Investigation of the structure and function of ion channels, pumps, and receptors that are vectorially inserted into a lipid bilayer, is often hampered by the complexity of the cell membrane. Therefore, usually as a first approach, the membrane protein of interest is solubilized with detergents, isolated, and purified.

The subsequent study of the protein in the mixed detergent-lipid-protein micelle gives only restricted answers, mainly for two reasons. In the first place, the new microenvironment has chemical and physical properties quite different from the native one, and might affect the structure and activity of the protein. (Additives such as a combination of phospholipid and glycerol can restore part of the function, as has been demonstrated for the solublized aspartate receptor of chemotaxis from Salmonella typhimurium (1)). In the second place, since pumps and gated channels create and regulate, respectively, vectorial solute gradients, an intact membrane phase separating two compartments is required for functional studies. Reconstituted protein-lipid vesicle systems provide a more appropriate experimental system in this respect. Various approaches have been previously developed for functional reconstitution of membrane proteins into lipid vesicles as illustrated for the light-energized proton pump bacteriorhodopsin in Table I. (The field of receptor reconstitution is reviewed in ref. 2). All of these procedures require harsh treatments such as prolonged sonication, detergents, organic solvents, freezing and thawing, etc., that may be harmful for the membrane protein to various degrees. A novel technique for successful membrane protein reconstitution avoiding any harsh treatment is presented (6). Mixing aqueous suspensions of long-chain lecithins (soybean phospholipids, DMPC, DPPC) with the short-chain lecithin diheptanoylphosphatidylcholine (20 mol% of total lipid) in the presence of purple membranes (containing bacteriorhodopsin as the sole protein) leads to the spontaneous formation of reconstituted bacteriorhodopsin-lipid vesicles. Bacteriorhodopsin is inserted into the lipid bilayer and is highly active as a proton pump. Since the procedure is easy, fast, and particularly has no harmful effect on the membrane protein, it might be the method of choice for functional reconstitution of other membrane pumps, channels and receptors as well.

Table I. Reconstitution Procedures Commonly Applied to Bacteriorhodopsin

| | |
|---|---|
| Sonication | (3,4,5,6) |
| Freeze-thaw sonication | (4,7) |
| Reverse phase evaporation | (8) |
| Detergent-mediated reconstitution: | |
| removal by dilution | (9,10,11) |
| dialysis | (3,4,5,11,12,13) |
| gel filtration | (14,15) |
| adsorption | (12,14) |

Transmembrane Reconstitution of Bacteriorhodopsin

The integral membrane protein bacteriorhodopsin of the purple membrane can be reconstituted into lipid vesicles by several procedures, the commonly applied ones are listed in Table I.

Sonication. This is the most often used, but unfortunately also most unsuitable procedure. Purple membrane patches are incorporated into preformed small sonicated lipid vesicles by prolonged sonication with a powerful tip-sonicator. The reconstituted vesicles obtained are quite small and therefore less suitable for transport studies. Furthermore, they are very heterogeneous with respect to the protein-to-lipid ratio; a high percentage of the vesicles (up to 50%) does not contain bacteriorhodopsin at all (5). During prolonged sonication, part of the bacteriorhodopsin is destroyed.

Freeze-thaw sonication. Purple membrane patches are inserted into preformed small sonicated lipid vesicles by slowly cooling the sample to about -70°C in a refrigerator or by rapid freezing in liquid nitrogen (- 196°C). Thereafter the sample is warmed up to room temperature and then shortly sonicated to convert multibilayer vesicles into unilamellar vesicles. To increase the amount of incorporated bacteriorhodopsin, the freeze-thawing step should be repeated

2-3 times. We are currently using this technique for functional co-reconstitution of bacteriorhodopsin and a $H^+$-ATPase of yeast plasma membrane (15).
Reverse phase evaporation. Phospholipid in diethylether is mixed (3:1,$^v$/v) with aqueous purple membrane suspension. The resulting two-phases system is sonicated for 3 minutes and thereafter the organic solvent is removed under reduced pressure (8). Since many membrane proteins will not tolerate the organic solvent, application of this procedure is limited.
Reconstitution by aid of detergents. Using various detergents (e.g., octyl-β-glucopyranoside (octylglucoside), Triton X-100, deoxycholate/cholate) intact purple membrane patches as well as monomeric bacteriorhodopsin can be reconstituted into lipid vesicles upon detergent removal by different methods.
**Detergent dilution:** Bacteriorhodopsin in purple membrane sheets can be incorporated into phospholipid vesicles by a detergent dilution method (10,11). Lipids (e.g., 27 mM soybean phospholipids) are sonicated to clarity in a bath-type sonicator. 1.1 mg of the vesicles obtained are mixed with 30-300 µg of bacteriorhodopsin (purple membrane) in a final volume of 400 µl containing buffer (e.g., 1 mM HEPES, pH 7.4, and 75 mM KCl), and 1.25% octylglucoside. Two minutes prior to the addition of the lipid vesicles, purple membrane is mixed with the detergent solution and sonicated for 20 sec. The bacteriorhodopsin-phospholipid-octylglucoside mixture is incubated in the dark at 20°. After 10-180 min, 40-µl samples are diluted with 1 ml buffer, and the vesicles are ready for use.
**Detergent dialysis:** Monomeric bacteriorhodopsin can be reconstituted into phospholipid vesicles by mixing lipid and detergent-solubilized protein together and removing the detergent by dialysis (11,13). Bacteriorhodopsin is solubilized to the state of monomers in the nonionic detergents Triton X-100 or octylglucoside (12). For DMPC and DPPC the procedure works best with Triton X-100. Soybean phospholipid, diphytanoyl PC, and phosphatidylserine vesicles can be prepared only with bacteriorhodopsin solubilized in octylglucoside. Monomeric bacteriorhodopsin (at a concentration required to achieve the desired lipid-to-protein ratio after mixing) is added to the lipids and incubated with occasional shaking at a temperature above the lipid-phase transition for 20 min. The mixture is poured into a dialysis bag and dialyzed for at least 2 days or 8 days in the case of octylglucoside and Triton X-100, respectively, as detergent. In order to remove residual traces of detergent, Bio-Beads SM-2 are added to the dialysis buffer. The vesicles are fractionated by centrifugation on a 5-40% (w/w) sucrose gradient (250,000 g for 5 hr). They are unilamellar, with radii between 35 and 300 nm.

**Gel filtration:** Reconstituted vesicles can be obtained in 2-5 minutes by passing a mixture of bacteriorhodopsin/lipid/detergent through a short Sephadex G-25 or G-50 column (14,15). The detergent, e.g., octylglucoside, is nearly completely removed and the vesicles formed are eluted with the void volume. If dye molecules such as the hydrophilic, pH-sensitive probe pyranine are present in the initial mixture, the dye is entrapped in the internal aqueous compartment of the vesicles and the external free dye molecules are separated (11).
**Adsorption:** Rapid removal of detergent from mixtures of bacteriorhodopsin/lipid/detergent and vesicle formation in the time-course of minutes can be achieved by adsorption to nonpolar polymeric adsorbents, e.g., Bio-Beads SM-2 (Bio-Rad) or Amberlite XAD-2 (Sigma). Either a short column made of this resin is used or the adsorbents are added directly to the sample (12,14).

Spontaneous insertion of bacteriorhodopsin into lipid vesicles facilitated by the short-chain phospholipid diheptanoylphosphatidylcholine (DHPC). Reconstitution proceeds via the following steps: The long-chain and the short-chain phospholipids are dissolved in a small volume of chloroform and separately spread as a thin film on the wall of two glass test tubes by evaporation of the solvent under a stream of nitrogen. Residual traces of solvent are removed under vacuum ($< 10^{-3}$ Torr, 5-15 h) at room temperature. The dried lipid films are hydrated in an appropriate aqueous solvent, e.g., 150 mM KCl solution. This step can be assisted by 10 s sonication. The aqueous suspension of the respective long-chain phospholipid (DMPC, DPPC, or soybean phospholipid SBPL), final concentration of 20 mM after addition of all constituents, is mixed with a concentrated aqueous suspension of purple membranes. The purple membranes should be sonicated prior to mixing to reduce the size of the membrane sheets, however, sonication is not essential. Sonication of the purple membranes for about 60 s, depending on the power of the sonicator, is recommended to obtain an optimum in the extent of incorporation of bacteriorhodopsin (BR) as well as in functional activity. To this mixture of long-chain phospholipid and purple membranes, the aqueous micellar 50 mM DHPC (Figure 1) solution is added, yielding a final DHPC concentration of 5 mM (20 mol% of total lipid), and the sample is immediately vortexed. Finally, this lipid-purple membrane mixture is sonicated in the bath-sonicator for 30 s. This sonication step is only required for SBPL and can be omitted with DMPC and DPPC. All manipulations should be performed at temperatures above the lipid phase transition of the respective long-chain phospholipids, e.g., room temperature for SBPL, 30°C for DMPC, and 44°C for DPPC. Transmembrane insertion of BR into the lipid vesicles occurs immediately upon addition of DHPC (and 30 s sonication in the case of

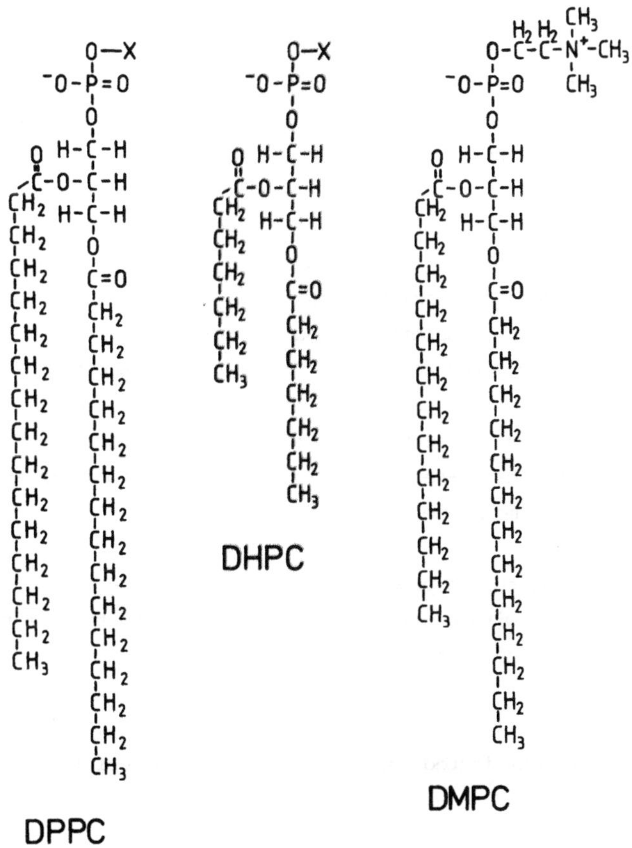


Figure 1. Structural comparison of the short-chain phospholipid diheptanoylphosphatidylcholine (DHPC, fatty acid chain length of 7 carbons) with the long-chain phospholipids dimyristoylphosphatidylcholine (DMPC, chain length of 14 carbons) and dipalmitoylphosphatidylcholine (DPPC, chain length of 16 carbons).

SBPL). Usually, the samples are incubated at room temperature or 30°C for 3-8 h and thereafter subjected to density gradient centrifugation. Stable BR-lipid vesicles are spontaneously formed upon mixing all constituents. The large alterations in the light-scattering properties of the sample allow detection of vesicle formation. In accordance with a previous report for pure lipid systems (16), the observed light-scattering changes reveal that DHPC facilitates the formation of stable unilamellar vesicles from aqueous supensions of preexisting multibilayers of long-chain lecithins and purple membrane. Transmembrane insertion of BR into the lipid bilayer is verified by means of density gradient centrifugation, circular dichroism measurements, and vectorial $H^+$-transport. Reconstitution efficiency and general properties of the vesicles depend on the physical and chemical state of the long-chain lecithins. The majority of the SBPL-DHPC-BR vesicles have diameters between 35 and 100 nm, whereas the DMPC-DHPC-BR vesicles are much larger, ranging from 100 to 450 nm in diameter. The reconstituted BR-lipid vesicles are highly active in light-energized vectorial $H^+$-translocation. Steady-state values corresponding to a net inward transport of about 11 $H^+$/BR are observed for SBPL-DHPC-BR vesicles, as compared to <0.16 $H^+$/BR in the absence of DHPC. Both, the reconstitution procedure and the properties of the vesicles obtained are described in more detail in refs 6 and 17. Recently, this procedure has been successfully applied for the co-reconstitution of bacteriorhodopsin and a $H^+$-ATPase of yeast plasma membrane (15).

Another gentle reconstitution procedure utilizes myristate or cholesterol as fusogen in combination with cooling to temperatures below the gel to liquid -crystalline phase transition (18).

## Bacteriorhodopsin Reconstituted into Unilamellar Lipid Vesicles

In the reconstituted vesicle systems, bacteriorhodopsin is active as a light-driven proton pump: up to 35 protons per bacteriorhodopsin are transported into the vesicle during illumination. The light-induced fluorescence quenching of the dye 9-aminoacridine demonstrates that bacteriorhodopsin in soybean phospholipid vesicles (molar SBPL to BR ratio of 262) is able to generate a large transmembrane pH-gradient, inside acidic (Figure 2). Calibrating this fluorescence quenching signal by creating pH gradients of known magnitude

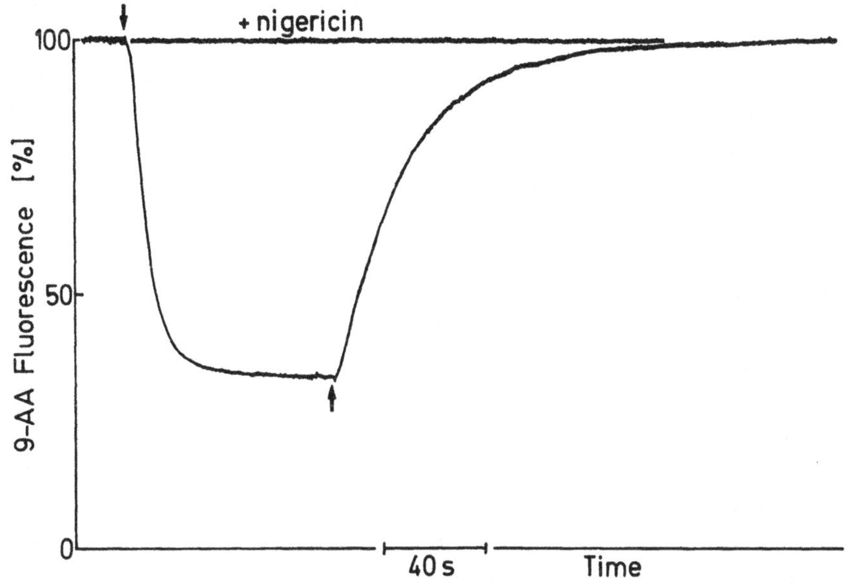


Figure 2. Light-induced generation of a pH-gradient across reconstituted soybean phospholipid vesicles by monomeric bacteriorhodopsin. SBPL-bacteriorhodopsin vesicles (molar lipid-to-protein ratio of 262, average vesicle diameter of 105 nm) were prepared by the octylglucoside dialysis procedure. The vesicles were suspended in 40 mM phosphate buffer, pH 7.5, containing 150 mM KCl and 1 µg/ml valinomycin to collapse the membrane potential. Temperature: 20.2°C. 9-Aminoacridine (5 µM) was excited at 403 nm and the fluorescence monitored at 460 nm. In the subsequent measurement the pH-gradient was abolished with the $K^+/H^+$ antiporter nigericin (1 µg/ml). The maximum fluorescence quenching corresponds to a pH-gradient of 2.4 units according to the applied calibration procedure with pH-gradients of known magnitude. Arrows depict onset and termination of the illumination period, about 25 $mW/cm^2$. (Experiment performed in collaboration with Dr. R. Casadio).

leads to an estimate for the steady-state ΔpH of 2.4 units if the membrane potential is abolished by valinomycin (Figure 2) and of 2.2 units in the absence of this ionophore (data not shown). The $K^+/H^+$ antiporter nigericin inhibits formation of a pH gradient. (It should be mentioned, however, that various experimental results challenge the application of 9-aminoacridine as accurate monitor of both the magnitude and kinetics of ΔpH changes (11). Calculating the transmembrane ΔpH according to ref. 19 for the data depicted in Figure 2 would result in an overestimate by 1 pH-unit). A net inside-out orientation of 70-90% for the bacteriorhodopsin molecules, depending on the vesicle system, is determined by selective proteolysis with pronase, papain, or chymotrypsin and subsequent gel electrophoresis. The state of aggregation of bacteriorhodopsin in the vesicle membrane (i.e., either monomeric or aggregated as trimers in a hexagonal lattice) is controlled by the physical state of the lipid phase and/or the lipid-to-protein ratio. It is worth mentioning that even if vesicles are reconstituted with purple membrane, bacteriorhodopsin can be present as monomer at a high lipid-to-protein ratio (i.e., above a molar ratio of about 70).

Structural and functional properties of bacteriorhodopsin are either studied directly in reconstituted vesicles by means of various biochemical and biophysical techniques, or the vesicles are used as starting material for the formation of planar lipid bilayers with transmembrane inserted bacteriorhodopsin suitable for electrical methods (20). By aid of reconstituted BR-lipid vesicles it could be demonstrated that the functional unit responsible for bacteriorhodopsin's photocycle and for proton transport is the monomer itself (20,21,22). Monomeric bacteriorhodopsin is an effective proton pump (Figure 2). Experiments with reconstituted vesicles showed that the chromophore retinal itself blocks the $H^+$-conducting pathway across the transmembrane protein bacteriorhodopsin or indirectly controls this path by inducing conformational changes in the protein upon binding (11,23). Bacteriorhodpsin-DMPC vesicles, which allow the reversible disaggregation of bacteriorhodopsin by merely changing the temperature, are an attractive model system to study protein-protein and protein-lipid interactions (22,24,25).

Acknowledgement

This work was supported by the Deutsche Forschungsgemeinschaft (SFB 312/B4, Heisenberg Grant De 300/1).

References

1. Bogonez, E. and D.E. Koshland, Jr.. 1985. Proc. Natl. Acad. Sci. USA 82, 4891-4895.

2. Levitzki, A. 1985. Biochim. Biophys. Acta 822, 127-153.

3. Hwang, S.-B. and W. Stoeckenius. 1977. J. Membr. Biol. 33, 325-350.

4. Racker, E. 1979. Methods Enzymol. 55, 699-711.

5. Van Dijck, P.W.M. and K. van Dam. 1982. Methods Enzymol. 88, 17-25.

6. Dencher, N.A. 1986. Biochemistry 25, 1195-1200.

7. Casadio, R. and W. Stoeckenius. 1980. Biochemistry 19, 3374-3381.

8. Rigaud, J.L., A. Bluzat, and S. Buschlen. 1983. Biochem. Biophys. Res. Commun. 111, 373-382.

9. Racker, E., B. Violand, S.O'Neal, M. Alfonzo, and J. Telford. 1979. Arch. Biochem. Biophys. 198, 470-477.

10. Abdulaev, N.G., N.A. Dencher, A.E. Dergachev, A. Fahr, and A.V. Kiselev. 1984. Biophys. Struct. Mech. 10, 211-227.

11. Dencher, N.A., P.A. Burghaus, and S. Grzesiek. 1986. Methods Enzymol 127, 746-760.

12. Dencher, N.A. and M.P. Heyn. 1982. Methods Enzymol. 88, 5-10.

13. Heyn, M.P. and N.A. Dencher. 1982. Methods Enzymol. 88, 31-35.

14. Krupinski, J. and G.G. Hammes. 1985. Biochemistry 24, 6963-6972.

15. Dencher, N.A. and A. Wach. (unpublished experiments).

16. Gabriel, N.E. and M.F. Roberts. 1984. Biochemistry 23, 4011-4015.

17. Dencher, N.A. 1987. Methods Enzymol., in press.

18. Scotto, A.W. and D. Zakim. 1986. Biochemistry 25, 1555-1561.

19. Schuldiner, S., H. Rottenberg, and M. Avron. 1972. Eur. J. Biochem. 25, 64-70.

20. Bamberg, E., N.A. Dencher, A. Fahr, and M.P. Heyn. 1981. Proc. Natl. Acad. Sci. USA 78, 7502-7506.

21. Dencher, N.A. and M.P. Heyn. 1979. FEBS Lett. 108, 307-310.

22. Dencher, N.A., K.-D. Kohl, and M.P. Heyn. 1983. Biochemistry 22, 1323-1334.

23. Burghaus, P.A. and N.A. Dencher. 1986. Biochim. Biophys. Acta, in press.

24. Heyn, M.P., R.J. Cherry, and N.A. Dencher. 1981. Biochemistry 20, 840-849.

25. Rehorek, M., N.A. Dencher, and M.P. Heyn. 1985. Biochemistry 24, 5980-5988.

# USE OF MONOCLONAL ANTIBODIES TO STUDY BOVINE RHODOPSIN

N.G. Abdulaev, E.R. Eganyan, Yu.A. Ovchinnikov
Shemyakin Institute of Bioorganic Chemistry USSR Academy of Sciences, Moscow 117871, USSR

## Introduction

Rhodopsin is a photoreceptor protein of the visual cell of vertebrates. The protein (1) and its structural gene (2) were analyzed to determin the amino acid sequence of bovine rhodopsin. A light-sensitive antenna is 11-*cis* retinal bound to the ε-amino group of Lys 296. Photon absorption isomerizes 11-*cis* retinal to the all-*trans* form. Biochemical data available show isomerization to be the cause of protein conformational changes followed by activation of a few soluble enzymes (3) that leads to the cell hyperpolarization. Enzymatic changes are blocked by phosphorylation of the bleached rhodopsin molecule. Enzymes of the amplifying cascade interact with rhodopsin in the regions located on the cytoplasmic surface of the photoreceptor disk. Here of great importance is elucidation of topography of polypeptide chain fragments which provide the system functioning upon interaction with soluble proteins.

Membrane folding of the rhodopsin polypeptide chain was earlier elaborated on the basis of experiments on the limited proteolysis and chemical modification (Fig. 1) (4, 5). The model revealed that the rhodopsin molecule consisted of seven segments each spanning the lipid bilayer, besides it permitted localization of these transmembrane segments and the N- and C-terminal sites of the protein. To refine the hypothesis we applyed immunochemical methods, earlier used for investigating acetylcholine receptor topography (6), myoglobin (7), bacteriorhodopsin (8) etc. The rhodopsin molecule was studied by monoclonal antibodies (9, 10).

Receptors and Ion Channels

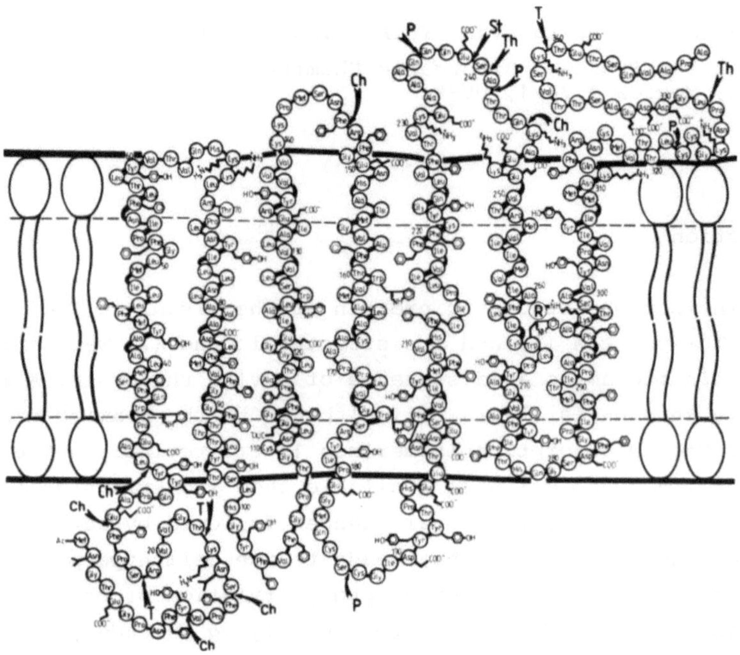

Fig. 1. Topography of rhodopsin molecule in the membrane.

Results

Tatle 1 presents two schemes for interperitoneal immunization of BALB/c mice. The animals were divided into two groups. The first group was injected with the suspension of photoreceptor disks with complete Freund's adjuvant (100 γ per mouse). Then they were given two injections of an antigen with incomplete Freund's adjuvant separated by an interval of two weeks. No adjuvant was used at the final stage of the immunization procedure. The spleens of mice were hybridized 2-4 days after the fourth injection. A 15-day scheme was introduced to immunize the second group of mice (11):15 and 8 days before hybridization the injection dose was 50 γ of suspension of photoreceptor disks with complete Freund's adjuvant per mouse, 5 days before fusion daily injection dose was 25 γ of anti-

Table 1. Schemes for Immunization

| The day before fusion | Amount of antigen ($\gamma$) | The buffer |
|---|---|---|
| I | | |
| 36 | 100 | Freund's adjuvant (complete) |
| 22 | 100 | Freund's adjuvant (incomplete) |
| 18 | 100 | " - " - " - " - " - " - " |
| 4 | 100 | PBS |
| 0 (fusion) | | |
| II | | |
| 15 | 50 | Freund's adjuvant (complete) |
| 8 | 50 | " - " - " - " - " - " - " |
| 5 | 25 | PBS |
| 4 | "-" | " - " - " - " - " - " - " |
| 3 | "-" | " - " - " - " - " - " - " |
| 2 | "-" | " - " - " - " - " - " - " |

gen in the isotonic phosphate buffer, pH 7.4 (PBS). The fusion was performed one day later according to Kohler and Milstein (12) with some modification, splenocyte myeloma ratio ranges from 10:1 to 1:1. Fusion agents were 45% polyethylene glycol (M 4000) and 15% DMSO. Ten-fourteen days later supernatants from cloning wells were tested for specificity of antibodies to rhodopsin and its fragments (Table 2) by immunoenzymatic assay. Cloning was performed as described in (13). To produce monoclonal antibodies in preparative amounts hybridimas were injected into BALB/c mice, then transferred to large-scale culture. Antibodies were precipitated from ascites liquids or cultures by 35% ammonium sulfate, a higher degree of purity was obtained by ion exchange chromatography on Sephacryl S-200 in 0.1 M Tris-HCl, 1 M NaCl, pH 7.5 and on Protein-A-Sepharose (14). The purified antibodies were characterized by polyacrylamide gel electrophoresis (15) and thin layer electrofocusing (16).

Monoclonal antibodies to rhodopsin were obtained and characterized. Native (adaptive to the darkness) photoreceptor disks isolated

Table 2. Fragments of Visual Rhodopsin

| Peptide name | Peptide sequence |
| --- | --- |
| B1 | $Asn^{2}$-$Met^{39}$ |
| B4 | $Leu^{50}$-$Met^{86}$ |
| B5+B6 | $Val^{87}$-$Met^{155}$ |
| T7 | $Phe^{148}$-$Arg^{177}$ |
| B8 | $Ala^{164}$-$Met^{183}$ |
| B9 | $Gln^{184}$-$Met^{207}$ |
| B10 | $Phe^{208}$-$Met^{253}$ |
| B12+B13 | $Val^{258}$-$Met^{309}$ |
| B15 | $Val^{318}$-$Ala^{348}$ |

from bovine retina were used as antigens upon immunization of BALB/c mice. Five independent hybridizations generated the lybrary of hybridomas (∿40) which produced monoclonal antibodies to rhodopsin. Some of them interacting with rhodopsin fragments of tryptic hydrolysis and cyanogen bromide cleavage were chosen for further study. The fragments taken together covered the whole length of the polypeptide chain (Table 2).

Almost all hybridomas produced antibodies to linear determinants, majority of monoclonal antibodies interacted with two cyanogen bromide fragments B1 and B5+B6. Obviously, amino acid sequences of these peptides incorporate the main immunogenic regions of the rhodopsin molecule. It is noteworthy the library contains hybridomas producing monoclonal antibodies to the polypeptide chain fragments exposed to the intradisk space in accordance with the proposed model, inaccessible to proteolytic enzymes upon treatment of native photoreceptor disks. Antigen is known to split, by enzymes on macrophages during the immune response (17), that under certain conditions breaks intactness of photoreceptor disks and makes the polypeptide chain fragments exposed to the intradisk space inaccessible (18).

Five monoclonal antibodies with various specifity were selected for further experiment (Table 3). Antibody affinity was established

Table 3. Monoclonal Antibodies Rhodopsin

| Antibody name | Sunclass of IgG | $K \cdot M^{-1}$ |
|---|---|---|
| $R_1$ | γ3 | $6.2 \cdot 10^8$ |
| $R_2$ | γ1 | $0.8 \cdot 10^8$ |
| $R_3$ | γ1 | $1.1 \cdot 10^8$ |
| $R_5$ | γ2a | $3.0 \cdot 10^8$ |
| $R_6$ | γ1 | $1.2 \cdot 10^9$ |

by the Scatchard technique (19). Delipidated rhodopsin served as antigen. Binding constant values appeared high enough to define antigenic determinants.

## Locatization of antigenic determinants, their amino acid composition

To investigate interaction of monoclonal abtibodies with rhodopsin and its fragments, immunoenzymatic assay was applied with modification which allowed peptides to be used in small amounts (20 pm).

As described above all the hybridomas produced were tested in the rhodopsin fragments overlapping the complete sequence. The approach provided an opportunity for selecting hybrid clones which produced antibodies to the sites of interest. Thus the following hybridomas were detected, their specifity given in brackets: $R_1$ (BI), $R_2$ and $R_3$ (B5+B6), $R_5$ (B8, B9), and $R_6$ (B15). Then we studied interaction of each antibody with the overlapping peptides, which composed a large fragment (Fig. 2). Antibodies $R_1$ interact with the N-terminal cyanogen bromide fragment (2-39) of the protein molecule. Three peptides of the rhodopsin N-terminal region were isolated from the apomembrane tryptic hydrolyzate: AcMet$^1$-Lys$^{16}$, Thr$^{17}$-Arg$^{21}$, and Ser$^{22}$-Lys$^{66}$, but the antibodies were observed to interact only with the first peptide listed. Consequently, the antigenic determinant recognized by antibodies $R_1$ is in region Asn$^2$-Lys$^{16}$. Earlier when stusying bacteriorhodopsin tophography to identify amino acid residues in antigenic determinants we used shortened peptides formed at the

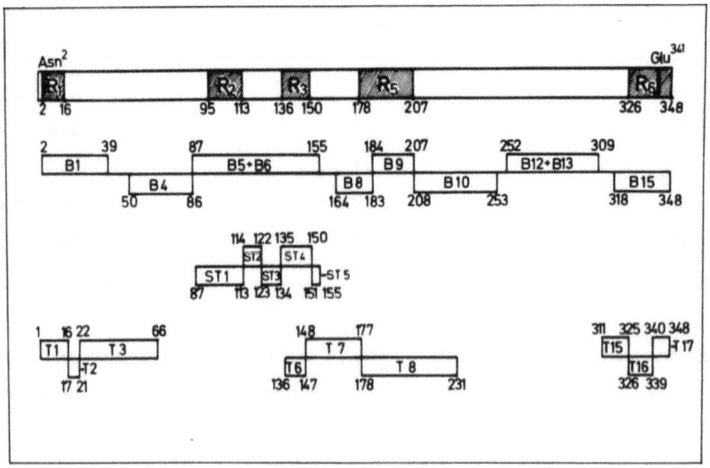


Fig. 2. Rhodopsin fragments used at localization of antigenic determinants.

cleavage of the N-terminal residues by the Edman degradation (20), the same approach was applied to establish antigenic determinants. Degradation of fragment was performed, interaction of the shortened peptides with monoclonal antibodies $R_1$ was studied (Fig. 3a), intrestingly, the interaction sharply decreases, after cleavage of $Asn^2$, so, this amino acid residue is important to antigenic determinant formation.

Antibodies $R_2$ and $R_3$ interact with cyanogen bromide fragment B5+B6. To refine the antigenic determinants recognized with these antibodies we cleaved fragment B5+B6 with protease *St. aureus*, the peptides obtained were separated by HPLC (Fig. 4). Analysis of the newly formed short fragments ($Val^{87}$-$Glu^{113}$, $Glu^{114}$-$Glu^{122}$, $Ile^{123}$-$Glu^{134}$, $Arg^{135}$-$Glu^{150}$, $Asn^{151}$-$Met^{155}$) revealed that antigenic determinant interacting with antibodies $R_2$ is located within peptide $Val^{87}$-$Glu^{113}$, and that interacting with antibodies within peptide $Arg^{135}$-$Glu^{150}$. Antibodies $R_3$ are bound to tryptic fragment $Tyr^{136}$-$Arg^{147}$, thus the overlapping region of the polypeptide chain $Tyr^{136}$-

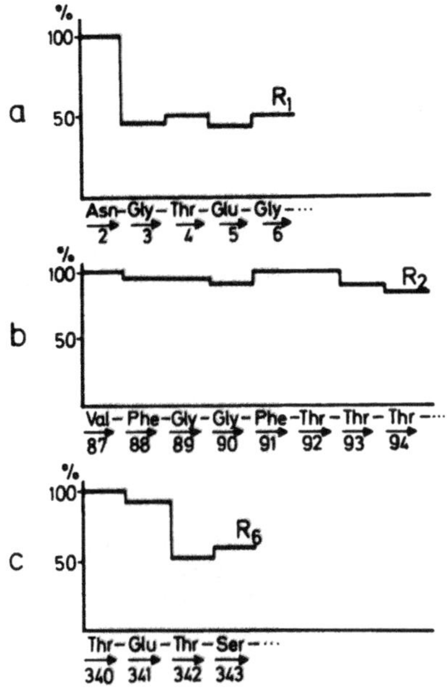


Fig. 3. Interaction of antibodies with Edman degradation products (results of immunoenzymatic assay).

$Glu^{150}$ contains the antigenic determinant. Efficiency of monoclonal antibodies $R_2$ interaction did not change upon cleavage of eight amino acid fragments B5+B6 (Fig. 3b), that indicated the antigenic determinant location recognized with these antibodies in region $Leu^{95}$-$Glu^{113}$.

Antibodies $R^5$ interact with peptides B8 and B9 as well as with tryptic fragment $Tyr^{178}$-$Lys^{231}$, all the three fragments have overlapping region $Tyr^{178}$-$Met^{207}$ where the antigenic determinant should lie.

Specifity of antibodies $R_6$ is locatized within the C-terminal cyanogen bromide fragment of rhodopsin. Interaction does not change with shorter peptides from tryptic hydrolyzate $Asn^{236}$-$Lys^{339}$, $Thr^{340}$-$Ala^{348}$ and, consequently, the antigenic determinant recog-

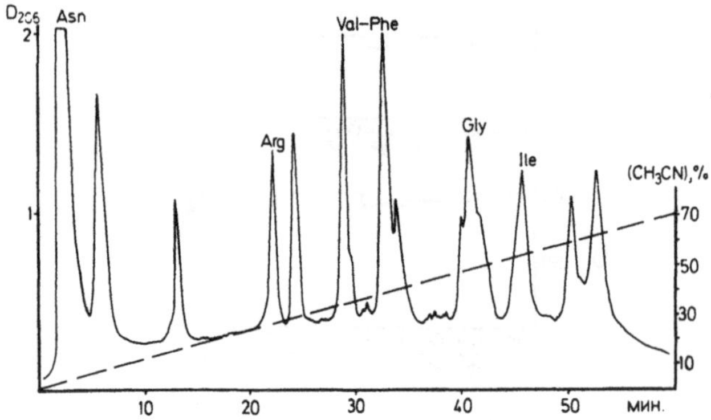


Fig. 4. Separation of peptides obtained after at *St. aureus* cleavage of fragment B5+B6. HPLC on a Nucleosil $C_8$ column (0.46x25 cm), gradient of acetonitrile in 0.1% trifluoroacetic acid, flow rate 0.8 ml/min.

nized with antibodies $R_6$ is within these fragments. Cleavage of amino acid residue $Glu^{341}$ ($Thr^{340}$-$Ala^{348}$) decreases sharply interaction of antibodies $R_6$ (Fig. 3c), so the given amino acid residue is important for antigenic determinant formation.

Results on limited proteolysis of native and bleached photoreceptor disks showed the C-terminal fragment and the fragments between the third and fourth as well as between the fifth and sixth segments to be exposed outside (21). The enzymatic reactions on inside out disks permitted mapping of two other outside membrane fragments (the N-terminal region of the protein and the fragment between the fourth and fifth segments) (18). Thus at least five of seven membrane segments were proved to be outside the membrane sufrace.

Immunochemical research into rhodopsin by monoclonal antibodies revealed the fragments exposed to cytoplasm and to intradisk space that confirmed the preceding results. For the first time, the frag-

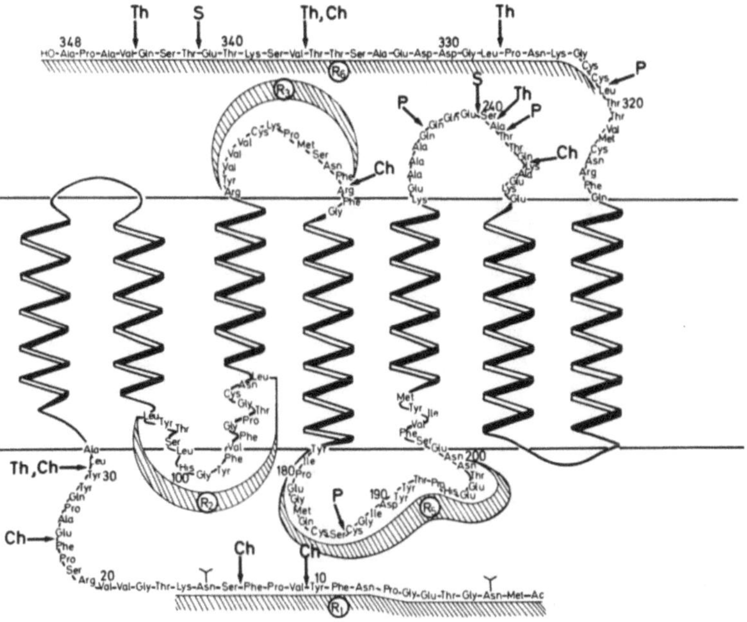


Fig. 5. Model for arrangement of the rhodopsin polypeptide chain with designated antigenic determinants. Arrows indicate the points of enzymatic cleavage.

ment between the second and third transmembrane segments in the native rhodopsin was established to be exposed.

Therefore imminochemical assay results and those of limited proteolysis evidence in favour of the rhodopsin model with seven transmembrane segments (Fig. 5).

At the next step of our experiments the attempts were made to apply monoclonal antibodies for detecting the conformational changes of the protein upon illumination. We obtained and characterized several monoclonal antibodies to the bleached membranes as an antigen. The same strategy was used to localize the epitopes: $A_6$ ($Leu^{50}$-$Met^{86}$), $A_1$ ($Asn^{151}/Phe^{148}$-$Met^{163}$), $A_3$ ($His^{152}/Phe^{148}$-$Met^{163}$) et al. It is interesting that, for instance, monoclonal antibodies $A_6$ interact only with the bleached membranes.

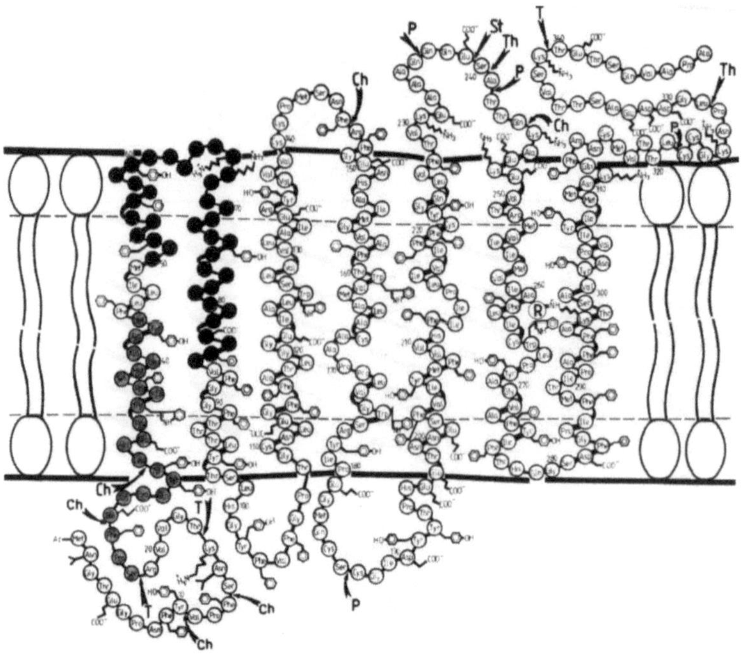

Fig. 6. The model of the moving of bovine rhodopsin.

Polyclonal antibodies to native and bleached rhodopsin molecules and to its several large fragments were isolated and compared in interaction with the peptides listed (Table 2). Now we can say, that upon illumination the red-colored region (Fig. 6) protrudes out of the membrane, whereas the green-one gets inside. It may be closely connected with the functioning of rhodopsin. We intend to study this problem in our future research.

## References


1. Ovchinnikov, Yu.A., N.G.Abdulaev, M.Yu. Feigina, I.D. Artamonov, A.S. Zolotarev, M.B. Kostina, A.S. Bogachuk, A.I. Miroshnikov, V.I. Martynov, A.B. Kudelin. 1982. Bioorg. Khim. 8, 1424

2. Nathans, J., D.S.Hogness. 1983. Cell. 34, 807.

3. Pellicone, C., N.J.Cook. G. Nullans, N.Virmaux. 1985. FEBS Lett. 181, 184.

4. Ovchinnikov, Yu.A., N.G. Abdulaev, M.Yu. Feigina, I.D. Artamonov, A.S. Bogachuk, A.S. Zolotarev, E.R. Eganyan, P.V. Kostetsky. 1983. Bioorg. Khim. 9, 1331.

5. Hargrave, P.A., S.-L. Fong, J.H. McDowell, M.T.Mass, D.R.Curtis, J.K. Wang, E.Juszczak, D.P. Smith. 1980. Neurochem. Int. 1, 231.

6. Lindstrom, J., S. Tzartos, B. Gullick. 1981. Ann. N.Y. Acad. Sci. 377, 1.

7. Atassi, M.Z. 1975. Immunochem. 12, 423.

8. Ovchinnikov, Yu.A., N.G. Abdulaev, R.G.Vasilov, I.Yu. Vturina, A.B. Kuryatov, A.V. Kiselev. 1985. FEBS Lett. 179, 343.

9. MacKenzie, D., A. Arendt, P.A. Hargrave, J.H. McDowell, R.S. Molday. 1984. Biochemistry. 23, 6544.

10. De Grip, W.J. 1985. In: Progress in Retinal Research (N.N.Osborne and G.J.Chander, eds.) Pergamon Press. N.Y. 4, 137.

11. Shevchevchenko, T.F., G.R. Kalamkarov, M.A. Ostrovsky. 1980. Biophisika. 25, 462.

12. Artamonov, I.D., A.S. Zolotarev, M.B. Kostina, N.I. Khoroshilova, M.Yu. Feigina, N.G. Abdulaev. 1983. Bioorg. Khim. 9, 1317.

13. Ovchinnikov, Yu.A., N.G. Abdulaev, A.S. Bogachuk, 1985. Biolog. Membr. 2, 962.

14. Koshland, D.E., K.E. Neel. 1968. Ann. Rev. Biochem. 37, 359.

15. Cianfriglia, M., D. Armellini, A. Massone, M. Mariani. 1984. Hybridoma. 3, 104.

16. Fazekas, de S.G., R.N. Scheideggar. 1980. J.Immunol.Meth. 35, 1.

17. Mishell, B.B., S.M. Shiigi. 1980. In: Selected Methods in Cellular Immunology (W.H.Freeman and Co. eds.). San Francisco, 17, 351.

18. Ey, P.L., S.J. Prouse, C.R. Senkin. 1978. Immunochem. 15, 429.

19. Laemmli, U.K. 1970. Natufe. 277, 680.

20. Winter, A., K.Ek, U.V. Anderson. 1977, LKB Application Note 250.

21. Greenwood, F.C., W.M. Hunter, J.S. Glover. 1963. Biochem. J. 89, 114.

22. Masson, D.W., A.F. Williams. 1980. Biochem. J. 187, 1.

23. Davies, D.R., H.Metzger. 1983. Ann. Rev. Immunol. 1, 87.

24. Martynov, V.I., M.B. Kostina, M.Yu. Feigina, A.I. Miroshnikov. 1983. Bioorg. Khim. 9, 737.

25. Trucco, M., S. de Petris. 1983. In: Immunological Methods (I. Levkovits and Perhis B., eds.). 12.

26. Vturina, I.Yu., A.B. Kuryatov, A.V. Kiselev, N.I. Khoroshilova, G.V. Ovechkina, N.G. Abdulaev, V.I. Tsetlin, R.G. Vasilov. 1984. Biolog. Membr. 1, 1161.

4. Ovchinnikov, [illegible] Mongin, [illegible] Kiselev, [illegible]
[illegible] 1983, [illegible]

5. [illegible] 1980, [illegible]
[illegible] 1979, [illegible]

6. Lindstrom, [illegible]

7. [illegible] 12, [illegible]

8. Ovchinnikov, [illegible]
[illegible] 1983, [illegible]

9. [illegible] A. Kargapolov [illegible]
[illegible] 23, [illegible]

10. [illegible]

11. [illegible]

12. [illegible]

13. [illegible] Abdulaev, [illegible]

14. [illegible] 1965. Ann. Rev. Biochem. [illegible]

15. [illegible] A. Kiselev, [illegible]

16. [illegible] 1980. [illegible]

17. [illegible] 1981. [illegible]

18. [illegible] 1983. Immunol. [illegible]

19. [illegible] Nature, 321, 580.

20. Winter, [illegible] Anderson. 1977. LKB Application Note [illegible]

21. Greenwood, F.C., [illegible] Hunter, J.S. Glover. 1963. [illegible]
89, [illegible]

22. Masson, D.W., A.F. Williams. 1980. Biochem. J. [illegible]

23. Davies, D.R., [illegible] 1983. Ann. Rev. Immunol. 1, [illegible]

24. Kargapolov, [illegible] Kostina, M.Yu. Feldina, A.I. [illegible]
1983. [illegible] 9, [illegible]

25. Franco, M., S. de Petris. 1981. In: Immunological Methods
(I. Lefkovits and Pernis B., eds.), 12.

26. Vturina, I.Yu., A.S. Kuryatov, A.V. Kiselev, N.I. Khoroshilova,
G.V. Ovechkina, [illegible] Abdulaev, V.I. Tsetlin, [illegible] 1984
Bioorg. Khim. [illegible]

# $Na^+$, $K^+$-PUMP: STRUCTURAL ORGANISATION

N.N. Modyanov, N.M. Arzamazova, E.A. Arystarkhova, N.M. Gevondyan, E.E. Gavrylyeva, K.N. Dzhandzhugazyan, S.V. Lutsenko, N.M. Luneva, G.I. Shafieva, E.N. Chertova

Shemyakin Institute of Bioorganic Chemistry USSR Academy of Sciences, USSR, Moscow

Nowadays research into structural bases of functioning of the systems of the active ion transport across biological membranes or ion pumps is being intensely developed. This is rather understandable, for ion transport plays one of the key roles in mechanism of action of bioenergetic and receptor systems, in transmission of nerve impulses, and in other processes in the organism. Among the ion pumps $Na^+,K^+$-ATPase, an obligatory component of plasma membranes of animal cells, is the best studied system. It translocates sodium and potassium ions against electrochemical potential gradients; this process coupled with the ATP hydrolysis provides nonequilibrium distribution of monovalent ions between the cell and medium (1,2).

The enzyme molecule consists of equimolar amounts of two subunits, α and β (for the studied enzyme from outer medulla of pig kidney their Mr ∿112 and ∿44 kDa, respectively). Its carbohydrate moiety (Mr ∿9 kDa) consists of three chains linked to the β-subunit by N-glycosidic bonds (3). The α-subunit is a functionally main component. The ATP-hydrolysing catalytic site being located in the cytoplasmic region of its polypeptide chain. Protein molecule regions exposed to the membrane outer side make up the binding site for cardiac glycosides - enzyme specific inhibitors (1,2). The transmembrane organisation of the α-subunit indicates the possible participation of its polypeptide chain in formation of a cation-conducting pathway in the $Na^+,K^+$-ATPase molecule (4). A role of β-glycoprotein is unknown.

To investigate into the principles of this enzyme functioning at the molecular level one should know the complete amino acid sequence of both subunits. The catalytic and glycoprotein subunits of the

Receptors and Ion Channels

enzyme from pig kidney were established to contain 1.016 and 302 amino acid residues, respectively (5,6). Since both proteins are integral membrane components and have rather extended regions exposed outside the membrane (4), the knowledge of their topography in the membrane is indispensable for revealing the mechanism of the protein action. Here we discuss how the protein may be arranged in the membrane judging by information procured from proteolytic cleavage, chemical modification and immunochemical assay.

A model for the α-subunit organisation in the membrane follows from results on limited proteolysis of the enzyme and theoretical calculation of its hydrophobicity profile as well. Selective tryptic digestion of the native membrane-bound $Na^+$,$K^+$-ATPase under the conditions for extensive hydrolysis of exposed regions of the α-subunit at complete retention of glycoprotein integrity was performed (7). As a result peptide amino acid sequences covering almost all the exposed regions of the catalytic subunit polypeptide chain were established. Considering the hydrophobicity profile of the protein calculated by two independent methods (Fig. 1) we singled out eleven hydrophobic regions, which could serve, in principle, as intramembrane segments. However, comparing the above data and those on amino acid sequences of the hydrophilic peptides of the α-subunit, covering mainly the 143-283 and 342-778 regions, we positioned segments 89-114, 123-142, 284-306 and 313-341, but not 530-553 and 569-597, inside the membrane. The two latter rather hydrophobic stretches cannot be transmembrane, as the lipid bilayer would include sequences $Arg^{544}$-$Val^{545}$ and $Arg^{589}$-$Ala^{590}$ hydrolyzed by trypsin (7).

It is hard to predict the arrangement of the remained more hydrophobic portion of the polypeptide chain. The extracellular domain of the α-subunit is to be large enough since it forms the main part of the binding site of the cardiac glycosides (it is supposed to be 20-30 % of the cytoplasmic portion according to chemical modification with impermeable reagents (8,9,10). This domain is substantially larger at the odd rather than even number of transmembrane segments.

Therefore we assume that of five potential transmembrane fragments only three (780-803, 842-867, and 946-972) are localized inside

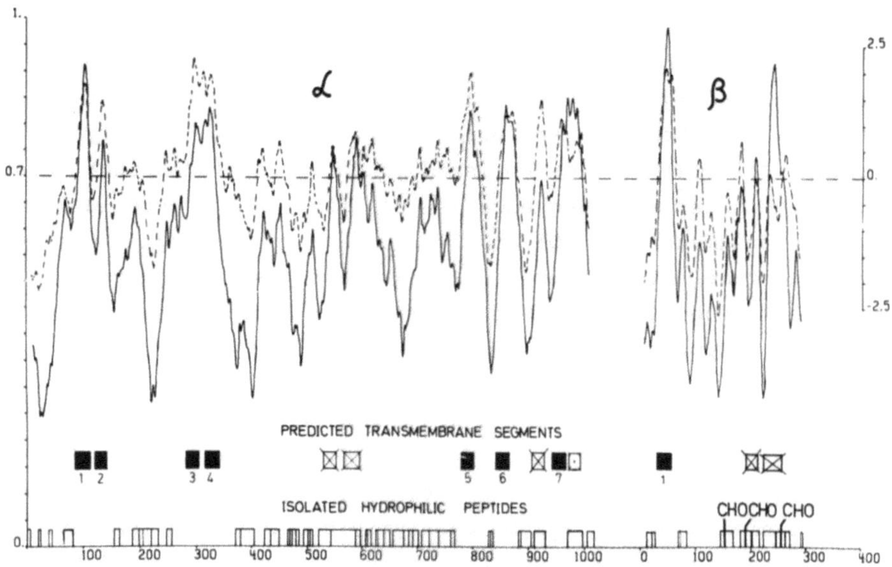


Fig.1. Hydrophobicity profiles of $Na^+,K^+$-ATPase α- and β-subunits. Dotted line - (19); solid line - (20).

the membrane, the rest two, shorter and less hydrophobic (909-930, 979-994) are exposed outside.

Not long ago (11) we also mentioned another possible way for the polypeptide chain arrangement, namely, one of the two latter fragments spaned the lipid bilayer twice, since it was essentially extended (768-817) preserving rather a high level of hydrophobicity. Just this pathway was proposed for the analogous part of $Ca^{2+}$-ATPase (12). Here segment (909-930) should be considered as transmembrane. However, it contradicts the results of the immunochemical assay. We obtained several hybridomas producing monoclonal antibodies to different parts of the polypeptide chain. The antibodies were characterized relative to their binding to the membrane-bound $Na^+,K^+$-ATPase, individual subunits and peptide fragments derived from limited trypsinolysis (7). The clones were divided into two groups by their ability to interact with both living and fixed cells of pig kidney embryo line. One of them contains monoclonal antibodies which interact with cytoplasmic portions of the molecule (e.g. clones $IIC_9$, $IIF_2$), the second group is composed of those bound to extracellular regions (clones $IIF_6$, $IE_1$). By affinity chromatography (clone $IIC_9$-a part of an immunosorbent) the peptide containing the antigenic determinant was isolated from the tryptic hydrolysate. Its structure and position in the α-subunit polypeptide chain (887-904) were established. Thus we concluded that this region of the amino acid sequence is localized in the cytoplasm and hydrophobic fragments 780-803 and 842-867 can run through the lipid bilayer only once. All the above data suggest that the polypeptide chain of the α-subunit traverses the membrane seven times and its C-terminus is exposed outside (Fig. 2).

The proposed model suggests three loops in the cell cytoplasm in addition to the N-terminal part of the molecule, the largest (431-780) linking the fourth and fifth intramembrane rods contains all the known elements of the enzyme catalytic site. A functionally important aspartic acid residue phosphorylated upon the acylphosphate intermediate formation is localized in position 369. The Cys-Ser-Asp-Lys sequence surrounding this residue completely agrees with that reported in (13). The 368-375 region is assumed to be a common structural element for the catalytic site found in all known transport ATPases (including $F_0F_1$-ATPases) (14). Another region (496-506) of the α-subunit, apparently, a part of the enzyme catalytic site, contains lysine residue (501), which can be modified with an irreversible inhibitor of the enzyme - fluoresceine isothiocyanate (15). To find out other regions of the catalytic α-subunit involved into the active site formation, the enzyme was modified with substrate analogs. As previously shown, alkylating analogue of ATP γ-4(N-2 chloroethyl-N-methylamono) benzyl-amidate ATP (ClR-ATP) yields a covalent compound with the α-subunit (16) thus completely inhibiting the $Na^+$,$K^+$-ATPase activity. For isolation of the peptide containing covalently and specifically bound ClR-ATP the modified protein ($K^+$-form) was hydrolysed with pepsin at pH 1.5 providing stability of the lable. Determination of the (706-718) peptide structure allowed us to reveal that between the protein and the ATP molecule the ester bond is formed through one of two residues of aspartic acid 710 or 714. Interestingly, the same region of the polypeptide chain was identified at affinity modification of

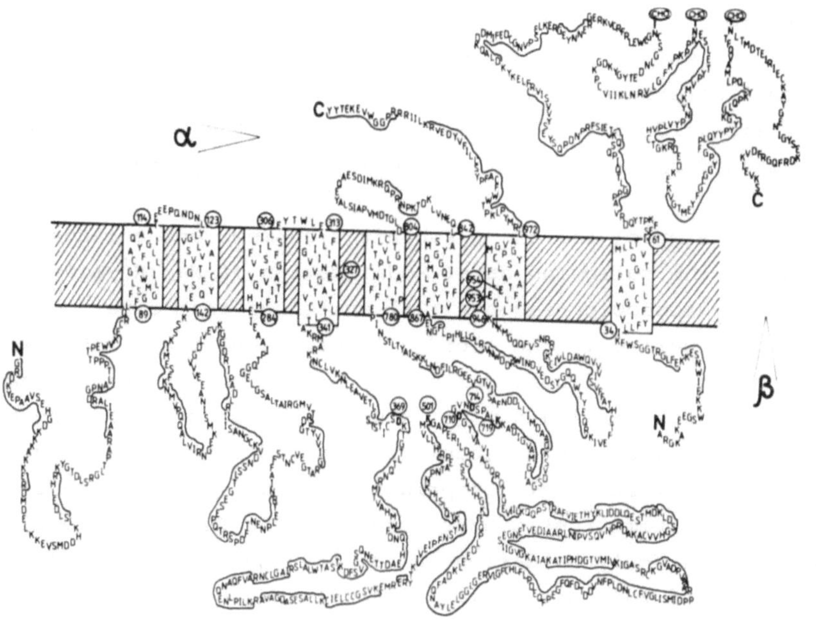

Fig. 2. Model for spatial organisation of the enzyme molecule. N-Glycosylation sites marked with CHO.

the enzyme with another ATP analogue - 5-(p-fluorosulfonyl)benzoyl-adenosine (FSBA) (17). The reactive group in this case is, apparently, $Lys^{725}$. The isolated peptide is a part of the large homologous region of amino acid sequences of $Ca^{2+}$-ATPase and the α-subunit of $Na^{+},K^{+}$-ATPase (645-744), it, probably, participates in formation of the region of the active site in the vicinity of γ-phosphate of the ATP-molecule in both enzymes.

The secondary structure of the α-subunit region localized in the cytoplasm has a number of "tension points", that is confirmed by the results of limited proteolysis of the membrane-bound enzyme(7). There were found fifteen trypsin-unspecific splits, such as Asp-His, Ala-Ala, Pro-Asp, etc., marked by arrows in Fig. 2. Apparently, these parts of the sequence are situated on the surface of the protein globula in bends of the polypeptide chain and are the first targets for the proteolytic attack.

However, the α-subunit may be of more complex organisation than in Fig. 2. Even according to this model the ratio of outer and inner hydrophilic regions is smaller than it was predicted from chemical labelling (8,9,10). Also one cannot exclude, e.g., the presence of additional stretches in the lipid bilayer, since the three residues of glutamic acid (327, 953, 954) situated in the membrane are, probably, insufficient to form a cation-conducting pathway.

To build up a model for the β-subunit transmembrane arrangement we based on the following data. Modification of $Na^+,K^+$-ATPase with permeable hydrophobic reagents (18) evidences that a part of the β-subunit is buried in the lipid bilayer. Labelling of the exposed enzyme portion with fluorescamine (9) or the Bolton-Hunter reagent (8) and immunochemical assay (4) showed that practically the whole hydrophilic part of the β-subunit is exposed on the outer surface of the membrane. Three glycopeptides (152-169, 182-202 and 253-272) were isolated from tryptic hydrolyzate of the βsubunit. So all canonic sites of N-glycosylation in the β-subunit (asparagine residues 157, 192 and 264) are really glycosylated, consequently these regions of the polypeptide chain are exposed on the extracellular side of the membrane.

Calculation of local hydrophobicity of the β-subunit polypeptide chain revealed three, probably, intramembrane hydrophobic segments 23-67, 197-214 and 223-260 (Fig. 2). If the central part of the first stretch (made up of 28 uncharged residues) forms a single-transmembrane rod (34-61), the considerable portion of the N-terminal region of 7-8 amino groups is in cytoplasm. Inaccessibility of the latter to modification with impermeable reagents might be due to the protection by the cytoplasmic portion of the α-subunit. Fragment 23-67 involving 75% of hydrophobic residues has the length enough to span the hydrophobic part of the lipid bilayer twice in a hairpin shape.

Thus several models of β-subunit polypeptide chain organisation in the membrane can be considered. The first one suggests the subunit having one transmembrane rod (34-61). The N-terminus is oriented into the cytoplasm. The second model considers the 23-67 region as a hairpin in the membrane, the N-terminal region is localized outside the membrane. Also one could assume the presence of additional intramembrane hairpin structure - 197-214, and 223-260.

However, at proteolysis of the membrane-bound β-subunit the peptides, which compose these fragments, were found in the water-soluble portion of the hydrolyzate. There was also peptide EFLGR (22-26) that indicates the first hydrophobic region to be shorter as compared to its theoretically proposed length. Apparently, the membrane part of the β-subunit consists of the sole α-helical rod (34-61).

Determination of the primary structure of $Na^+,K^+$-ATPase and design of the preliminary model for its transmembrane arrangement paved the way for elucidation of the comprehensive spatial organisation and molecular mechanism of functioning of this universal system for active ion transport.

Acknowledgement

The authors are grateful to Professor Ovchinnikov for helpful advice and stimulating discussion.

References

1. Jørgensen, P.L. 1982. Biochem. Biophys. Acta 694, 27-68.

2. Cantley, L.C. 1981. Curr. Top. Bioenerg. 11, 201-237.

3. Dzhandzhugazyan, K.N., N.N. Modyanov, Yu.A. Ovchinnikov. 1981. Bioorgan, Khimia 7, 847-857.

4. Dzhandzhugazyan, K.N., N.N. Modyanov, Yu.A. Ovchinnikov. 1981. Bioorgan, Khimia 7, 1790-1800.

5. Ovchinnikov, Yu.A., S.H. Arsenyan, N.E. Broude, K.E. Petrukhin, A.V. Grishin, N.A. Aldanova, N.M. Arzamazova, E.A. Arystarkhova, A.M. Melkov, Yu.V. Smirnov, O.S. Guryev, G.S. Monastyrskaya, N.N. Modyanov. 1985. Dokl. Akad. Nauk SSSR 285, 1490-1495.

6. Ovchinnikov, Yu.A., N.E. Broude, K.E. Petrukhin, A.V. Grishin, N.I. Kiyatkin, N.M. Arzamazova, N.M. Gevondyan, E.N. Chertova, A.M. Melkov, Yu.V. Smirnov, I.V. Malyshev, G.S. Monastyrskaya, N.N. Modyanov. 1986. Dokl. Akad. Nauk SSSR 287, 1491-1496.

7. Arzamazova, N.M., E.A. Arystarkhova, G.I. Shafieva, I.V. Nazimov, N.A. Aldanova, N.N. Modyanov. 1985. Bioorgan. Khimia 11, 1598-1606.

8. Dzhandzhugazyan, K.N., P.L. Jorgensen. 1985. Biochem. Biophys. Acta 817, 165-173.

9. Dzhandzhugazyan, K.N., N.N. Modyanov. 1985. In: The Sodium Pump (Glynn, I. and Ellory, C., eds). The Company of Biologists Ltd., Cambridge, UK, p. 129-134.

10. Sharkey, R. 1983. Biochim. Biophys. Acta 730, 327-341.

11. Ovchinnikov, Yu.A., N.N. Modyanov, N.E. Broude, K.E. Petrukhin, A.V. Grishin, N.M. Arzamazova, N.A. Aldanova, G.S. Monastyrskaya, E.D. Sverdlov. 1986. FEBS Letters 201, 237-245.

12. MacLennan, D.H., C.J. Brandel, B. Korczak, N.M. Green. 1985. Nature 316, 696-700.

13. Walderhaug, M.O., R.L.Post, G. Saccomani, R.T. Leonard, D.P. Briskin. 1985. J. Biol. Chem. 260, 3852-3859.

14. Modyanov, N.N., N.M. Arzamazova, E.A. Arystarkhova, N.M. Gevondyan, Yu.A. Ovchinnikov. 1985. Biol. Membrany 2, 844-848.

15. Farley, R.A., C.M. Tran, C.T. Carilli, D. Hawke, J.E. Shively, 1984. J. Biol. Chem. 259, 9532-9535.

16. Dzhandzhugazyan, K.N., S.V. Lutsenko, N.N. Modyanov. 1986. Biol. Membrany 3, 858-868.

17. Ohta, T., K. Nagano, M. Yoshida. 1986. Proc. Natl. Acad. Sci. USA 83, 2071-2075.

18. Giradet, M., R. Geering, B.C. Rossier, J.P. Krahenduhl, C. Bron. 1983. Biochemistry 22, 2296-2300.

19. Capaldi, R.A., G. Vanderkooi. 1972. Proc. Natl. Acad. Sci. USA 69, 930-932.

20. Kyte, J., R.F. Doolitle. 1982. J. Mol. Biol. 157, 105-132.

# ATP-DEPENDENT ELECTRIC CURRENTS OF THE PURIFIED $Na^+K^+$ PUMP

K. Fendler, G. Nagel, E. Grell and E. Bamberg
Max-Planck-Institut für Biophysik, Heinrich-Hoffmann-Str. 7
D-6000 Frankfurt am Main

## Summary

The transport activity of purified $Na^+K^+$ ATPase was investigated by measuring the electrical pump current induced on black lipid membranes. Discs containing purified $Na^+K^+$ ATPase from pig kidney were attached to planar lipid bilayers in a sandwich-like structure. ATP was released by an UV-light flash, which converted caged ATP to ATP. This led to a transient current in the system. The transient photoresponse indicates that the discs and the underlying membrane are capacitively coupled. Stationary pump currents were obtained after the addition of the $H^+$,$K^+$, $Na^+$ exchanging agent monensin together with the protonophore 1799 to the membrane system, which increased the membrane permeability. In the absence of ADP and $P_i$ the half saturation for the maximal photoeffect is obtained at 2 µM released ATP. Pump activity was obtained only in the presence of $Mg^{2+}$ together with $Na^+$ or $Na^+$ and $K^+$. No pump current was obtained in the presence of $Mg^{2+}$ together with $K^+$. The electrical response was blocked completely by the $Na^+K^+$ ATPase specific inhibitors vanadate and ouabain. The method described offers the possibility to investigate directly pump currents of $Na^+K^+$-ATPase with a large variety of different parameters. It turned out, that ATP dependent continuous $Na^+$ pumping in the absence of $K^+$ is electrogenic.

## Introduction

$Na^+K^+$ transporting ATPase (EC 3.6.1.3), the $Na^+K^+$ ATPase, from mammalian cells, is an electrogenic pump where three $Na^+$ ions are exchanged for two $K^+$ ions in the presence of $Mg^{2+}$. The energy for the pump is obtained from hydrolysis of ATP. Electric pump currents of the $Na^+K^+$-ATPase have been observed in intact cells (1, 2, 3). The transport activity of $Na^+K^+$ ATPase has

Receptors and Ion Channels

been studied in red cells (4, 5) as well as in reconstituted vesicles (6, 7, 8). Time resolved studies with a photolabile ATP derivative ($P^3$-1-(2-nitro)phenylethyladenosine 5 -triphosphate, caged ATP) have been reported on red cells and reconstituted proteoliposomes as well (6, 9). Recently we described a method to observe ATP-driven electrial pump currents in reconstituted systems (10).

Purified $Na^+K^+$ ATPase membranes in form of cup-shaped discs (0.1 - 0.6 µm diameter) were associated in a sandwich-like structure to a planar lipid bilayer. The pump was activated by photolysis of caged ATP by an UV-flash, leading to a concentration jump of ATP of about 10 µM. The resulting pump current was measured by the capacitive coupling between the discs and the supporting lipid bilayer. (Fig. 1).

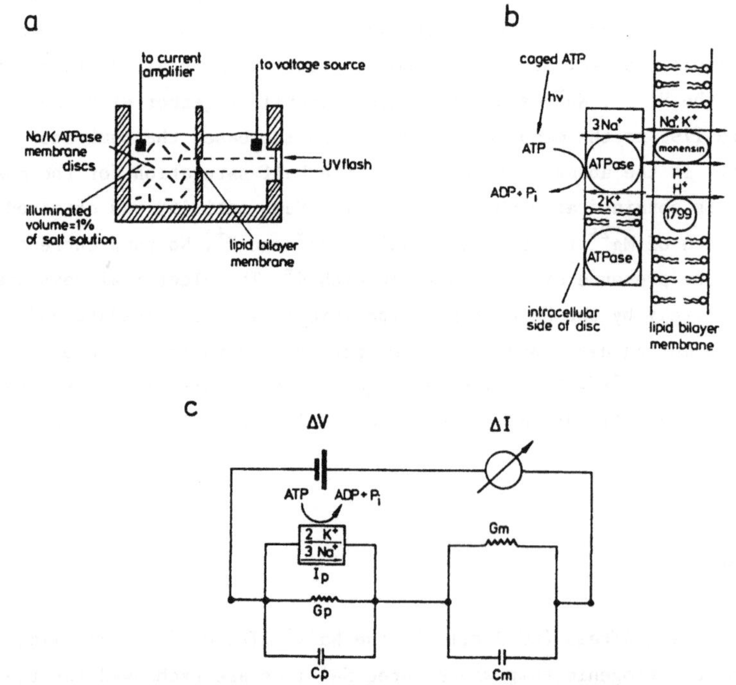


Fig. 1: Schematic representation of the bilayer setup. a: Teflon chamber with black lipid membrane (BLM) and adsorbed $Na^+K^+$-ATPase discs. b: Proposed sandwich-like arrangement of discs and underlying lipid membrane. The two membranes are capacitively coupled. c: Equivalent circuit diagramm of the two membranes in series. $G_m$, $G_p$ refer to conductance of the BLM and the disc membrane, respectively; $C_m$ and $C_p$ to the capacitance of BLM and discs, respectively. $I_p$ designates the pump current generator. For small values of $G_m$ only transient currents are observable, whereas for large values of $G_m$ in the presence of 1799 and monensin stationary pump currents are obtained.

Results and Discussion

A record of the short-circuit current obtained 30 min after the addition of the protein and caged ATP to the lipid bilayer is shown in Fig. 2a. The sign of the current in all experiments was same. Under identical conditions different experiments gave current amplitudes with a variation of 50 %. During the same experiment, however, the current amplitude can be reproduced with an accuracy of 5 %. The direction of the current corresponds to a movement of positive charges to the protein free side of the membrane system, indicating that the periplasmic side of the ion transporting discs is faced with lipid bilayer, whereas the cytoplasmic side is directed to the electrolyte of the cis-chamber of the cuvette.

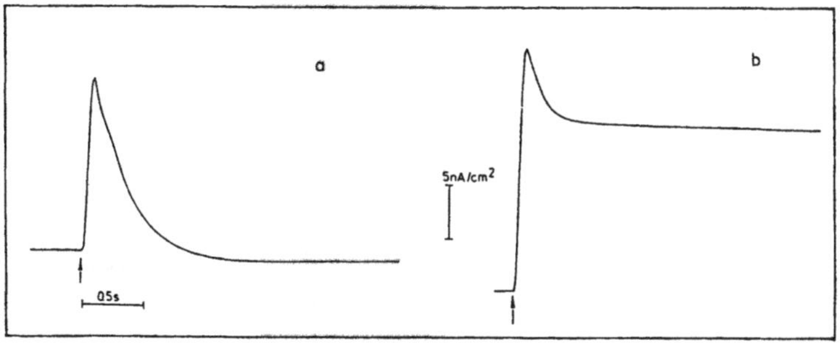


Fig. 2: Short circuit currents on the lipid bilayer system under different experimental conditions. The membrane bathing solution contained 130 mM NaCl, 20 mM KCl, 3 mM $MgCl_2$, 25 mM imadazole-HCl pH 7.5. The arrows indicate opening of the shutter.
a: 100 µM caged ATP, no addition of ionophores.
b: Same membrane system after addition of monensin and 1799 to a concentration of 10 µM and 0.6 µM, respectively.

The discs are apparently not integrated into the black film, because in case of continuous pump activity of the $Na^+K^+$ ATPase stationary pump currents should result in a short circuit experiment, as long as liberated ATP is available for the enzyme. That the $Na^+K^+$ ATPase acts on the combined discs-bilayer system as a pump was demonstrated by stationary pump currents.

The underlying lipid bilayer membrane was made permeable to $Na^+$ and $K^+$ when the $H^+/Na^+$, $K^+$ exchanging agent monensin was added to the system together with the $H^+$ carrier 1799. As can be seen from Fig. 2b, the current induced by a UV-flash became nearly stationary after a transient component and disappeared after minutes (not shown), indicating that all deliberated ATP is hydrolysed.

The addition of 1 mM vanadate abolished the electrical pump current. Ouabain did not block the pump if it was added to the lipid bilayer system at a concentration of 1 µM. If, however, the $Na^{+}K^{+}$-ATPase was pre-incubated for 10 min with 4 mM ouabain and then added to the lipid bilayer, no electrical response was obtained. It can be concluded that the binding site for ouabain is not accessible to those of the attached discs, which contribute to the pump current.

Fig. 3 summarizes the results obtained with different electrolyte compositions. Trace d shows the electrical signal under normal conditions (3 mM $Mg^{2+}$, 20 mM $K^{+}$, 130 m $Na^{+}$). Removing $Mg^{2+}$ by addition of 10 mM EDTA abolished the pump current (trace b), showing the well known requirement of $Mg^{2+}$ for the $Na^{+}K^{+}$-ATPase activity. In another set of experiments only either $Na^{+}$ or $K^{+}$ were present together with 3 mM $Mg^{2+}$. Trace c shows that $K^{+}$ does not give any electrical response, while in the presence of $Na^{+}$ an ATP dependent electrical signal was measured (trace a).

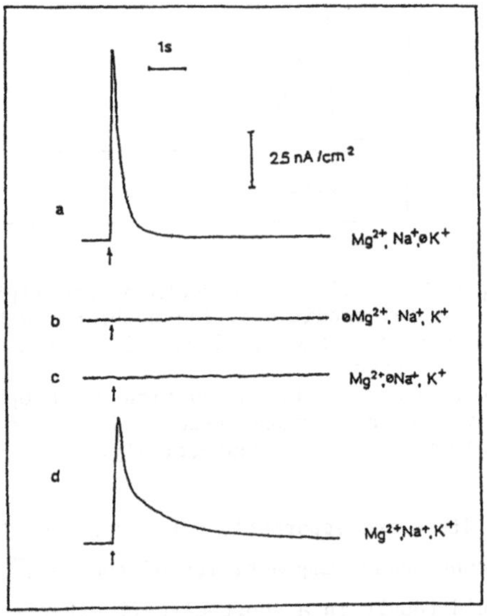


Fig. 3: Ion specificity of the $Na^{+}K^{+}$-ATPase signal.
Conditions: 35 µM caged ATP,
25 mM imidazole HCl pH 7.5 plus
a: 3 mM $MgCl_2$, 130 mM NaCl
b: 10 mM EDTA, 130 mM NaCl, 20 mM KCl
c: 3 mM $MgCl_2$, 20 mM KCl
d: 3 mM $MgCl_2$, 130 mM NaCl, 20 mM KCl
The arrows indicate the opening of the shutter, flash duration 0.125 s.

The pump activity was measured at different concentrations of released ATP (Fig. 4). The peak current was half-maximal at 1.7 uM in the presence of 130 mM $Na^{+}$, 20 mM $K^{+}$ and 3 mM $Mg^{2+}$. Omittance of $K^{+}$ led to the same result. Because an inhibition by caged ATP was observed, the true $K_{0.5}$ was calculated to be 2 uM for ATP, whereas the $K_I$ for caged ATP is 30 µM. This aspect is discussed in more detail in a forthcoming paper (11).

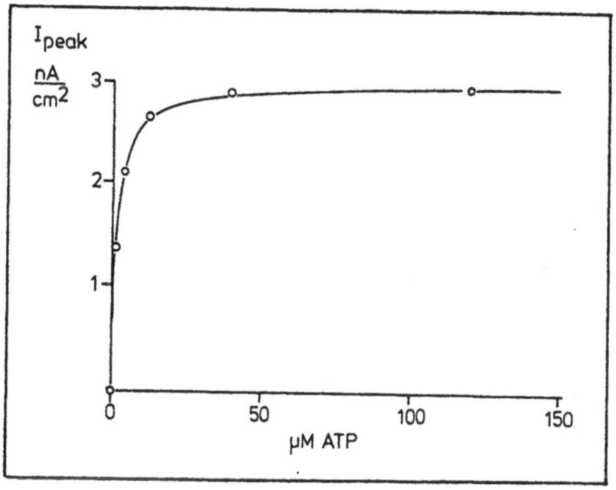


Fig. 4: ATP dependency of the peak current, measured by successive addition of caged ATP. Electrolyte composition as in Fig. 2. Omittance of $K^+$ did not change the result. Conversion rate was always 34 %. Fit curve according to the equation: $I_{peak} = I_{peak\ max} * \frac{c_{ATP}}{K_{0.5} + c_{ATP}}$

The permeabilization of the bilayer with the protonophore 1799 in combination with monensin made it possible to study stationary pump currents. It turned out, that even in the absence of $K^+$ (6 µM residual $K^+$ concentration) a distinct stationary current could be measured, which could be further increased by the addition of $K^+$ (Fig. 5).

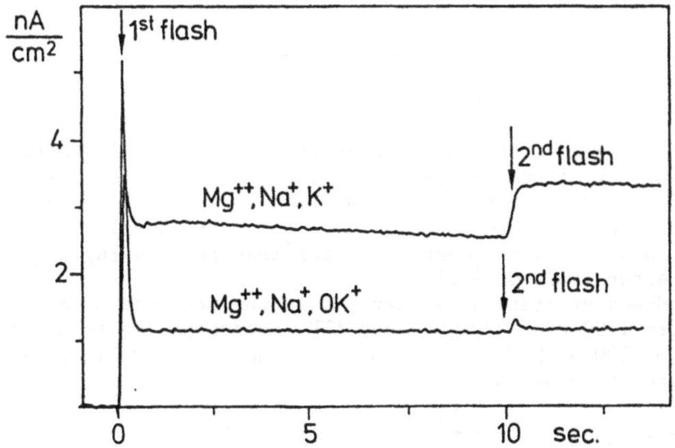


Fig. 5: Demonstration of ATP stimulation of pump currents in the presence and absence of $K^+$. Caged ATP concentration = 50 µM corresponding to 15 µM released ATP with the first flash and additional 10 µM ATP with the second flash. a: 100 mM NaCl, 3 mM $MgCl_2$, 25 mM imidazole-HCl pH 7.5. b: Same membrane and electrolyte as in a) after addition of 10 mM KCl.

Fig. 5 shows in addition, that a second flash, which increased the ATP concentration in the irradiated volume, led to an even higher stationary current in the presence of $K^+$, whereas in the absence of $K^+$ a second flash had nearly no effect. This fits to the current conception of the enzyme, i.e. ATP accelerates the $E_2$ to $E_1$ conformational change in the presence of $K^+$, thereby acting at a low affinity site and speeding up the turnover rate.

Fig. 6a shows the dependency of the stationary current on the $Na^+$ concentration. For the peak current only a high affinity was obtained (10), whereas the stationary current shows a high (< 1 mM) and a low affinity to $Na^+$ (≥ 0.2 M). Additional potassium added to the same membrane stimulates the pump current with an $K_{0.5}$ of 700 µM, according to a simple Michaelis Menten formalism (Fig. 6b).

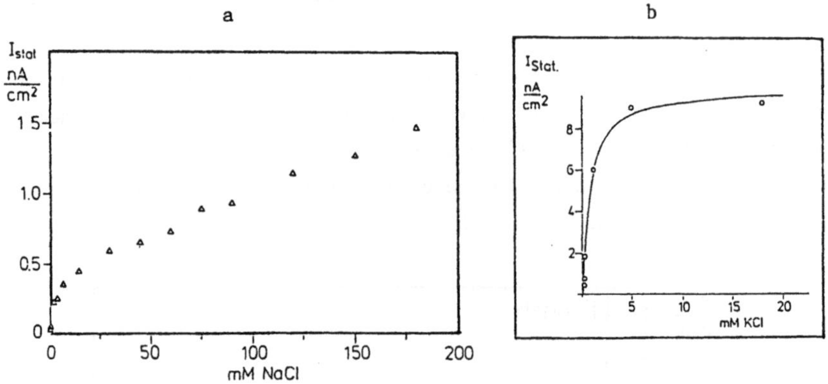


Fig. 6: Dependency of stationary currents on $Na^+$ and $K^+$, respectively.
a: $Na^+$ dependency of stationary currents in the presence of monensin and the protonophore 1799. Electrolyte: 25 mM imidazole-HCl, 3 mM $MgCl_2$ pH 7.5, residual $K^+$ concentration = 6 uM. The 1 M $Na^+$ stock solution for titration contained 10 uM $K^+$. Three membranes were measured showing the same affinities within an error limit of ± 25 %.
b: $K^+$ dependency of stationary currents in the presence of monensin and the protonophore 1799 with 270 µM caged ATP, corresponding to 81 µM ATP. Electrolyte: 130 mM NaCl, 25 mM imidazole-HCl, 3 mM $MgCl_2$ pH 7.5. Fit curve according to the equation:

$$I_{stat.} = I_{stat.max} * \frac{c_{K^+}}{K_{0.5} + c_{K^+}}$$ leading to a $K_{0.5}$ of 0.7 mM.

The addition of $K^+$ speeds up dephosphorylation of the enzmye and therefore increases the stationary current (Fig. 6b). The fact, that in the presence of $K^+$ the reaction cycle involves a second, low affinity ATP binding site is clearly demonstrated by the increase of the stationary current after a second ATP releasing flash (Fig. 5).

The affinity of $K^+$ stimulation of the stationary current has been measured at high ATP concentrations in order to avoid limitation of the signal by the slow $E_2K$ - $E_1K$ step. The $K_{0.5}$ for $K^+$ stimulation is in good agreement with data reported in the literature for $K^+$ binding at the extracellular side of the pump (12, 13).

From the fact, that $Na^+$ at high concentrations can stimulate the stationary pumping, we conclude, that $Na^+$ can replace $K^+$, but binds with a very low affinity, as postulated for the ATP hydrolysing activity of the $Na^+$-ATPase (7, 14). Analogous to $Na^+/K^+$ pumping this ATP dependent $Na^+/Na^+$ exchange is electrogenic.

Acknowledgements

The authors wish to thank A. Hüby, E. Lewitzki and G. Schimmack for excellent technical assistance, E. Müller and Dr. Pusch for help on determination of the $K^+$ concentration. Work was supported partially by the Deutsche Forschungsgemeinschaft (SFB 169).

References


1. Abercrombie, R. and De Weer, P. (1978) Am. J. Physiol., 44, 389-400

2. Gadsby, D.C., Kimura, J. and Noma, A. (1985) Nature, 315, 63-65

3. Lafaire, A.V. and Schwarz, W. (1986) J. Membr. Biol., 91, 43-51

4. Glynn, I.M. and Karlish, S.Y.D. (1976) J. Physiol. London, 256, 465-496

5. Hoffmann, J.F., Kaplan, J.H. and Callahan, T.J. (1979) Fed. Proc., 38, 2440-2441

6. Forbush III, B. (1984) Proc. Natl. Acad. Sci. USA, 84, 5310-5314

7. Cornelius, F. and Skou, J.C. (1985) Biochim. Biophys. Acta, 818, 211-221

8. Apell, H.J., Marcus, M.M., Anner, B.M., Oetliker, H. and Läuger, P. (1985) J. Membr. Biol., 85, 49-63

9. Kaplan, J.H., Forbush III, B. and Hoffmann, J.F. (1978) Biochemistry (Wash.), 17, 1929-1935

10. Fendler, K., Grell, E., Haubs, M. and Bamberg, E. (1985) EMBO J., 4, 3079-3085

11. Nagel, G., Fendler, K. Grell, E. and Bamberg, E. (1987) submitted

12. Bashford, C.L. and Pasternak, C.A. (1985) Eur. Biophys. J., 12, 229-235

13. Gache, C., Rossi, B., Leone, F.A. and Lazdunski, M. (1979) in Skou, J.C. and Nørby, J.G. (eds.), Na,K-ATPase Structure and Kinetics, Academic Press, London, 301-314

14. Garrahan, P.J., Horenstein, A. and Rega, A.F. (1979) in Skou, J.C. and Nørby, J.G. (eds.), Na,K-ATPase Structure and Kinetics, Academic Press, London, 261-274

# V NEUROTOXINS

ARGIOPIN - A NATURALLY OCCURRING BLOCKER OF GLUTAMATE-SENSITIVE SYNAPTIC CHANNELS

L.G. Magazanik, S.M. Antonov, I.M. Fedorova

Sechenov Institute of Evolutionary Physiology and Biochemistry Academy of Sciences of the USSR, Leningrad, USSR

T.M. Volkova, E.V. Grishin

Shemyakin Institute of Bioorganic Chemistry, Academy of Sciences of the USSR, Moscow, USSR

## Introduction

The advances in the study of the molecular nature and function of nicotinic cholinoreceptor to a great extent are owing to the discovery and wide employment of its highspecific ligand - α-bungarotoxin. This prompts to search for some neurotoxins which could block selectively the glutamatergic receptor.It was found by Kawai et al. in Japan and by Tashmukhamedov et al. in the USSR that venoms of spiders from Araneidae family do lower sensitivity of arthropods muscles and some vertebrate neurons to l-glutamate(1-3). Usherwood and coworkers (4) tried to identify the main molecular component of these venoms, responsible for antiglutamate action. They assumed that it is a substance with a low molecular weight (500-1000 D) which is capable of blocking the glutamate-sensitive channels.

The individual substance referred to as argiopin was isolated in our laboratories from the venom of Argiope lobata spider by high performance liquid chromatography. It turned out to be a peculiar

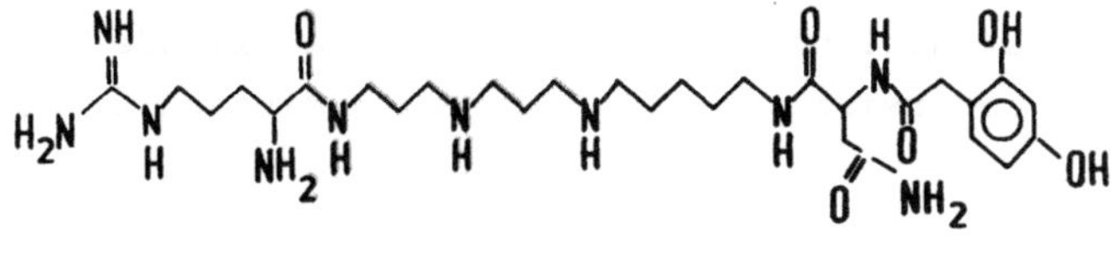

Receptors and Ion Channels

compound of 636 D molecular weight identified by $^{1}H$- and $^{13}C$-NMR-spectroscopy, mass-spectroscopy, elementary and aminoacid analysis (5).

The results of detalied study concerning the mode of argiopin action on glutamate and acetylcholine postsynaptic receptors are presented below.

## Results

Experiments were made on the isolated neuro-muscular preparations from the blowfly larvae Calliphora vicina and frog Rana temporaria for comparison of the argiopin effects on glutamatergic and cholinergic transmission, respectively. Changes in the amplitude and time course of excitatory postsynaptic potentials (EPSP) and currents (EPSC), as well as in the glutamate induced noise were estimated. The methods have been described in detail previously (6).

Unlike the crude venom, argiopin reduced to the same extent the amplitude of miniature EPSP's and multiquantal EPSP's, evoked by motor nerve stimulation. It means that argiopin reveals only a postsynaptic blocking effect. On the frog preparations it was 36 times weaker, compared to that of insects: 50% fall of EPSC amplitude was produced by argiopin at $4.4 \times 10^{-7}$M concentration in insect and $1.6 \times 10^{-5}$M in frog preparations. Being exponential in control the decay of EPSC's in both preparations in the presence of argiopin became biphasic (Fig. 1).

The initial and final segments of the decay curve could be approximated by two exponents: $\tau_1$ (fast) and $\tau_2$ (slow), correspondingly. Both effects of argiopin (changes in EPSC amplitude and time course) were reversible, i.e. could be eliminated by longlasting washing.

Such phenomenology of the argiopin effect on glutamate and acetylcholine receptors seems to be similar to that of some blockers on postsynaptic ion channels, which allows application of

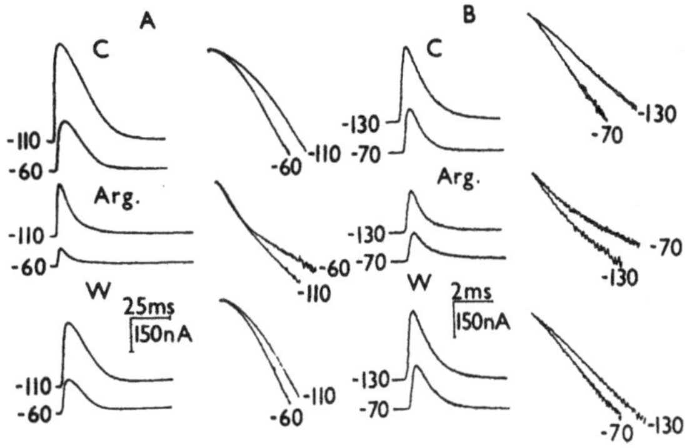


Fig. 1. The effect of argiopin on excitatory postsynaptic currents (EPSC) recorded in (A) blowfly larvae muscle (4.4 x $10^{-7}$M) and (B) frog muscle (4.7 x$10^{-5}$M). Left - EPSC's recorded on certain potential levels (indicated). Right - semilogarithmic plots of EPSC decay 100% to 5% of their amplitude. C - control; Arg. - after 30 min treatment by argiopin; W - after 60 min washing. Each curve is the result of averaging of 16 responses.

the sequential model of the open channel block (7):

$$2T + R \underset{k_{-1}}{\overset{k_1}{\rightleftharpoons}} T_2R \underset{\alpha}{\overset{\beta}{\rightleftharpoons}} T_2R^* + B \underset{k_b}{\overset{k_f}{\rightleftharpoons}} T_2R^*B,$$

where T - transmitter molecule, R - receptor in rest state (channel is closed; R* - activated receptor (channel is open); B - blocker molecule; $k_1$, $k_{-1}$, $\beta$ and $\alpha$,$k_f$ and $k_b$ - rate constants of respective reactions. According to this scheme, the blocker (in our case - argiopin) has the affinity only to the open state of channels, and the complex $T_2R^*B$ loses conductivity for cations. This leads to shortening of the life time of open channel and thereby to modifing the synaptic current time course. The dependence of EPSC decay changes on argiopin concentration allowed to estimate both the rate constants of argiopin interaction with either open glutamate or acetylcholine channels ($k_f$ and $k_b$) and dissociation constants ($K_d$). The results are given in Table. Under the same conditions (resting potential and room temperature) $K_d$ of argiopin interaction with open glutamate channels was found to be 36 times lower, compared to that of open acetylcholine channels, due to higher association and lower dissociation rate constant of the argiopin-channel complex. It means that argiopin has preferential affinity to glutamate receptors.

Table. Interaction of Argiopin With the Open Synaptic Channels

| | | Concentr. M | °C | mV | $k_f \times 10^8$ $M^{-1}s^{-1}$ | $k_b$ $s^{-1}$ | $K_d \times 10^{-7}$ M |
|---|---|---|---|---|---|---|---|
| Channels activated by glutamate | EPSC | 3.1-23.4 x $10^{-7}$ | 21 | -50 | 1.0±0.3(6) | 55±12(6) | 6.7±1.5(6) |
| | | | 21 | -120 | 2.0±0.3(4) | 72±10(4) | 3.5±0.4(4) |
| | noise | 4.4x$10^{-7}$ | 8 | -60 | 4.3±0.2(14) | 36± 2(14) | 0.8±0.3(14) |
| Channels activated by acetylcholine | EPSC | 1.6-4.7 x $10^{-5}$ | 21 | -80 | 0.19±0.04(5) | 409±68(5) | 238±33(5) |
| | | | 21 | -120 | 0.34±0.1(7) | 558±73(7) | 222±44(7) |

Means ± s.e., number of experiments in parenthesis

The specific effect of argiopin on the open glutamate channels was confirmed by the analysis of current fluctuations induced by iono-phoretic application of glutamate (glutamate noise). Argiopin produced not only a fall of integral glutamate-induced current but the changes in power density spectrum. In control spectrum could be adequately described by a single Lorentzian. But in the presence of argiopin 4.4 x $10^{-7}$M it was fitted by two Lorentzians (Fig. 2). However, $K_d$ of argiopin interaction with the open glutamate channels obtained from the fluctuation analysis gave a value even 8 times lower (Table). This disagreement may be ascribed to different experimental conditions.

Interaction of argiopin with open glutamate or acetylcholine channels is likely to be dependent on membrane potential. The time constants of fast decay component are markedly decreases by hyperpolarization, which reflects the increase of the association rate of the argiopin molecule with open channels (Fig. 3). It occurred, however, that the differencies in $K_d$ values obtained at the different MP levels were non-significant (Table).

In the presence of argiopin the analysis of current-voltage relationship brought up distinct differences in the effects on glutamate

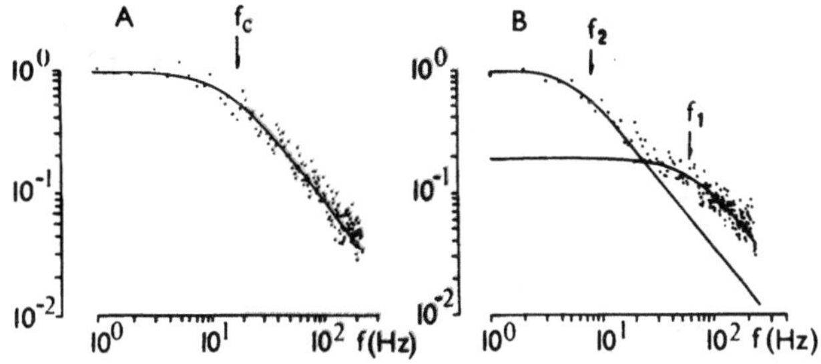


Fig. 2. The effect of argiopin on the mean life-time of open glutamate channel. Normalized current spectral densities of glutamate-induced currents in blowfly larvae muscle in control (A) and in the presence of argiopin 4.4 x $10^{-7}$M (B). The continuous lines were obtained by least-squares fits of the points to single Lorentzian (A) and to two ones (B). The arrows denote the cut-off frequences $f_c$= 14 Hz in control, $f_1$= 48 Hz and $f_2$= 7 Hz (corresponding time constants are 11 ms, 3.3 ms and 23 ms) and after treatment by argionin. MP = -60 mV, temp. 8°C.

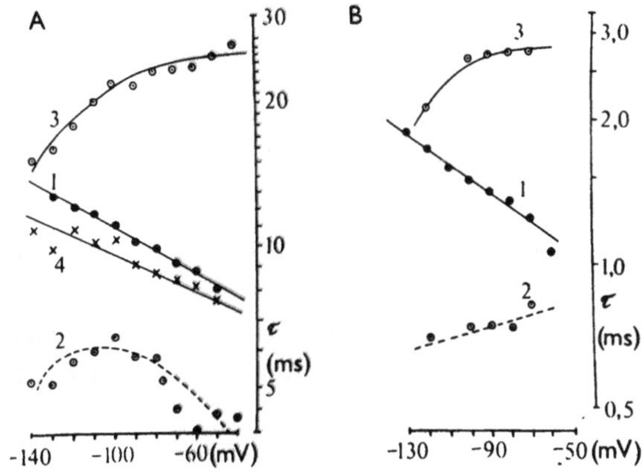


Fig. 3. The effects of voltage on the duration of EPSC decay before (1), after addition of argiopin (2 fast and 3 slow components of decay), and after washing (4). A. - blowfly larvae muscle (argiopin 4.4 x $10^{-7}$M); B. - frog muscle (argiopin 3.1 x $10^{-5}$M). Direct lines represent least-squares fits. Abscissa - MP in mW. Ordinate - time in ms. Temper. 21°C.

and acetylcholine receptors (Fig. 4). In frog muscle liniarity of the dependence of EPSC amplitude on the membrane potential was not changed by argiopin. However, in blowfly larvae muscle the fall of EPSC amplitude induced by argiopin was much more pronounced at the

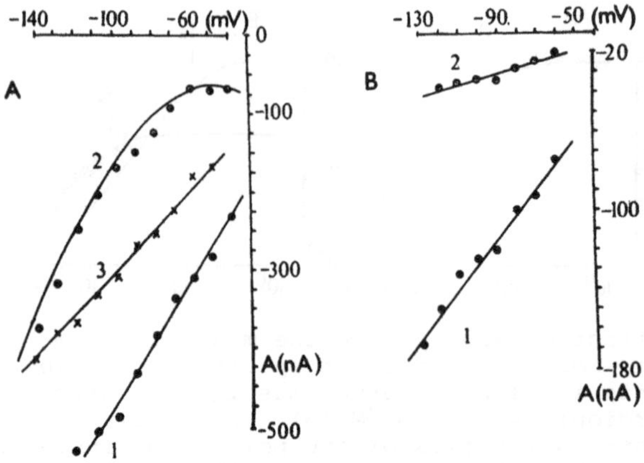


Fig. 4. The effects of voltage on the amplitude of EPSC's before (1), after addition of argiopin (2), and after 60 min washing (3). A - blowfly muscle (argiopin 4.4 x $10^{-7}$M); B - frog muscle (3.1 x x $10^{-5}$M). Abscissa - MP in mV, ordinate - EPSC amplitude in nA.

resting potential level (-50 mV) than after hyperpolarization. It means that the changes of glutamergic EPSC's in the presence of argiopin may be the result of different processes. Since the interaction of argiopin with open glutamate channel was not weakened by hyperpolarization, the decreasing effect of argiopin on the EPSC amplitude at -50 mV can be due to its interaction with closed glutamate channels. Being weakened by hyperpolarization, the potential dependence of this kind of interaction is in this particular case oppositely directed. This assumption was specially checked (Fig. 5).

In the presence of argiopin 4.4 x $10^{-7}$M, EPSC's were evoked by motor nerve stimulation in different time intervals after jump-like change in the membrane potential level from -130 mV to -40 mV. This allowed to estimate the rate for another equilibrium state to be achieved by the complex of closed glutamate channel - blocking drug (argiopin) at a new level of membrane potential. It follows it is possible to calculate the rate constant of argiopin binding to closed glutamate channel to be 2.7 ± 0.5 x $10^{8}$ $M^{-1}s^{-1}$. The amplitude of EPSC turned out to be exponentially decreasing with the time constant 4.5 ± ± 0.7 ms (n=4), as the time interval between the potential jump and EPSC increased. The argiopin concentration (4.4 ± 1.4 x $10^{-7}$M)

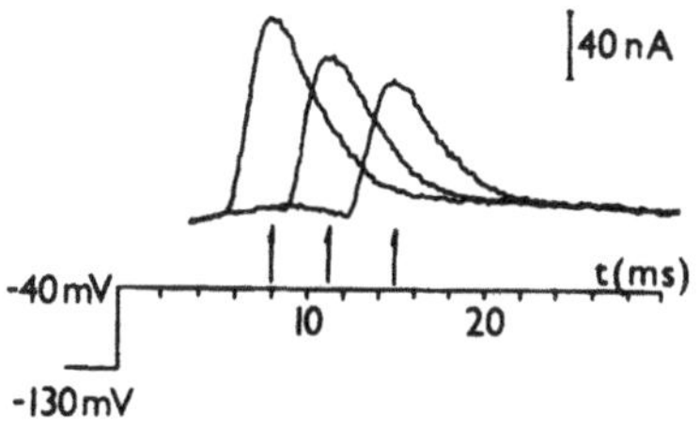


Fig. 5. The potential dependent effect of argiopin on the EPSC amplitude. EPSC's were recorded within different time intervals (indicated by arrows) after the membrane potential from -130 to 40 mV in the presence of 4.4 x $10^{-7}$M argiopin. Blowfly larvae muscle.

that induced a half-fall of EPSC amplitude under equilibrium conditions (at MP = -40 mV) was taken as a minimal value of $K_d$. Dissociation rate constant found to be 116 ± 68 $s^{-1}$. The obtained data shows that argiopin can also interact with a resting glutamate receptor to prevent its sequential activation (transition from $T_2R$ to $T_2R^*$ in the above scheme). $K_d$ of argiopin interaction with open or closed states of glutamate channel is quite similar at the resting potential -50 mV. But the fact that the potential dependence of interaction with these two states is differentialy directed speaks in favour that there are two different binding sites on the glutamate receptor for argiopin.

## Conclusion

The main active component of Argiope lobata venom producing a strong postsynaptic effect is the substance of low molecular weight, argiopin. The action of argiopin appears to be relatively specific and is directed preferentially to glutamate receptors It is realized by two molecular mechanisms: blocking effect on open and closed states of glutamate channel. $K_d$ for open channel is 6.7 x $10^{-7}$M and 4.4 x $10^{-7}$M for closed one. Both kinds of this interaction are potentialy dependent, but the sign of this dependence is different in case of open and closed states. Hence, the existence of two binding sites for argiopin may be presumed.

One of them is functionally and structurally related to the open channel. The nature of the second is far from being determined. In particular, it is necessary to elucidate whether this binding is competitive.

Argiopin is also capable of interacting with acetylcholine receptors, but then it would have affinity (40-70 times weaker compared to glutamate receptor) only to the open channel.

Identification of the molecular structure and the mode of action of argiopin allows to hope that this natufally occurring substance and its synthesized analogs will serve as valuable tools for investigation of glutamate receptors.

References

1. Kawai, N., A. Niwa, T. Abe. 1983. Toxicon 21, 438.

2. Tashmukhamedov, B.A., P.B. Usmanov, J. Kasakov, D. Kalikulov, L.Ja.Jukelson, B.U. Atakuziev. 1983. In: Toxins as tools in Neurochemistry, Walter de Gruyter, Berlin, p. 312.

3. Kawai, N., A. Niwa, M. Saito, H.S. Pan-Hou, M. Yoshoka. 1984. J. Physiol. (Paris) 79, 228.

4. Bateman, A., P. Boden, A. Dell, J.R. Duce, D.L.J. Quice, P.N.R. Usherwood. 1985. Brain Research 339, 237.

5. Grishin, E.V., T.M. Volkova, A.S. Arsenjev, O.S. Reshetova, V.V. Onoprienko, L.G. Magazanik, S.M. Antonov, I.M. Fedorova. 1986. Bioorg. chemistry 12, 1121 (in Russian).

6. Magazanik, L.G., S.M. Antonov, V.E. Gmiro. 1984. Biol. membranes 1, 130 (in Russian).

7. Peper, K., R.S Bradley, F. Dreyer. 1982. Physiol. Rev. 62, 1271.

ISOLATION OF ISOTOXINS FROM THE SEA ANEMONE ANEMONIA SULCATA BY HPLC-CHROMATOGRAPHY

E. Wachter

Institut für Physiologische Chemie, Physikalische Biochemie und Zellbiologie der UNI. München, Goethestr. 33, 2000 München 2, West Germany

G. Klostermann, A. Binder and L. Béress

Klinikum der Christian-Albrechts-Universität Kiel, Abteilung Toxikologie, Hospitalstr. 4-6, 2300 Kiel 1, West-Germany

## Introduction

From the sea anemone *Anemonia sulcata* up to now 5 toxins were described - ATX I, II and III (1), ATX IV (2) and AS V (3) - all basic polypeptides whose sequences have been determined (4, 5, 6, 2, 7). With the exception of ATX III and ATX IV - the latter is a relative of ATX III lacking the last two amino acids - Lys-Val in its sequence - the toxins of the *Anemonia sulcata* are homologous polypeptides having only a few alterations in their sequences (see Table 1).

These alterations are responsible for their different isoelectric points for which they can be separated from each other by use of ion exchange chromatography (1, 3). Earlier sequence studies on ATX I (4), ATX II (5) and on AS V (7) indicated already that the named toxins had distinct microheterogeneities in their sequences. ATX I contains Ala-Pro in position 3, ATX II Ile-Val in Position 2 and AS V Pro-Gly in position 39 (see Table 1). This inhomogeneity could not be eliminated even by use of the finest classical chromatographic techniques.

Only the use of the HPLC-Chromatography on a RP C 18 Reverse Phase column enabled the further purification of the sea anemone toxins up to different isotoxins. Four isotoxins from ATX I, eight isotoxin fractions from ATX and also five isotoxins from ATX II have been isolated.

Receptors and Ion Channels

The two main isotoxins are ATX I (Ala) and ATX I (Pro), whereas ATX II can mainly be separated in ATX II (Val) and ATX II (Ile).

<u>Table 1:</u> Amino acid sequences of the sea anemone toxins ATX I, II, AS V and ATX III, IV

| | 1 | | | | 5 | | | | | 1o | | | | | 15 | | | | | 2o | | | |
|---|---|---|---|---|---|---|---|---|---|---|---|---|---|---|---|---|---|---|---|---|---|---|---|
| ATX I. | G | A | A/P | C | L | C | K | S | D | G | P | N | T | R | G | N | S | M | S | G | T | I | W |
| ATX II. | G | I/V | P | C | L | C | D | S | D | G | P | S | V | R | G | N | T | L | S | G | I | I | W |
| AS V. | G | V | P | C | L | C | D | S | D | G | P | S | V | R | G | N | T | L | S | G | I | L | W |
| ATX III. | R | S | C | C | P | C | Y | W | G | G | C | P | W | G | Q | N | C | Y | P | Q | G | C | S |
| ATX IV. | R | S | C | C | P | C | Y | W | G | G | C | P | W | G | Q | N | C | Y | P | Q | G | C | S |

| | | 25 | 26 | | | | 3o | | | | | 35 | | | | | 4o | | | | | | 47 |
|---|---|---|---|---|---|---|---|---|---|---|---|---|---|---|---|---|---|---|---|---|---|---|---|
| ATX I. | V | F ' | ' G | C | P | S | G | W | N | N | C | Q | G | R | A | | I | I | G | Y | C | C | K | Q |
| ATX II. | L | A ' | ' G | C | P | S | G | W | H | N | C | K | K | H | G | P | T | I | G | W | C | C | K | Q |
| AS V. | L | A ' | ' G | C | P | S | G | W | H | N | C | K | K | H | K | P/G | T | I | G | W | C | C | K | |
| ATX III. | G | P ' | ' K | V | | | | | | | | | | | | | | | | | | | | |
| ATX IV. | G | P ' | ' | | | | | | | | | | | | | | | | | | | | | |

Material and Methods

The isolation of the sea anemone toxins ATX I, ATX and ATX II has been achieved with a slight modification of the methods described earlier (1, 3, 8). Five kg wet <u>Anemonia sulcata</u> were homogenized and extracted with five liter ethanol at pH 4,5. After centrifugation (2000 g for ten minutes) the supernatant was collected and the residue reextracted with five liter 50% watery ethanol and centrifuged again.
The two supernatants were combined and concentrated at reduced pressure (rotavapor) to one liter and the toxin was precipitated by adding of ten liter aceton at room temperature.
After the precipitation was completed at -20°C within twelve hours, the aceton was discarded and the toxin precipitate redissolved in two liter distilled water and dialysed against 2 x 20 liter water for eight hours in a visking tube.
The non dialysable tube content was centrifuged and the supernatant, containing the toxins, was passed through a column filled with SP-Sephadex C 25 (column size 7 x 50 cm) at pH 3.5 and at

conductivity of 3 mS, whereby the toxins with different other basic polypeptides were adsorbed. Afterwards the column was washed with distilled water and the adsorbed proteins were released in one step with a 1 molar solution of ammoniumacetate at pH 9.0. The eluate was dialysed against 20 liter distilled water for five hours and concentrated at reduced pressure.

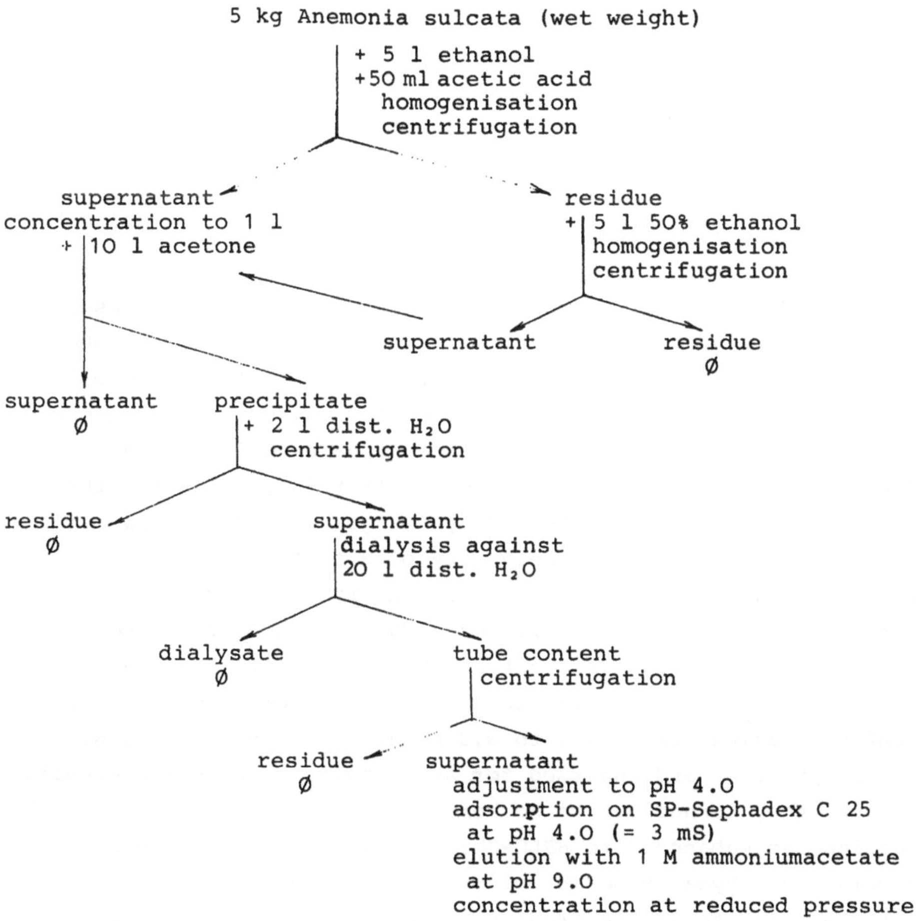


Fig. 1: A schema for the modified isolation of the toxins of the sea anemone *Anemonia sulcata*

The concentrated eluate was filtered on a Sephadex G 50 column (7 x 140 cm). The sea anemone toxins ATX I, ATX and ATX II were concentrated together in the third chromatographic fraction (see Fig. 2 A3) which was concentrated and lyophilized. This procedure resulted in 9 g of greybrown crude toxin. This material was dissolved in 500 ml distilled water and the pH was adjusted with a diluted $NH_3$ solution to pH 8.0. The precipitated impurities were eliminated by centrifugation and the crude toxin solution was chromatographied on a QAE-Sephadex A 25 column (3 x 40 cm) equilibrated with a 0,05 molar ammoniumacetate buffer solution pH 8.0 in order to eliminate the coloured nontoxic contaminations, which were adsorbed on the column.

One half of the eluated basic toxins were separated at pH 6.0 on a SP-Sephadex C 25 column (3 x 40 cm) by use of an ammoniumacetate buffer with a concentration gradient of 0,05 to 0,3 molar. With this gradient all sea anemone toxins were eluted successively (Fig. 2 C1, 3, 5). The non toxic strongly basic sea anemone proteins were eluted by use of a buffer concentration from 0,3 to 1,0 molar. The toxic fractions were collected, concentrated under reduced pressure and gelfiltered on a Sephadex G 25 column (3 x 50 cm) in 0,5 molar acetic acid. After lyophilization the purity of the samples was tested by PAA-gel electrophoresis at pH 8,6 which indicated the necessity of a further purification step for each toxin. For this reason the fractions were subjected to rechromatography on CM-Cellulose (Whatman CM-C 52) using an ammoniumacetate buffer gradient at pH 6.0. For ATX I a gradient from 0,01 m to 0,1 m was used.ATX and ATX II were repurified with a buffer gradient from 0,05 to 0,3 molar. The toxin fractions were lyophilized and analysed for homogeneity by electrophoresis. Although they turned out to be homogeneous by this criteria, each fraction was subjected to HPLC-Chromatography at reversed phase material on a Vydac RP C 18 column by use of a 10 mM triflouracetic acid/acetonitrile gradient to get a further proof for purity. The toxicity was tested on the shore crab carcinus maenas by intramuscular injection (8).

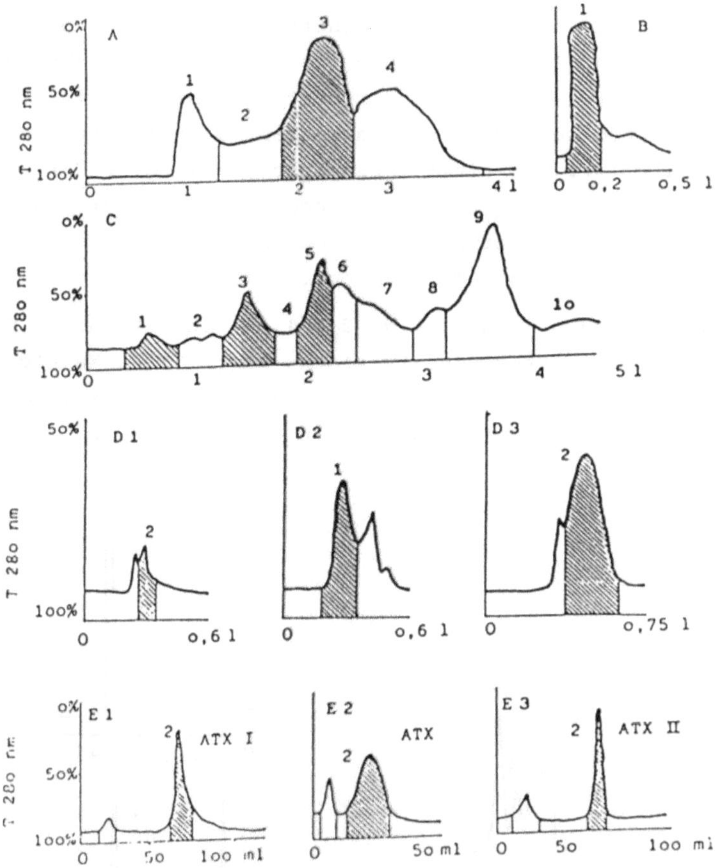


Fig. 2: Chromatographic purification of the Anemonia sulcata toxins ATX I, ATX and ATX II

A Gelfiltration on a Sephadex G 50. Column: 7 x 140 cm. Solvent: 0,5 m acetic acid

B Chromatography of A3 on QAE-Sephadex A 25 at pH 8.0 and = 6 mS. Column: 3 x 40 cm. Solvent: 0,05 m $NH_4$-acetate.

C Chromatography of B1 on SP-Sephadex C 25 at pH 6.0 Gradient: $NH_4$-acetate 0,05-0,3 1 m. Column: 3 x 40 cm.

D Gelfiltration of C1, C3, C5 on Sephadex G 25. Column: 3 x 40 cm

E Rechromatography of D 1,2, D 2,1, D 3,2 on CM-cellulose (Whatman C52at pH = 6.0.
Gradient: $NH_4$-acetate 0,01-0,1 m for E 1 and 0,05-0,3 for E 2 and E 3. Column: 0,5 x 10 cm for 5 mg toxin.

In contrast to our earlier studies where we have found only two toxins (Toxin I and Toxin II) during the ion exchange chromatography (1, 8), here we have found repeatedly three toxin fractions following this protocol. This is in agreement with the results of Schweitz et al. (3). The first toxin fraction (Fig. 2 C1) turned out to contain the ATX I group, the second (Fig. 2 C3) a so ar structurally not characterized ATX group and the third fraction (Fig. 2 C5) contained the ATX II group.

HPLC-Chromatography of ATX I (Fig. 2 E 1, 2) on a Vydac RP C 18 column revealed the heterogeneity of the pure ATX I. Mainly four components could be isolated using a 10 mM triflouracetic acid/ acetonitrile gradient from 10-50% organic solvent (Fig. 3).

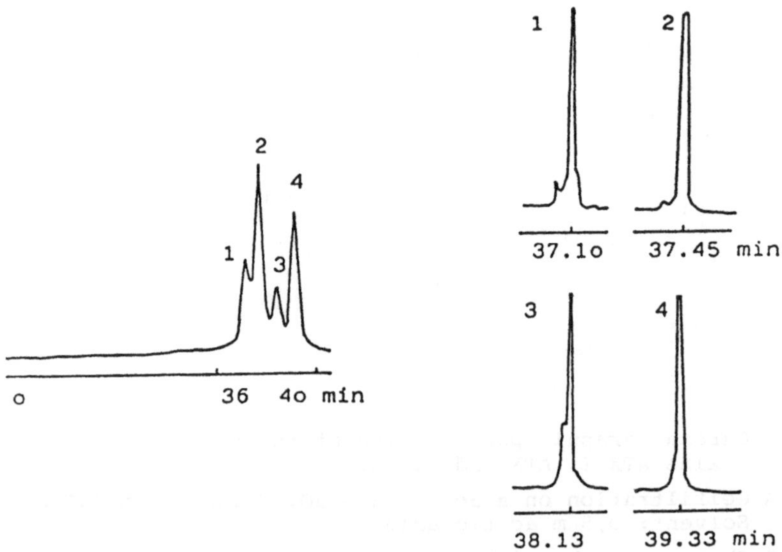


Fig. 3: HPLC-Chromatography of ATX I on an analytical Vydac 10 TPRP C 18 column (4,5 x 250 mm), $CH_3CN$-TFA (0,1%) gradient 10-50% in 60 min, flow rate 1,0 ml/min, detection 0,05 AUFS, 278 nm and rechromatography of the isolated fractions with their retention times

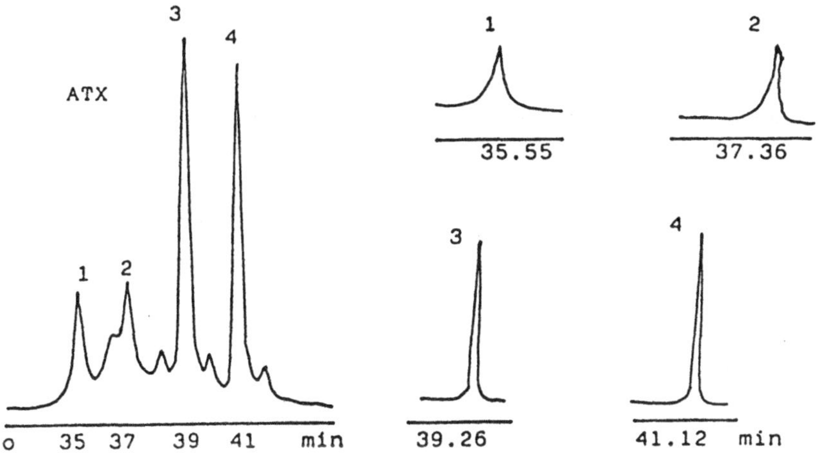


Fig. 4: HPLC-Chromatography of ATX on analytical Vydac 10 TPRP C 18 column (4,6 x 250 mm), $CH_3CN$-TFA (0,1%) gradient 10-50% in 60 min, flow rate 1,0 ml/min, detection 0,05 AUFS, 278 nm and rechromatography of the isolated fractions with their retention times

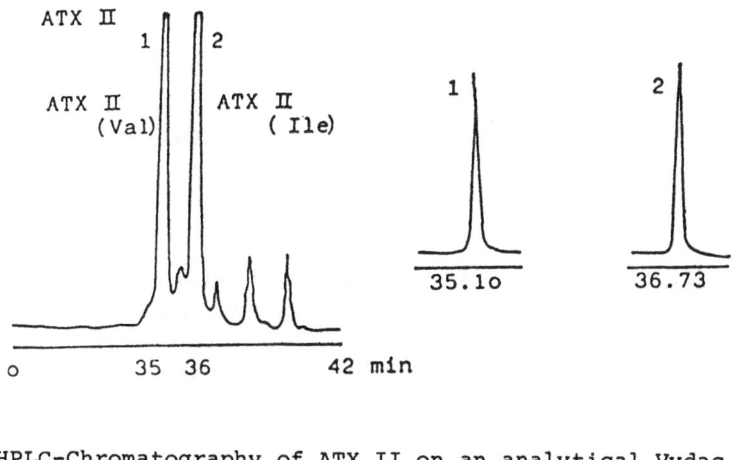


Fig. 5: HPLC-Chromatography of ATX II on an analytical Vydac 10-50% in 60 min, flow rate 1,0 ml/min, detection, 0,05 AUFS, 278 nm and rechromatography of the isolated fractions with their retention times

The two major components of ATX I (Fig. 3, Fr. 2 and Fr. 4) were subjected to amino acid analysis. The first of them (Fr. 2) turned out to contain an increased amount of alanine and a lowered amount of proline compared to our earlier results (9). The second (Fr. 4) revealed increased amount of proline and lowered alanin values. To substantiate these findings both fractions were subjected to solid phase Edman degradation (10). The two isotoxins were immobilized at p-phenylene-diisothiocyanate porous glass beads and degraded. The analysis of the resulting phenylthiohydantoins demonstrated alanin in the position 3 of the sequence in the case of the first major isotoxin of ATX I, whereas the same position is occupied by proline in the case of the second major isotoxin of ATX I. The two minor isotoxins of ATX I (Fig. 3 Fr. 1 and Fr. 3) have not yet been structurally characterized up to now because of lack of sufficient material. The new fraction ATX (see Fig. 2 E 2,2) was purified by HPLC-Chromatography in the same way as ATX I resulting in eight fractions (see Fig. 4). However electrophoretic studies on PAA-gel gave a hint that these isotoxins especially B 5, 6, 7, 8 are closely related to those of the isotoxins of the ATX II group (see Fig. 6), the lack of the amino acid analysis and sequence studies do not allow any further identification.

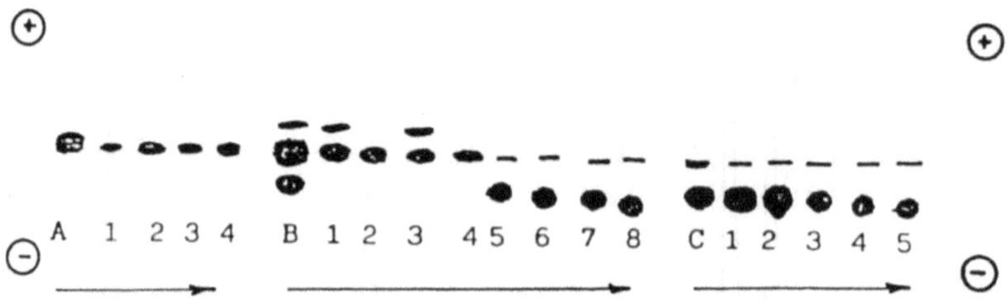


Fig. 6: Electrophoresis on PAA-gel at pH 8.6

A: ATX I with the related 4 HPLC purified isotoxin fractions

B: ATX with the related 8 HPLC purified isotoxin fractions

C: ATX II with the related 5 HPLC purified isotoxin fractions

The two major components of ATX II after its separation with the HPLC-Chromatography (see Fig. 5 Fr. 1 and Fr. 2) were analysed and degradated in the same way as described for ATX I. The result was that ATX II HPLC Fr. 1 has valin at the second position in the sequence whereas HPLC Fr. 2 contained isoleucin at the same position. In the case of ATX II the minor components of the HPLC fractions have also been investigated. All these subfractions can be attributed either to the ATX II (Val) or the ATX II (Ile) isotoxin group. ATX II Fr. 3 is ATX II (Ile), ATX II HPLC Fr. 4 is ATX II (Ile/Val) and ATX II HPLC Fr. 5 is ATX II (Ile).

## Discussion

The HPLC-Chromatography on reversed phase materials is an extremly useful tool for the separation of the microheterogeneous neurotoxins from the sea anemone Anemonia sulcata.
This can be demonstrated by the rapid and exact separation of the two isotoxins of ATX I with the only difference of an Ala/Pro exchange. As expected from theory the alanin derivative is eluted before the proline isotoxin from the column which is in accordance with the relative hydrophobicity of these two residues. This also holds true for the ATX II isotoxins where the slight difference in the hydrophobic character of valin and isoleucin is sufficient for an almost complete separation of these two isotoxins. The ATX II (Val) is eluated before the ATX II (Ile) isotoxin.
However, further investigations are necessary to clear up the occurence of the later eluting fractions of the ATX isotoxins. The toxicity of the two isotoxins ATX II (Val) and ATX II (Ile) is the same as estimated on the shore crab carcinus maenas and also on the guinea-pig heart. The same is true for the two main isotoxins of the ATX I group tested on the shore crab. Further investigations will reveal the nature of these varieties of isotoxins, whether they are already virgine products paralysing different prays, or simply they are enzymatic degradation products of the native toxins caused by the preparation procedures.

## Acknowledgement

The authors are very greatful to Prof. Dr. O. Wassermann, Kiel, for supporting our work and to Miss. G. Thurow, Mr. P. Somogyi and Mr. T. Panksy for scientific co-operation. Supported by the Deutsche

Forschungsgemeinschaft and the Fonds der Chemischen Industrie. This work is a part of the doctor thesis of Mr. A. Binder.

## References

1. Béress, L., R. Béress and G. Wunderer, 1975
Toxicon 13, 359-367

2. Wachter, E., unpublished results

3. Schweitz, H., J.P. Barhanin, C. Frelin, G. Hugues and M. Lazdunski, 1981
Biochemistry 20, 5245-5252

4. Wunderer, G. and M. Eulitz, 1978
Eur. J. Biochem. 89, 11-17

5. Wunderer, C., W. Machleidt and E. Wachter, 1976
Hoppe Seyler's Z. Physiol. Chem. 357, 239-248

6. Béress, L., G. Wunderer and E. Wachter, 1977
Hoppe Seyler's Z. Physiol. Chem. 358, 985-988

7. Scheffler, J.J., A. Tsugita, G. Linden, H. Schweitz and M. Lazdunski, 1982
Biochim. Biophys. Res. Comm. 107, 272-278

8. Béress, L. and R. Béress, 1971
Kieler Meeresforsch. 27, 117-127

9. Béress, L., R. Béress and G. Wunderer, 1975
FEBS Letters 50, 311-314

10. Wachter, E., W. Machleidt, H. Hofner and J. Otto, 1973
FEBS Letters 35, 97-102

# RECONSTRUCTION OF SOLUTION SPATIAL STRUCTURE OF NEUROTOXIN $M_9$ *BUTHUS EUPEUS* BY DISTANCE GEOMETRY ALGORITHM ACCORDING TO NMR SPECTROSCOPY DATA

V.N. Maiorov, V.S. Pashkov, V.F. Bystrov
Shemyakin Institute of Bioorganic Chemistry, USSR Academy of Sciences, Moscow 117871, USSR

## Introduction

"Long" scorpion polypeptide toxins form large group of compounds consisting of 60-70 amino acid residues and possessing four disulfide bridges (1). The toxins are able to interact with nerve tissue membranes provoking their functional changes. Difference in amino acid sequences correlates with changes in the specificity and toxicity of the molecules, so that the toxins are of interest for study of structure-function relashionships in globular proteins (1,2).

In present work the solution spatial structure of neurotoxin $M_9$ (66 amino acid residues) from the venom of scorpion *Buthus eupeus* (3) was elucidated by NMR spectroscopy and compared with the known spatial structures of other scorpion toxins. Some improvements of the distance geometry approach were implemented, which allow to consider dense packing of a globular molecule and *L*-isomerism of the protein amino acid residues in simplified presentation.

## Method

By means of distance geometry algorithm (4-8) the spatial structure of neurotoxin $M_9$ was solved with the use of interproton distance constraints resulting from nuclear Overhauser effect (NOE) contacts. Simplified presentation of amino acid residues by two spherical pseudoatoms (5) was employed to save computer memory and calculation time. The α-pseudoatom represents backbone atoms, while the β-pseudo-

Receptors and Ion Channels

atoms-all side chain atoms of a residue. Practice of spatial structure calculations (6-8) shows that such simplification works quite well for solving backbone polypeptide chain fold and to define side chains orientations of amino acid residues. NOE experimental data were taken into account as follows. If protons of two distant in primary structure residues demonstrate mutual NOE, then upper constraint on the distance between the surfaces of corresponding pseudoatoms are set to empirically determined in the test calculations value of 1.5 Å. To improve the quality of three dimensional structure modeling some modifications were implemented in the form of penalty function:

$$F = w_d \cdot \sum_{i<j} D_{ij} + w_c \cdot \sum_k C_k + w_r \cdot R, \qquad \text{(I)}$$

which is minimized for refinement of cartesian coordinates of pseudoatoms at the final step of distance geometry algorithm processing.

In equation (I)

$$D_{ij} = \begin{cases} (d_{ij}^2 - u_{ij}^2)^2, & \text{if } d_{ij} > u_{ij} \\ 0, & \text{if } l_{ij} < d_{ij} < u_{ij} \\ (l_{ij}^2 - d_{ij}^2)^2, & \text{if } d_{ij} < l_{ij} \end{cases}, \qquad \text{(II)}$$

where $d_{ij}$, $l_{ij}$ and $u_{ij}$ - distance between $i$ and $j$ pseudoatoms and its lower and upper constraints, correspondingly;

$$C_k = \begin{cases} (c_k - c_k^{(u)})^2, & \text{if } c_k > c_k^{(u)} \\ 0, & \text{if } c_k^{(l)} < c_k < c_k^{(u)} \\ (c_k^{(l)} - c_k)^2, & \text{if } c_k < c_k^{(l)} \end{cases}, \qquad \text{(III)}$$

$$c_k = \vec{r}(\alpha_k\beta_k) \cdot |\vec{r}(\alpha_k\alpha_{k-1}) \times \vec{r}(\alpha_k\alpha_{k+1})|, \qquad \text{(IV)}$$

where $c_k$ - chirality parameter, which value depends on the mutual arrangement of α- and β-pseudoatoms of the $k-1$, $k$ and $k+1$ amino acid resudues for all but the terminal residues, $c_k^{(l)}$ and $c_k^{(u)}$ - correspondingly, lower and upper constaints of chirality parameter, $\vec{r}(A,B)$ - radius-vector between $A$ and $B$ pseudoatoms;

$$R = (r_g^2 - r_{go}^2) \,, \tag{V}$$

where $r_g$ and $r_{go}$ are the calculated and the target gyratio radii, correspondingly.

Factors $w_d$, $w_c$ and $w_r$ perform weighting of $D$, $C$ and $R$ term contributions to the penalty function, thus allowing to control relative significance of the terms during minimization procedure. Their values were empirically adjusted in the computational tests.

The first term in equation (I) serves for keeping all interatomic distances within defined ranges of constraints (4).

The second term is responsible for the correct chirality of asymmetrical $C^{\alpha}$ centers and is aimed to arrange pseudoatoms in correct $L$- or $D$-amino acid isomers. The ranges of chirality parameter $c_k$ were defined as 6 to 21 $Å^3$ for $L$-residues, and -21 to -6 $Å^3$ for $D$-residues on the basis of analysis of sterically allowed amino acid conformations. In the simplified presentation of polypeptide chain the absence of this term would result in incorrect mutual arrangement of β-pseudoatoms of neighboring amino acid residues, so that wrong structural results may appear. The third term is introduced into the penalty function (1) to rich the native extent of packing density, because as a rule relatively swollen spatial structure corresponds to the distance constraints inferred from NMR data. The target value of gyratio radius $r_{go}$ is estimated from the known protein packing density and the total volume of the all atomic groups of the molecule (6).

## Results

A number of conformations of the solution spatial structure of neurotoxin $M_9$ was calculated according to the input NOE contacts shown on Fig. 1. Estimation of agreement of the conformations is made with the use of method (9). The value of the average root-

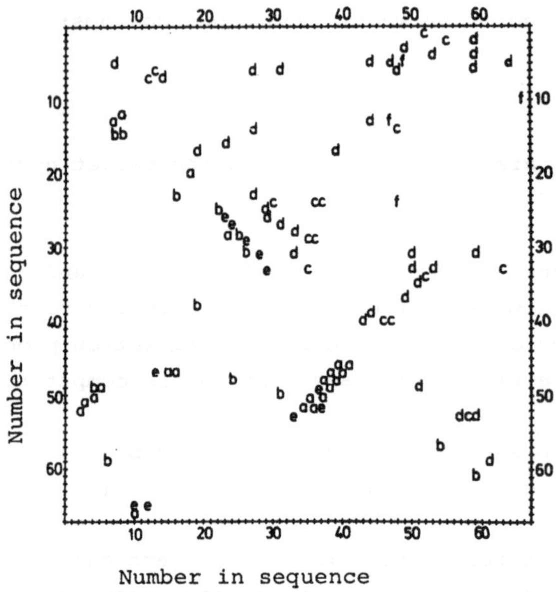


Fig. 1. NOE contact map of the neurotoxin $M_9$ used for calculation of spatial structure of the molecule. Along the axes amino acid sequence number are indicated. Each interproton NOE contact is assigned to the corresponding pseudoatoms ($\alpha$ or $\beta$) and is presented only once either over or bellow the diagonal. The letters denote the following types of contacts: a - $\alpha\alpha$; b - $\beta\beta$; c - $\beta\alpha$; d - $\beta\beta$; e - $\alpha\alpha+\alpha\beta$; f - $\beta\alpha+\beta\beta$.

mean-square deviation (RMSD) 2.1 Å for coordinates of backbone $\alpha$-pseudoatoms is low enough to indicate that all conformations are similar to each other and represent the only spatial structure of the molecule.

Identification of secondary structure fragments reveals two and a half turns of right-handed $\alpha$-helix (residues 22-31) and three stranded antiparallel $\beta$-structure (residue 1-5, 35-40 and 46-52). Changes in the direction of polypeptide chain fold occur in the region of residues 9-10, 19-20, 53-57 and 60-61.

On the Fig. 2 stereoscopic view of the neurotoxin $M_9$ spatial structure is shown.

Mutual arrangement of secondary structure fragments ($\alpha$-helix and

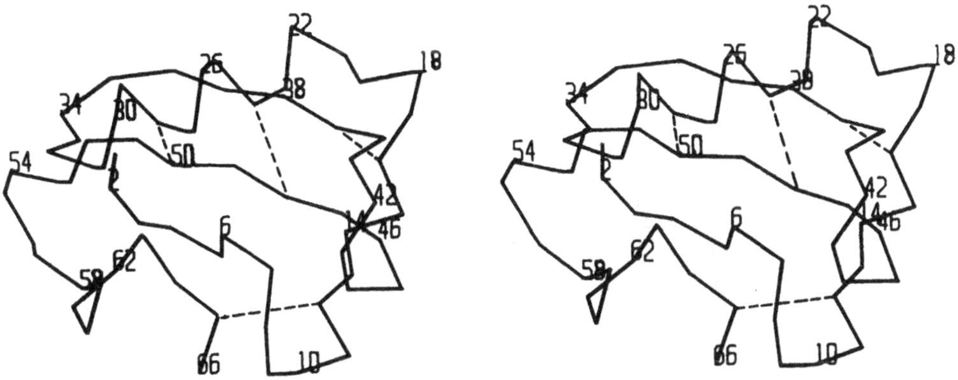


Fig. 2. Stereo drawings of the neurotoxin $M_9$ structure in α-pseudoatoms presentation. Each forth α-pseudoatom is numbered. Disulfide bridges are shown by dashed lines.

β-structure) and irregular fragments of molecule are well determined by taking into account NOE contacts between residues distant in the amino acid sequence, as well as disulfide bridges pattern (Fig. 3). The helical fragment 22-31 of the molecule follows by the reverse turn 31-35, after which the β-strand 35-40 is located. The residues 41-45 form loop connecting two other strands of the antiparallel β-structure (Fig. 3).

Neurotoxin $M_9$ is a third scorpion toxin, which three dimensional structure was established. Previously, the structure of the toxin V-3 *Centruroides sculpturatus* was determined by means of X-ray crystallography (2), and solution spatial structure of "short" insectotoxin (35 amino scid residues) $I_5A$ *Buthus eupeus* was determined by NMR spectroscopy (7). Thus there is an opportunity to compare their spatial organization and to discuss structure-functional relationships of these toxins.

Apparently the same structural motif in spatial organization of the molecules is evident (Fig. 4 a,b,c): α-helix, which is similarly oriented towards the β-structure (three strands in the $M_9$ (Fig. 4a) and v-3 (Fig. 4b) toxins and two strands in the insectoxin $I_5A$ (Fig. 4c)) and fixed against it by two disulfide bridges. On

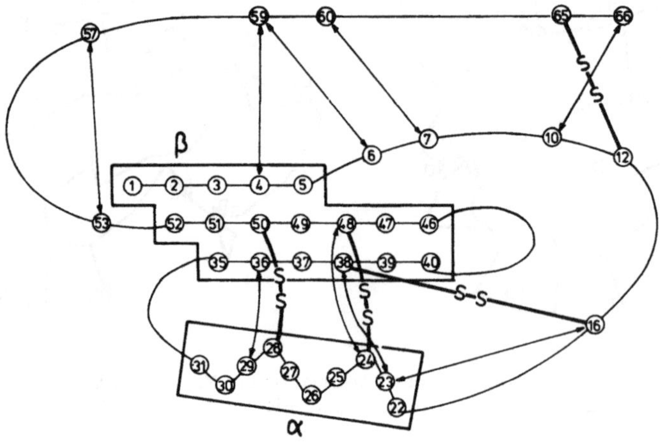


Fig. 3. Schematic representation of the neurotoxin $M_9$ spatial structure. Here α denotes the α-helix, and β denotes the β-structure. Arrows show longrange NOE contacts. Disulfide bridges are indicated.

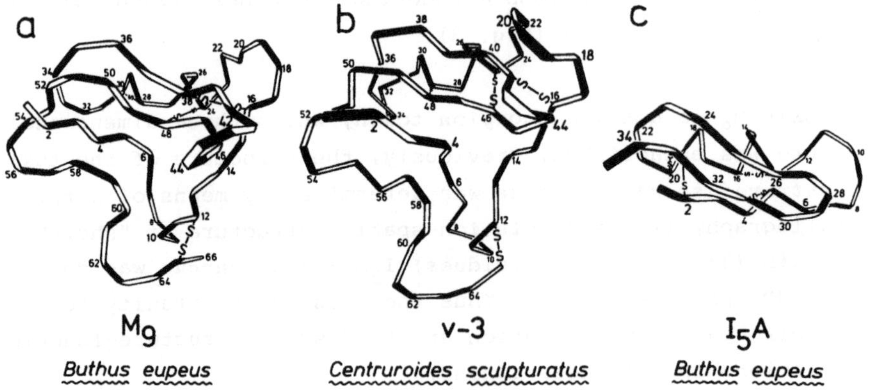


Fig. 4. Polypeptide chain folding of scorpion toxins: $M_9$(a) and $I_5$ (c) - according to NMR data, v-3 (b) - according to X-ray crystallography data.

the both termini of the helix two revese turns of polypeptide chain are located.

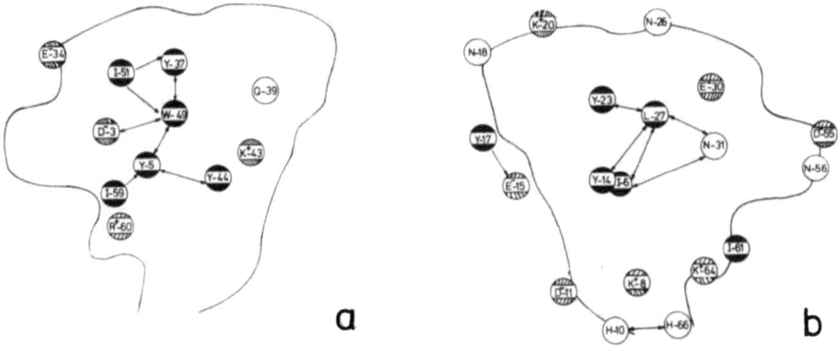


Fig. 5. Amino acid side chain distribution on the surface of the neurotoxin $M_9$ molecule (a) from the side of β-structure as presented on Fig. 4a and (b) from the back side. Hydrophobic side chains are darkned, while charged are shaded. Arrows indicate experimentally established NOE contacts between protons of corresponding side chains.

Even more considerable spatial structure resemblance is striking for the $M_9$ and v-3 toxins (Fig. 4 a,b), which have approximately equal number of amino acid residues. These molecules have many common structural features also outside of the described cluster of regular secondary structure: similar loops threading, similar mutual arrangement of fragments of irregular structure etc. The conformational similarity of toxins $M_9$ and v-3 in spite of their relatively poor primary structure homology leeds to the assumption that the revealed characteristic features of three dimensional structure might be in common for the whole group of "long" scorpion toxins.

Analysis of crystal structure of toxin v-3 reveals hydrophobic side chain clustering on the surface of the molecule. It was suggested that this cluster would be the site of interaction with receptor (2). The surface of the NMR structure neurotoxin $M_9$ also reveals two hydrophobic clusters on the opposite sides of the globule (Fig. 5). One of them is located on the β-structure side of the molecule and includes side chains of Tyr-5, Tyr-37, Tyr-44, Trp-49, Ile-51 and Ile-59 residues (Fig. 5a). Another, smaller cluster contains side chains of Ile-6, Tyr-14, Tyr-23 and Leu-27 residues (Fig.5b). It is noteworthy that about half of these residues are conservative in the primary structure of "long" scorpion toxins.

Biological activity of the toxins varies considerably in spite of common principle of spatial structure organization. Toxin v-3 manifests a weak toxical effect on cricets (10), while neurotoxin $M_9$ has no effect on insects, but affects mammals (3). "Short" insectotoxin $I_5A$, containing 30 residues less, acts only on the insects (11). Differences in the biological activity of toxins $M_9$ and $I_5A$ may be attributed both to the presence of additional residues in the $M_9$ primary structure and to the variations in the side chain properties of residues, which have the same position in the tertiary structures of these toxins. In the case of $M_9$ and v-3 the differences might be related to relatively small changes in the spatial structure and to the presence of unlike amino acid residues in the analogous position of the primary and tertiary structures.

For instance, in neurotoxin $M_9$ positively charged Arg-60 is situated near the larger hydrophobic cluster (Fig. 5a), while in toxin v-3 there is Tyr residue in this position.

References

1. Ovchinnikov, Yu.A. 1974. Pure and Appl. Chem. 56, 1049.

2. Fontecilla-Camps, J.C., R.J. Almassy, S.E. Ealick, I.L. Suddath, D.D. Watt, R.J. Feldmann, C.E. Rugg. 1981. Trends in Biochem. Sci. 6, 291.

3. Volkova T.M., A.F. Garsia, I.N. Telezhinskaya, N.A. Potapenko, E.V. Grishin. 1985. Bioorgan. Khimiya. 11, 1445.

4. Braun W., C. Bosch, L.R. Brown, N. Go, K. Wüthrich. 1981. Biochim. Biophys. Acta. 667, 377.

5. Braun W., N. Go, K. Wüthrich. 1981. Abstracts of VII International Biophysics Congress and III Pan-American Biochemistry Congress, p. 73.

6. Arseniev A.S., V.I. Kondakov, V.N. Maiorov, V.F. Bystrov, Yu.A. Ovchinnikov. 1983. Bioorgan. Khimiya. 9, 1667.

7. Arseniev A.S., V.I. Kondakov, V.N. Maiorov, V.F. Bystrov. 1984. FEBS Lett. 165, 57.

8. Maiorov V.N., A.S. Arseniev. 1984. J. Mol. Struct. 114, 339.

9. McLachlan A.D. 1979. J. Mol. Biol. 128, 49.

10. Babin D.R., D.D. Watt, S.M. Goos, R.V. Mlejnek. 1974. Arch. Biochem. Biophys. 164, 694.

11. Grishin E.V., T.M. Volkova, L.N. Soldatova. 1982. Bioorgan. Khimiya. 8, 155.

# STRUCTURAL AND FUNCTIONAL COMPARISON OF SNAKE NEUROTOXINS AND CURARE-LIKE ACETYLCHOLINE ANTAGONISTS. THE "ACTIVE TRIANGLE" HYPOTHESIS

W. Saenger

Institut für Kristallographie, Freie Universität Berlin, Takustr. 6, D-1000 Berlin 33, FRG

M.D. Walkinshaw

Department of Chemistry, University of Edinburgh, West Mains Road, Edinburgh EH9 3JJ, Scotland

A. Maelicke

Max-Planck-Institut für Ernährungsphysiologie, Rheinlanddamm 201, D-4600 Dortmund 1, FRG

## Introduction

In recent years, over 60 postsynaptic neurotoxins isolated from a wide variety of snakes have been sequenced (1). These studies suggest that two major classes of toxins exist, the "long" toxins with 71 to 74 amino acids cross linked by five disulfide bridges, and the "short" toxins with 60 to 62 amino acids cross linked by four disulfide bridges. Crystal structure analyses of both "short" and "long" toxins have been carried out (2-4) which can be used as prototypes for the respective neurotoxin families because the structural homologies within the families and also between the families are very strong. On the basis of these similarities and supported by chemical modification studies, it appears that the active site of the neurotoxins is located on one side of the long, central loop which also hosts the only tryptophan. If the distribution of charged and hydrophobic residues on this portion of the neurotoxins is further investigated, one finds triangles formed by positively charged and negatively charged residues and by hydrophobic patches. Since the spatial distribution of these sites is comparable in curare-like alkaloids, which also act as acetylcholine-antagonists in the

Receptors and Ion Channels

binding to the acetylcholine receptor, we looked at this class of compounds in more detail and came to the conclusion that there must be a triangle relationship which is described in the following.

## The definition of the active site of snake neurotoxins

In Fig. 1, we have illustrated schematically the molecular structures of α-cobratoxin (the "long" family) and of erabutoxin b (the "short" family) as α-carbon atom tracings. Both structures are essentially composed of three loops I, II, III which are tied together by the four invariant disulfide bridges in the globular head of the molecules. The "long" toxin family has one extra disulfide bridge at the lower tip of the long, central loop between amino acids 30 and 34. Besides these covalent bridges, the central loop is further stabilized by a number of hydrogen bonds which form a β-pleated sheet structure within this loop and between one strand of this loop and one strand of loop III.

If we look at the topologies of the two molecules more closely, we find that they superimpose almost identically at the lower tips of loop II and of loop III. Because both molecules have a comparable action on the acetylcholine receptor, this suggests that the active site must reside in these portions which overlap so remarkably.

Looking at the amino acid distribution which occurs in the "long" and in the "short" families, we find, as illustrated in Fig. 1, that there is very extensive exchange of amino acids in the globular head of both molecules and in loop I. The exchange is much less in the lower tip of loop II and of loop III, where the exchanges are also often type conserved. In Fig. 1, all the residues pointing towards the viewer in loops II and III are indicated by shading. These residues are the least varied and in many cases very strictly conserved like the Tyr25, Trp29, Glu/Asp42, Gly44.

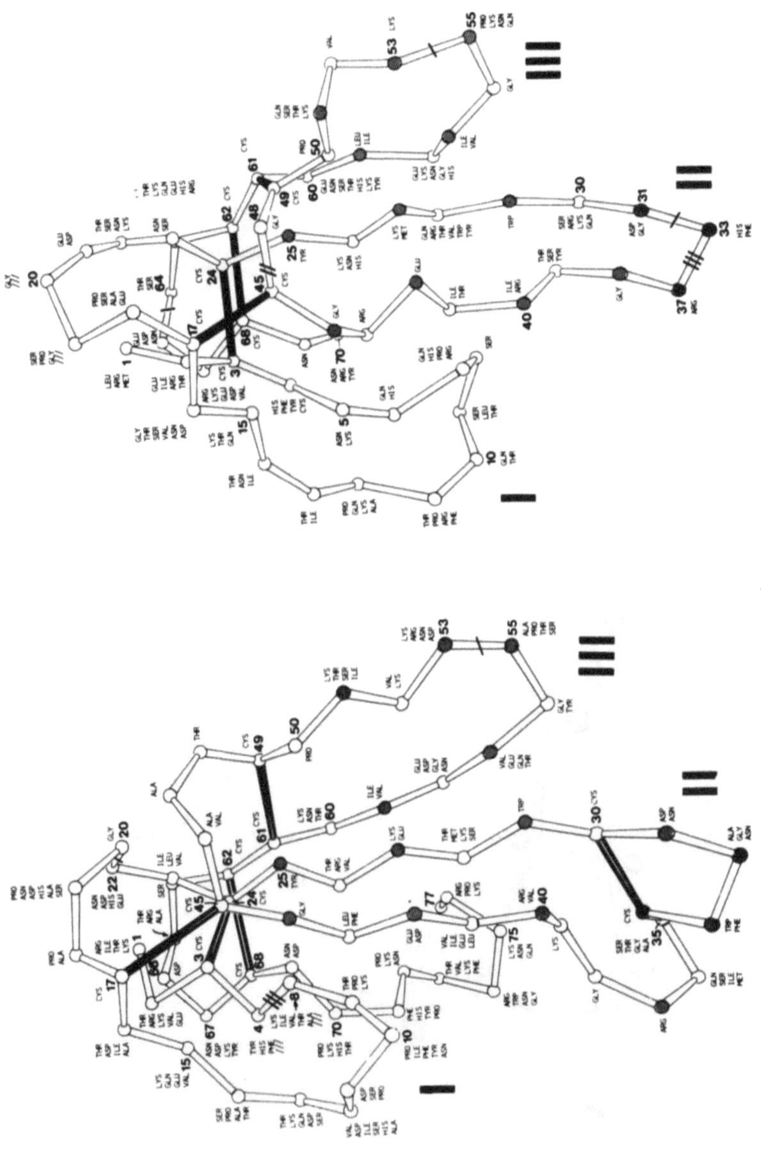

Fig. 1. Comparison of α-carbon tracings of α-cobratoxin (left), and erabutoxin b (right). The major loops are designated I, II, III, and deletions in amino acid sequences are indicated by slashes across bonds. Disulfide bridges are indicated by double-lines. Besides each α-carbon atom, the occurrences of amino acids in the available sequences (about 30 each) are indicated (23). Highly variable sites show many amino acids, and conserved sites show only one or few type-related residues. Amino acid residues pointing towards the viewer in loops II and III are indicated by shading.

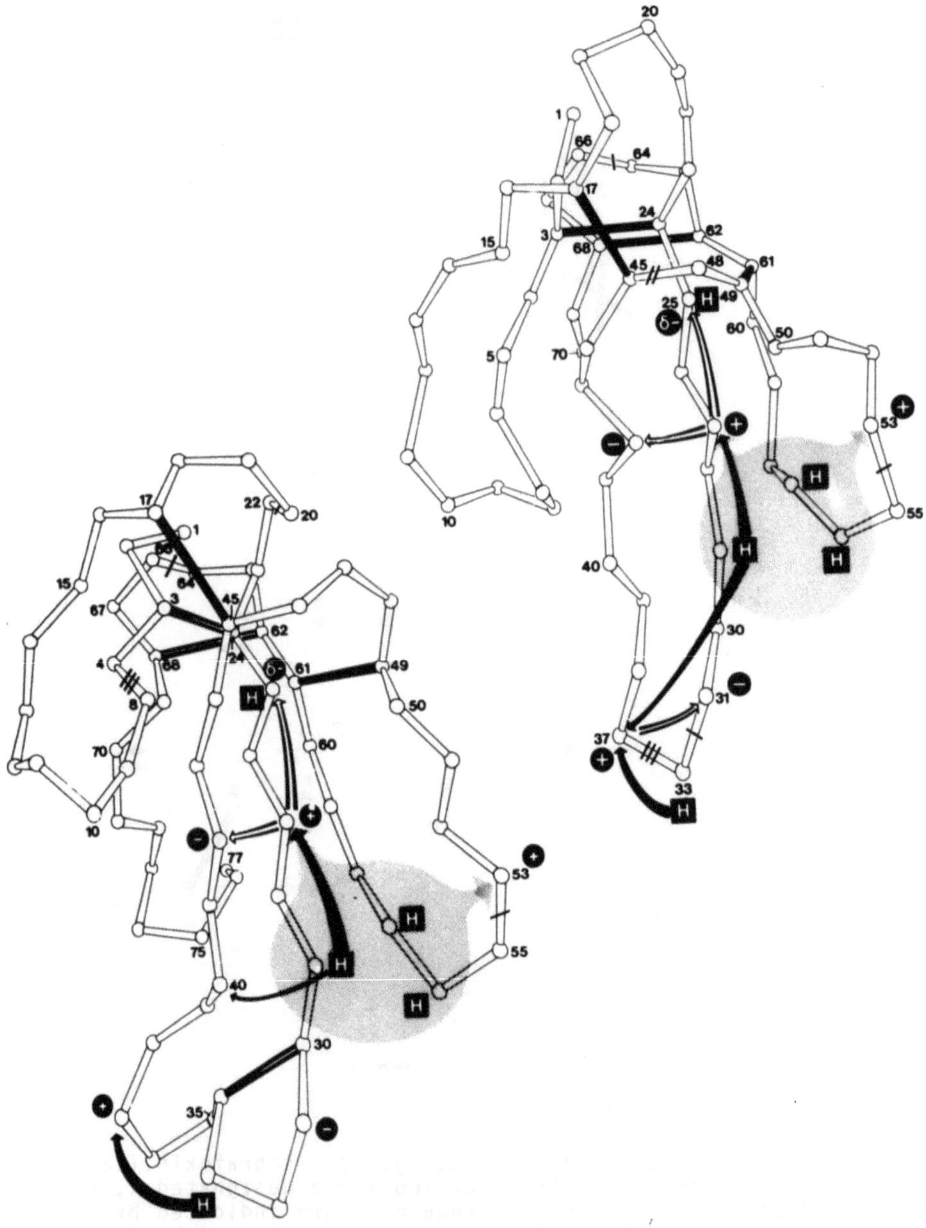

Fig. 2. Schematic representation of hydrophobic residues (H in squares), positive and negative charges (+ and - in circles) of α-cobratoxin (left) and erabutoxin b (right). Larger hydrophobic patches are indicated by shadowing, the arrows indicate distances between 5Å and 11Å.

If we further reduce the information to the essential points, we arrive at Fig. 2. We have only indicated the hydrophobic patches of the active site with H in black squares, and positive and negative charges in respective black circles. The arrows indicated in the figure mark distances between these sites which are of the order of 5Å to 11Å and also found in the curare-like alkaloids.

## The triangle hypothesis

To highlight the structural and functional similarities of α-cobratoxin and erabutoxin b, the central loop of the "long" toxin was modelled using only the α-carbon atoms of the invariant residues. In effect we have a "virtual bond" model which is illustrated in Fig. 3a,b. The amino acid side chain orientations in Fig. 3a,b are as observed in the crystal structure analyses. It is possible to rotate the more elongated side chains so that they superimpose.

Besides the structural similarity, the biochemical correspondence of a number of the conserved residues on the long, central loop is remarkable and has been reviewed in (1, 5-7).

It has been suggested previously that the mode of action of antagonists lies in their ability to mimic the acetylcholine molecule (8-13). A similar proposal for the action of erabutoxin b has been made based on the $N^+$---O distance of the invariant Asp31 and Arg37 residues which resembles the $N^+$---O distance in some non-peptide antagonists (9-11). An alternative mode of action of erabutoxin b has been suggested in which specific peptide side chains may act as mimics for the curareform non-depolarizing antagonists (9). A comparison of the structure of these agents showed the presence of two quaternary nitrogen atoms 11Å apart, separated by a concave hydrophobic surface (12), though some typical antagonists have only one quaternary nitrogen and the $N^+$---$N^+$ distance may vary between 7.5Å and 11.1Å.

The main classes of the curareform antagonists (11) are related to the naturally occurring alkaloids d-tubocurarine, toxiferine and erythroidine, and also to a number of synthetic analogues

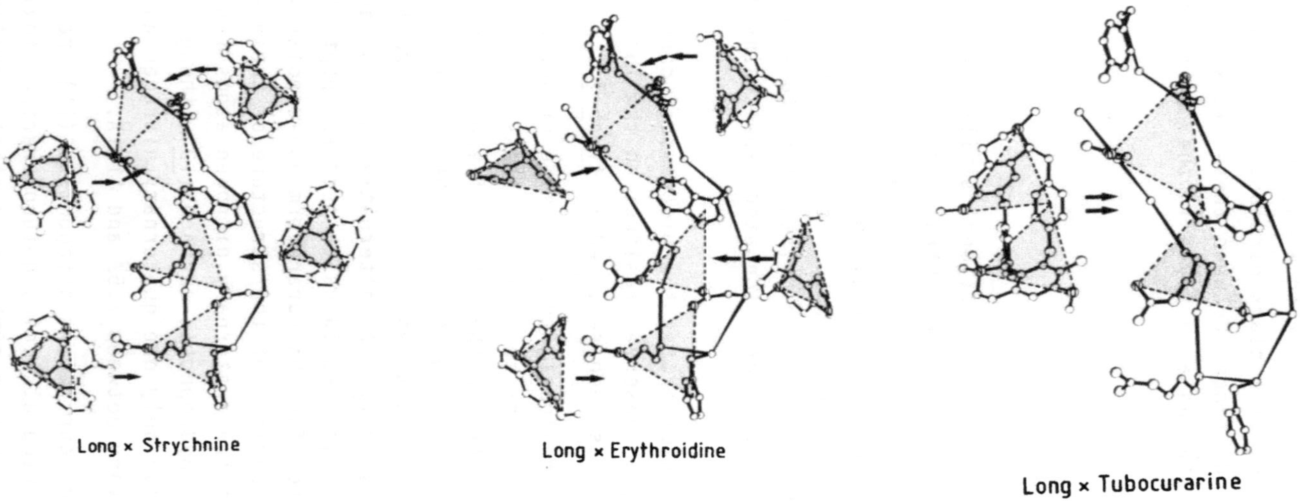


Fig. 3a,b. "Virtual bond" representations of the long, central loops of α-cobratoxin and erabutoxin b and structural comparison with strychnine, erythroidine, tubocurarine. In all cases except the larger tubocurarine, there are four possible correspondences of the small alkaloid molecules to the polypeptide loops as indicated by the shaded triangles.

For Fig. 3b, see next page.

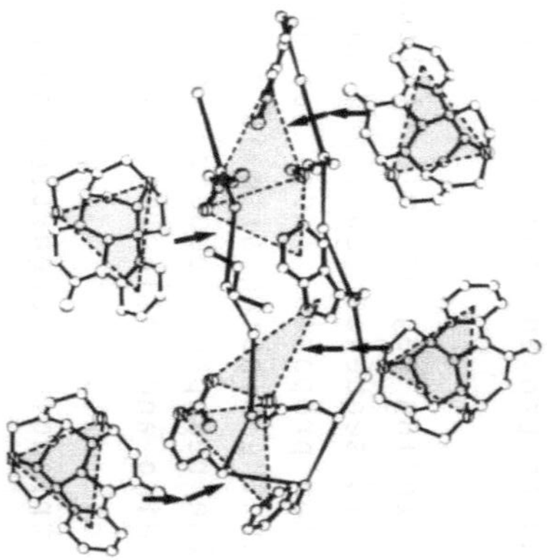

Short × Strychnine

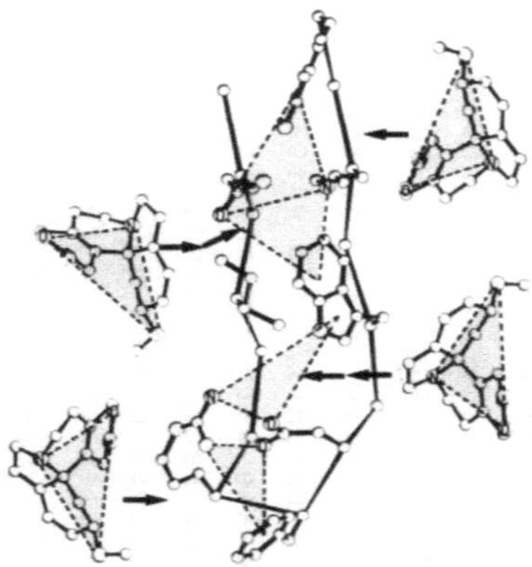

Short × Erythroidine

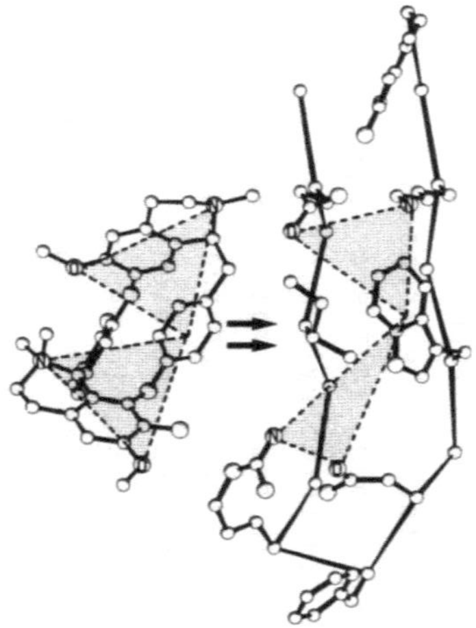

Short × Tubocurarine

like gallamine. Strychnine is also an antagonist with twenty times weaker toxicity than curare (14, 15). In strychnine, the quaternary nitrogen atom is 4.9Å from the ether oxygen and 4Å from the center of the aromatic ring (13, 16). This configuration is also found in the crystal structures of d-tubocurarine (17, 18), in trimethyltubocurare (19), and in the toxiferines. We have indicated the molecular structures of these alkaloids in Fig. 3a,b, and compared them with the analogous situations in the "virtual-bond" representations of the long central loops of the "long" and "short" neurotoxin families. In α-cobratoxin there are four sets of triplets (Asp42, Lys27, Trp29), (Asp42, Lys27, Tyr25), (Asp31, Arg37, Phe33), and (Asp31, Arg40, Trp29), as shown in Fig. 3a, and the corresponding triplets for erabutoxin b are displayed in Fig. 3b. In summary, this suggest that the very tight binding between toxin and receptor requires extensive subsidiary and perhaps less specific hydrophobic binding by the upper surfaces of loops II and III.

It is possible that it is not merely the hydrophobic character of Trp29 and Phe/His/Trp33 which is important, but more that these cooperate with a specific electrostatic interaction at the acetylcholine receptor binding site. The triplet arrangements of aromatic groups, hydrogen bond acceptors and positively charged Lys/Arg are situated on a region of polypeptide backbone exhibiting extreme conformational stability. Their geometrical positions are therefore well-defined. Only slight rotations of the side chains are required to bring them into a position to interact with the complementary recognition sites on the acetylcholine receptor and to provide for a multiplicity of simultaneous contacts.

A probable binding region on acetylcholine receptor, based on the amino acid sequence (20), and on site directed mutagenesis (21), has been proposed. Model building studies (22) further suggest that the binding site is related to a ß-turn in the acetylcholine receptor sequence Phe137-Asp138-Gln139-Gln140, with preceeding and following amino acids in ß-sheet arrangement. With all these data in mind, it appears possible in fact that there is a triangle recognition between the acetylcholine receptor and its agonists and antagonists which is based on a hydrophobic/positively charged/negatively charged configuration.

Acknowledgement

This work was supported by a short term EMBO fellowship awarded to M.D.W. and by Sonderforschungsbereich 312, Teilprojekt D 1.

References

1. Karlsson, E. 1979. Handbook of Experimental Pharmacology 52, 159.

2. Walkinshaw, M.D., W. Saenger, A. Maelicke. 1980. Proc.Natl. Acad.Sci.Wash. 77, 2400.

3. Kimball, M.R., A. Sato, J.S. Richardson, L.S. Rosen, B.W. Low. 1979. Biochem.Biophys.Res.Commun. 88, 950.

4. Tsernoglou, D., G.A. Petsko. 1976. FEBS Lett. 68, 1.

5. Chang, C.C., C.C. Yang, K. Hamaguchi, K. Nakai, K. Hayashi. 1971. Biochim.Biophys.Acta 236, 164.

6. Chibber, B.A., B.M. Martin, M.D. Walkinshaw, W. Saenger, A. Maelicke. 1983. In: Toxins as Tools in Neurochemistry (F. Hucho and Yu.A. Ovchinnikov, eds.). de Gruyter, Berlin, p.141.

7. Martin, B.M., B.A. Chibber, A. Maelicke. 1983. J.Biol.Chem. 258, 8714.

8. Beers, W.H., E. Reich. 1970. Nature 228, 917.

9. Tsernoglou, D., G.A. Petsko, R.A. Hudson. 1978. Mol.Pharmacol. 14, 710.

10. Dufton, M.T., R.C. Hider. 1980. Trends in Biochem.Sci. 5, 53.

11. Koelle, G.B. 1975. In: The Pharmacological Basis of Therapeutics (L.S.C. Goodman, A. Gilman, eds., 5th ed.). Macmillan, p. 575.

12. Pauling, P., T.J. Petcher. 1973. Chem.Biol.Interactions 6, 351.

13. Robertson, J.H., C.A. Beevers. 1951. Acta Cryst. 4, 270.

14. Karrer, P., C.H. Eugster, P. Waser. 1949. Helv.Chim.Acta 32, 2381.

15. Slater, N.T., D.O. Carpenter. 1982. Cell. Molecul.Neurobiol. 2, 53.

16. Cleasby, A., R.O. Gould, N. Moulden, M.D. Walkinshaw. 1981. Acta Cryst. A37, Suppl. C-72

17. Codding, P.W., M.N.G. James. 1973. Acta Cryst. B29, 935.

18. Reynolds, C.D., R.A. Palmer. 1976. Acta Cryst. B32, 1431.

19. Sobell, H.M., T.D. Sakore, S.S. Tavale, F.G. Canepa, P. Pauling, T.J. Petcher. (1972). Proc.Natl.Acad.Sci. 69, 2213.

20. Noda, M., H. Takahashi, T. Tanabi, M. Toyosato, Y. Furutani, T. Hirose, M. Asai, S. Inayama, T. Miyata, S. Numa. 1982. Nature 299, 793.

21. Mishina, M., T. Tobimatsu, K. Imoto, K. Tanaka, Y. Fujita, K. Fukuda, M. Kurusaki, H. Takahashi, Y. Morimoto, T. Hirose, S. Inayama, T. Takahashi, M. Kuno, S. Numa. 1985. Nature 313, 364.

22. Smart, L., H.-W. Meyers, R. Hilgenfeld, W. Saenger, A. Maelicke. 1984. FEBS Lett. 178, 64.

23. Mebs, B. 1979. Compilation of Amino Acid Sequences of Snake Venom Toxins. Zentrum der Rechtsmedizin, Universität Frankfurt, D-6000 Frankfurt.

# AUTHOR INDEX

# SUBJECT INDEX

Bei Fragen zur Produktsicherheit wenden Sie sich bitte an:
If you have any questions regarding product safety,
please contact:

Walter de Gruyter GmbH
Genthiner Straße 13
10785 Berlin
productsafety@degruyterbrill.com